Molecular Pathology Library

Creating a diagnostic, prognostic, and therapeutic treatment strategy precisely tailored to each patient's requirements is the fundamental idea behind precision medicine. The Molecular Pathology Library series integrates molecular biology with clinical data for treatment designed for the patient's individual genetic makeup. This approach is widely recognized as the future of medicine and it is vital for practicing pathologists to know the molecular biology, diagnostics and predictive biomarkers for specific forms of cancer or other diseases and their implications for treatment. Each volume focuses on a specific type of cancer or disease and provides concise essential information in a readily accessible, user friendly, convenient format. Each volume is oriented towards the pathologist who needs this information for daily practice, tumor boards, and conferences or for preparation for certification boards or other tests. Written by experts focusing on patient care, these books are indispensible aids to pathologists' participation in precision medicine in the 21st century.

Victor G. Prieto • Carlos A. Torres-Cabala
Editors

Precision Molecular Pathology of Melanocytic Lesions

Springer

Editors
Victor G. Prieto
Departments of Pathology and Dermatology
The University of Texas MD Anderson
Cancer Center
Houston, TX, USA

Carlos A. Torres-Cabala
Departments of Pathology, Dermatology,
and Translational Molecular Pathology
The University of Texas MD Anderson
Cancer Center
Houston, TX, USA

ISSN 1935-987X ISSN 1935-9888 (electronic)
Molecular Pathology Library
ISBN 978-3-032-18221-0 ISBN 978-3-032-18222-7 (eBook)
https://doi.org/10.1007/978-3-032-18222-7

This Springer imprint is published by the registered company Springer Nature Switzerland AG
The registered company address is: Gewerbestrasse 11, 6330 Cham, Switzerland

We dedicate this work to our families.
Without their support we would not have
been able to make this book possible.

Preface

In this time of emphasis on personalized medicine, it has become even clearer that Pathology plays an essential role in helping determine what therapy is most appropriate for a particular patient.

This book contains a summary of the current knowledge, and we refer our readers interested in a particular topic to also review the ever-growing corresponding literature.

Houston, TX, USA

Victor G. Prieto
Carlos A. Torres-Cabala

Acknowledgments

We would like to thank the Department of Pathology at the University of Texas- MD Anderson Cancer Center for their support and our colleagues in the multiple departments who provided many of the specimens that constitute the basis of this work.

Contents

Chapter 1
Introduction

Victor G. Prieto and Carlos A. Torres-Cabala

This book compiles an updated review of the newer information related to the molecular characteristics of melanocytic lesions. Although it is impossible to provide a comprehensive list of all the discoveries made in the last 10 years, the goal of the book is to provide a summary of the most important findings and their most relevant application to diagnosis, treatment, and prognosis of melanocytic lesions.

The book is subdivided into chapters by type of lesion and concludes with a chapter on biomarkers applied to diagnosis, prognosis, and treatment. Whenever appropriate, the chapters include clinical, histologic, and immunohistochemical images that illustrate the corresponding topic.

It is our goal to provide a useful tool, based on recent discoveries of the molecular features of these lesions, that can be used by pathologists, dermatologists, oncologists, and researchers when treating and studying patients affected by melanocytic tumors.

V. G. Prieto (✉)
Departments of Pathology and Dermatology, The University of Texas MD Anderson Cancer Center, Houston, TX, USA
e-mail: vprieto@mdanderson.org

C. A. Torres-Cabala
Departments of Pathology, Dermatology, and Translational Molecular Pathology, The University of Texas MD Anderson Cancer Center, Houston, TX, USA
e-mail: ctcabala@mdanderson.org

V. G. Prieto, C. A. Torres-Cabala (eds.), *Precision Molecular Pathology of Melanocytic Lesions*, Molecular Pathology Library,
https://doi.org/10.1007/978-3-032-18222-7_1

Chapter 2
Current Molecular Classification of Melanocytic Lesions (WHO 2025)

Victor G. Prieto and Carlos A. Torres-Cabala

The latest (fifth) edition of the World Health Organization's classification of skin tumors provides a summary of clinical, histological, and molecular findings of cutaneous neoplasms. This classification includes new entities and the recent contributions that molecular analysis has brought to the etiopathogenesis, diagnosis, prognostication, and treatment of cutaneous lesions. Among the most important updates is the subclassification into multiple pathways, e.g., traditional, Spitz, blue, etc., and the confirmation of a correlation between some of the molecular findings with histopathological diagnosis, prognosis, and response to treatment. This chapter and the rest of the book will highlight some of the most important ones.

Since the beginning of modern pathology in the nineteenth century, there have been several classifications aimed at studying melanocytic lesions. In 1969 and 1970, Dr. Wallace H. Clark [1] and Dr. Vincent G. McGovern [2] and subsequently together in 1973 [3] proposed a classification that has been used until today. This classification included mostly three types of malignant lesions: lentigo maligna, superficial spreading, and nodular melanomas. The first two ones are characterized by intraepidermal growth by melanoma cells (i.e., in situ melanoma) extending beyond the dermal component, while nodular melanomas lack that peripheral extension. Lentigo maligna was characterized by growth on actinically damaged skin (flat epidermis, loss of rete ridges, significant solar elastosis) as a confluent growth of atypical melanocytes arranged in single cells and nest along the dermal-epidermal

V. G. Prieto (✉)
Departments of Pathology and Dermatology, The University of Texas MD Anderson Cancer Center, Houston, TX, USA
e-mail: vprieto@mdanderson.org

C. A. Torres-Cabala
Departments of Pathology, Dermatology, and Translational Molecular Pathology, The University of Texas MD Anderson Cancer Center, Houston, TX, USA
e-mail: ctcabala@mdanderson.org

V. G. Prieto, C. A. Torres-Cabala (eds.), *Precision Molecular Pathology of Melanocytic Lesions*, Molecular Pathology Library,
https://doi.org/10.1007/978-3-032-18222-7_2

junction and skin adnexa. Superficial spreading melanoma had low-grade of actinic damage in the skin and mostly nests of atypical melanocytes with prominent involvement of the upper layers of the epidermis (pagetoid upward migration). Subsequent publications highlighted the presence of other morphologic patterns and subtypes: acral, desmoplastic melanoma, heavily pigmented lesions (blue nevus family and later deep penetrating lesions and pigmented epithelioid melanocytomas), spitzoid, melanomas arising on mucosalregions, etc. Most researchers and medical personnel accepted this classification although it was not universally followed.

After 2000, it became clear that many of the morphologic features described in these melanocytic lesions were associated with underlying molecular changes. Among others, the group at UCSF [4] described that acral lentiginous melanoma had copy number increases of chromosomes 5p, 12q, 4q, and 11q and losses involving 6q, 15q, and 16q. When comparing lentigo maligna and superficial spreading melanoma, the former lesions had more frequent gains on 15q and 17q while losses on 13q and 17p.

By 2018, the year when the WHO released the fourth edition of *Skin Tumours* [5], malignant melanocytic lesions were classified in different pathways. That classification was based on clinical, morphologic, and molecular findings. The main classifying criterion was location/degree of sun exposure. The current classification includes ten pathways (Fig. 2.1) [6]. The largest group was the one composed of lesions with some degree of solar damage (cumulative solar damage; CSD), including high CSD lesions (lentigo maligna), low CSD (superficial spreading), and desmoplastic melanoma. This group is considered the traditional pathway, since it comprises most melanomas. The second group included melanomas in areas not associated with significant solar exposure (Spitz, acral, mucosal, melanomas arising in congenital nevi, melanomas arising in blue nevi, uveal melanoma). These lesions show a spectrum of genetic abnormalities from uveal melanomas showing a relatively low number of changes to desmoplastic melanomas, which are among the tumors with the highest TMB (tumor mutation burden).

Melanomas arising in sun-exposed skin

- I: Low-CSD (cumulative sun damage) melanoma (superficial spreading melanoma)
- II: High-CSD melanoma (lentigo maligna melanoma)
- III: Desmoplastic melanoma

Melanomas without known associations with ultraviolet radiation exposure

- IV: Spitz melanoma
- V: Acral melanoma
- VI: Mucosal melanoma
- VII: Melanoma arising in congenital naevus
- VIII: Melanoma arising in blue naevus
- IX: Uveal melanoma
- X: Melanoma arising in the central nervous system

Fig. 2.1 Melanoma pathways included in the fifth edition of the WHO of Skin Tumours [6]

The classification also provides additional information on the types of genetic abnormalities and describes a progression from benign to malignant in some pathways. Thus, most nevi that are associated with superficial spreading/low CSD melanomas have *BRAF*^{v600E} mutations, and those mutations are also seen in most superficial spreading/low CSD melanomas. Detection of *BRAF* mutations plays a very important role since it describes most lesions from the traditional pathway. Furthermore, although *BAP1*-deficient lesions have cytologic features resembling Spitz lesions, the presence of *BRAF*^{v600E} mutations in such *BAP1*-deficient lesions resulted in their inclusion in the traditional pathway. Congenital nevi commonly have *NRAS* mutations, while the most common genetic mutation in Spitz nevi is in *HRAS*. Similarly, most blue nevi have *GNA11 or GNAQ* mutations, like some heavily pigmented melanomas from the skin, eyes, and central nervous system.

Another proposal from the classification is to include terminology to help describe the malignant potential of lesions that appear to fall in the boundary between benign and malignant behavior. In other organs, this concept may be described as “borderline” or “low malignant potential.” The WHO classification proposes the term “intraepidermal atypical melanocytic proliferation of uncertain significance (IAMPUS)” for melanoma lesions limited to the epithelium (melanoma in situ) and “superficial atypical melanocytic proliferation of uncertain significance (SAMPUS)” for melanoma lesions only involving the superficial dermis and lacking a vertical growth phase. “Melanocytic tumor of uncertain malignant potential (MELTUMP)” is proposed for thicker lesions with possible vertical growth phase. The WHO classification indicates that when using these acronyms, they should be spelled out and their meaning explained in the report. Similarly, to convey the expected clinical behavior, the WHO classification includes the revised Melanocytic Pathology Assessment Tool and Hierarchy for Diagnosis (MPATH-Dx version 2.0) schema [7]: lesions with low risk to progression to invasive melanoma (Class I low-grade and II high-grade), superficially invasive melanoma (Class III pT1a), and thicker melanoma (Class IV > pT1a).

In summary, the fifth edition of the WHO book on melanocytic lesions provides a framework that incorporates molecular pathology data and refines the concept of a spectrum of lesions from benign to malignant in at least some of the proposed pathways. Further studies will likely provide data to continue improving the classification in future editions.

References

1. Clark WH Jr, et al. The histogenesis and biologic behavior of primary human malignant melanomas of the skin. Cancer Res. 1969;29(3):705–27.
2. McGovern VJ. The classification of melanoma and its relationship with prognosis. Pathology. 1970;2(2):85–98.
3. McGovern VJ, et al. The classification of malignant melanoma and its histologic reporting. Cancer. 1973;32(6):1446–57.

4. Bastian BC, et al. Classifying melanocytic tumors based on DNA copy number changes. Am J Pathol. 2003;163(5):1765–70.
5. Elder DE, et al. The 2018 World Health Organization classification of cutaneous, mucosal, and uveal melanoma: detailed analysis of 9 distinct subtypes defined by their evolutionary pathway. Arch Pathol Lab Med. 2020;144(4):500–22.
6. Bastian BC, et al. Melanocytic neoplasms: introduction. In: Barnhill RL, et al., editors. WHO classification of tumours. Skin tumours. International Agency for Research on Cancer: Lyon; 2025. Internet; beta version ahead of print.
7. Barnhill RL, et al. Revision of the melanocytic pathology assessment tool and hierarchy for diagnosis classification schema for melanocytic lesions: a consensus statement. JAMA Netw Open. 2023;6(1):e2250613.

Chapter 3
Superficial Spreading (Low-CSD Melanoma) Melanoma

Dinesh Pradhan

Introduction

Superficial spreading melanoma (SSM) or "low CSD melanoma" is the most common subtype of cutaneous melanoma, accounting for approximately 70% of all melanoma cases [1, 2]. SSM mostly occurs at intermittently sun-exposed sites, such as legs in women and backs and shoulders in men. The term SSM was first described by Clark et al. in their seminal paper in 1969 [3]. It was described as pagetoid melanoma by McGovern et al. [4] and recently as "low-CSD melanoma" emphasizing the role of cumulative sun damage (CSD) in the fourth edition of the *WHO Classification of Skin Tumours*, published in 2018 [5]. SSM is the prototypic lesion of pathway I of the WHO 2018 classification of melanoma (that distinguishes nine melanoma families or pathways) [6]. The "precancerous melanosis" described by Dubreuilh as early as 1912 and "atypical melanocytic hyperplasia" by Sagebiel in 1979 [7] is termed now as "melanoma in situ, superficial spreading type (or low-CSD)" [6]. SSM is characterized by a prolonged horizontal or radial growth phase before vertical invasion. SSM typically presents as a flat or slightly elevated pigmented lesion with asymmetrical borders and variegated coloration. Early detection and treatment are critical, as prognosis significantly worsens with increasing tumor thickness and ulceration.

D. Pradhan (✉)
Departments of Pathology and Dermatology, University of Nebraska Medical Center, Omaha, NE, USA

V. G. Prieto, C. A. Torres-Cabala (eds.), *Precision Molecular Pathology of Melanocytic Lesions*, Molecular Pathology Library,
https://doi.org/10.1007/978-3-032-18222-7_3

Epidemiology

SSM is the most common melanoma subtype in young to middle-aged adults. The ratio of SSM to nodular melanoma (NM) in adolescence is 2:1, and in adults it is 5:1 [8]. The incidence of SSM rises until age 55 and then drops gradually [9, 10]. SSM shows an equal sex incidence [1]. SSM or low-CSD melanoma may arise at any cutaneous site, except palms and soles, that are intermittently exposed to the sun and are rare on areas unexposed to the sun (no CSD). SSM accounts for approximately 70% of cases in light-skinned individuals (Fitzpatrick skin phototypes I-III) [9]. It is significantly less common in the pigmented skin population [9, 10].

The incidence of melanoma has increased significantly over the last several decades, accounting for 1.7% of all cancers worldwide [11, 12]. SSM accounts for approximately 70% of these cases. In 2020, there were an estimated 325,000 new melanoma cases, with 57,000 deaths worldwide. In the United States, melanoma is the fifth most common cancer, with an estimated 104,960 new cases, of which an estimated 8430 people will die of the disease, according to the Surveillance, Epidemiology, and End Results (SEER) Program of the National Cancer Institute [13].

SSM is etiologically linked to sun exposure. The seminal study by Lancaster and Nelson in 1957 elucidated the role of sun exposure in the development of melanoma [14]. Holman et al. demonstrated that sun exposure during childhood is critical in developing the risk for melanoma [15]. Subsequently, it was found that the risk of developing melanoma is modified by sun exposure that persists in adult life too [16]. Studies also revealed that the melanomas on sun-exposed skin with little solar elastosis had distinct genetic alteration in comparison to those with marked solar elastosis, rationalizing the subclassification of melanoma based on CSD [10, 17]. In SSM or low-CSD melanoma, the cumulative sun exposure is low to moderate, mostly by intermittent acute exposure to sunlight on vacations or weekends, which mostly happens in recreational circumstances rather than continuous chronic exposure as seen in high-CSD melanomas [6]. Hence, SSM is common on the backs and shoulders in men and the backs of the legs or calves in women [18]. The association of SSM with ultraviolet (UV) radiation exposure through indoor tanning, mostly in young female individuals, was shown by Burbidge et al. [19] Hair, eye, and skin color, propensity to sunburn, history of sunburns in infancy, degree of freckling, number of solar lentigines, and number of melanocytic nevi were all found to be associated with melanoma risk [20]. Although the number of nevi proved to be the strongest risk factor for development of SSM (>45 nevi with 9.5 fold increased risk), fair skin and blue eyes had a two-fold increased risk each [20]. The odds ratio for developing SSM was 2:1 for individuals that burn frequently versus those that never burn, and also 2:1 for those that burn before 15 years of age versus after 15 years [20]. Other risk factors that apply particularly to SSM in epidemiological studies include the presence of dysplastic nevi, total number of nevi, and large size of nevi [21]. Increased number of small nevi (two-fold higher risk), increased numbers of both small and large nondysplastic nevi (four-fold higher risk), 1 clinically dysplastic nevus (two-fold higher risk), 10 or more clinically dysplastic nevi (12-fold higher risk), single histologically dysplastic nevus (four-fold higher risk), and lesion more than 4.4 mm (five-fold higher risk) [22–25]. Although SSM was earlier shown to be the most common in hereditary melanoma kindreds, the association of melanoma risk with hereditary nevus susceptibility genes is not clear [26, 27].

Clinical Features

SSM is the most common and prototypic subtype of melanoma in which the ABCDE criteria is most helpful for diagnosis [28]. The traditional ABCD rule created in 1985 emphasized the classic clinical characteristics for early detection of SSM—*A*symmetry, *B*order irregularity, *C*olor variation, and *D*iameter greater than 6 mm [29, 30]. Subsequently, *E* was added to the ABCD acronym, emphasizing the importance of recognizing *E*volution or change in the size, shape, color, surface, and symptoms [31–34]. Some variations to the ABCD (EFG) rule were published leading to uncertainty [35, 36].

SSM mostly presents as an irregular flat scaly pigmented macule (Fig 3.1a) or slightly elevated plaque. The initial plaque has an irregular outline, palpable border, and demonstrates greater variation in color than a dysplastic or benign nevus. The color varies from tan, brown, pink, gray, blue, to black. There is often characteristic scalloping of the border of the lesion. Subsequently, the initial macule or plaque develops into a black nodule of invasive melanoma (Fig 3.1b, c), signifying the development of tumorigenic vertical growth. Later, some cases may also develop ulceration (Fig 3.1d). Areas of regression are identified as hypopigmented, gray to white areas (Fig. 3.2a). Erythematous foci correspond to prominent vascularity and inflammation. Amelanotic or hypopigmented variants are tan to erythematous and difficult to diagnose [37]. The presence of a verrucous surface can cause difficulty

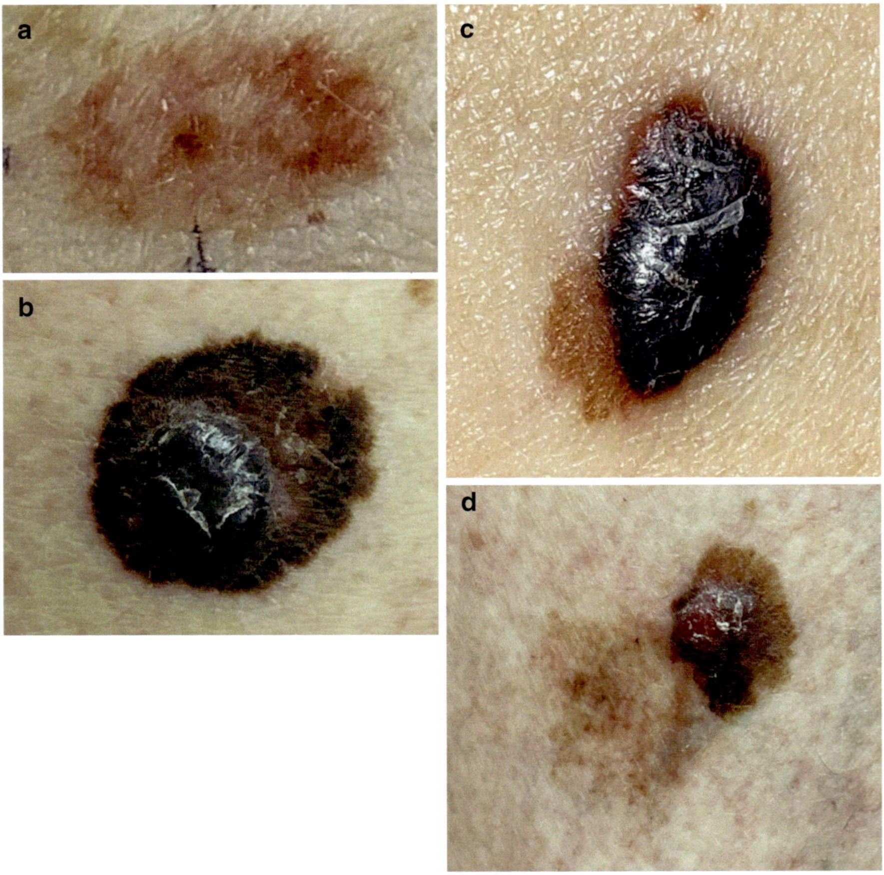

Fig. 3.1 (**a**) Superficial spreading melanoma: clinical finding—asymmetric pigmented macule with variegated colors and irregular borders on the abdomen. (**b**) Large black nodule of vertical growth phase in the center of the irregularly pigmented radial growth phase on the back of an elderly male. (**c**) Large black nodule of invasive component with surrounding macule on the left upper back. (**d**) Ulcerated pigmented nodule with surrounding large, variegated macule having irregular borders on the lower leg of an elderly female

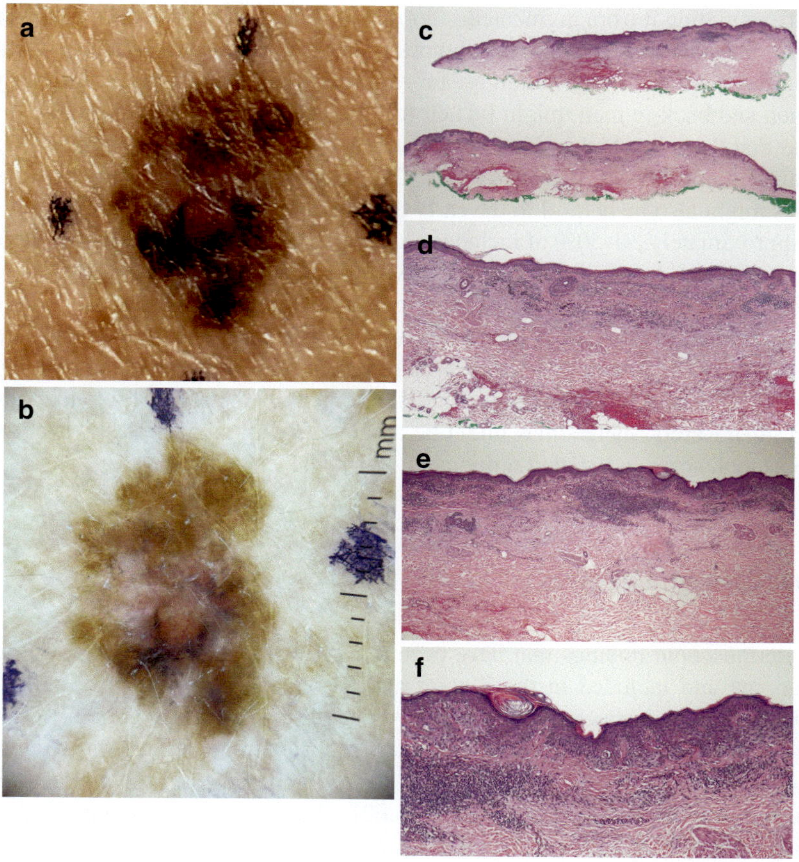

Fig. 3.2 (**a**) Superficial spreading melanoma: clinical finding—large irregular asymmetric slightly elevated plaque with variegated color. (**b**) Dermoscopic findings— asymmetry, atypical pigment network, atypical peripheral blotches, focal blue-gray veil, and polymorphous vessels. (Courtesy Kassidy M Bruhn, UNMC). (**c**) Histopathologic findings—asymmetric broad melanocytic proliferation with a central partial regression area and slightly elevated area on the upper right corresponding to blue-grey veil (H&E, 10×). (**d**) Area with partial regression corresponding to the polymorphous vessels in the dermoscopic image (H&E, 40×). (**e**) Predominantly intraepidermal component with bridging large junctional nests of atypical melanocytes on the right half corresponding to blue-gray veil in the dermoscopic image (H&E, 40×). (**f**) Higher magnification of blue-gray veil area in the dermoscopic image demonstrating lymphocytic infiltrate and fibrosis (H&E, 100×)

in differentiating it from pigmented seborrheic keratosis [38]. The differentiation of SSM from other histopathologic subtypes might be challenging; however, the anatomic distribution in intermittently sun-exposed sites, such as lower extremity in women and back in men, might be helpful [39, 40]. In a multicentric study, it was found that there is a higher frequency of melanoma on the left side by about 15%, possibly due to driving habits [41, 42]. Dermoscopy and other non-invasive techniques might also be helpful in the early detection of SSM.

Approximately 30–50% of melanomas are associated with a benign melanocytic nevus, although mostly SSM arise de novo [43]. The probability of developing an SSM in any nevus, including dysplastic nevus, is exceptionally low, and with current knowledge, it is impossible to determine confidently which nevus will transform. The "ugly duckling" sign denoting pigmented lesion that stands out in the midst of numerous other banal pigmented lesions is also very helpful in diagnosing SSM [44]. Rarely, melanomas might be associated with paraneoplastic syndrome, such as melanoma-associated retinopathy [45–47].

Dermoscopic Features

The dermoscopic findings that have been most sensitive for the detection of early melanoma and included in the 7-point and 3-point checklists for melanoma are atypical pigment network, blue-whitish veils, atypical vascular pattern, irregular streaks, irregular dots/globules, irregular pigmentation, regression structures, Chrysalis/crystalline structures/shiny white streaks, peripheral brown structureless area, and irregular blotches (Fig. 3.2) [48–62]. Most of these dermoscopic findings are identified in SSM; however, atypical pigment network, irregular streaks, irregular blotches, and peripheral brown structureless areas are most specific to the SSM subtype (Fig. 3.3) [48–62]. Dermoscopic (epiluminescence microscopy, ELM) findings and clinical information are helpful in the diagnosis of histologically challenging cases. Recently, reflectance confocal microscopy was found to have superior diagnostic accuracy to dermoscopy in a meta-analysis, especially in terms of specificity of differentiating melanoma from nevus [63]. Other non-invasive techniques that have shown promise include optical coherence tomography, infrared spectroscopy, Raman spectroscopy, and infrared thermography [64–66]. However, none of the techniques were able to provide a definitive diagnosis to completely replace histopathologic examination [67].

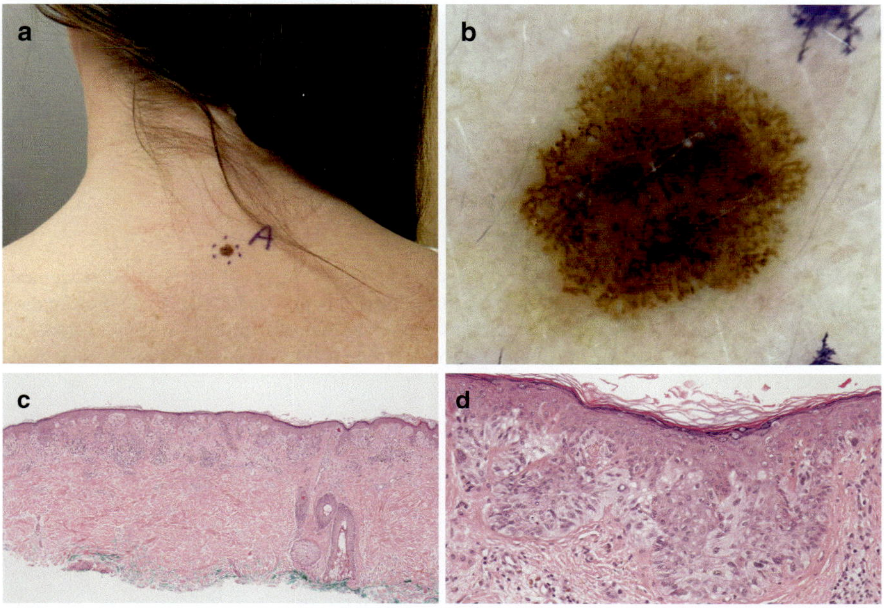

Fig. 3.3 (**a**) Clinical finding—asymmetric 6 mm pigmented macule on the upper back of a middle-aged female. (**b**) Dermoscopic findings—atypical pigment network, asymmetric peripheral radial streaming with focal "pseudopods" (at 4 o'clock and 9 o'clock) and focal "negative network" with atypical globules centrally. (Courtesy Megan R Arthur, MD). (**c**) Histopathologic findings—asymmetric nested melanocytic proliferation with pagetoid scatter even at the edges (H&E, 40×). (**d**) Higher magnification demonstrating enlarged epithelioid melanocytes with abundant amphophilic cytoplasm, focal dusty melanin pigment, enlarged irregular nuclei, and conspicuous nucleoli (H&E, 200×)

Histopathology

The gold standard for the diagnosis of SSM is histopathology, in conjunction with clinical correlation, immunohistochemical findings, and molecular results in some cases [3]. The classic histopathologic findings include asymmetric, poorly circumscribed, broad, atypical compound melanocytic proliferation, often with confluent lentiginous spread, prominent nesting, and pagetoid upward migration of the atypical melanocytes (Fig. 3.4) [68, 69]. In a proportion of cases, regression (focal or extensive), lymphocytic infiltrate (brisk or non-brisk), ulceration, lymphovascular

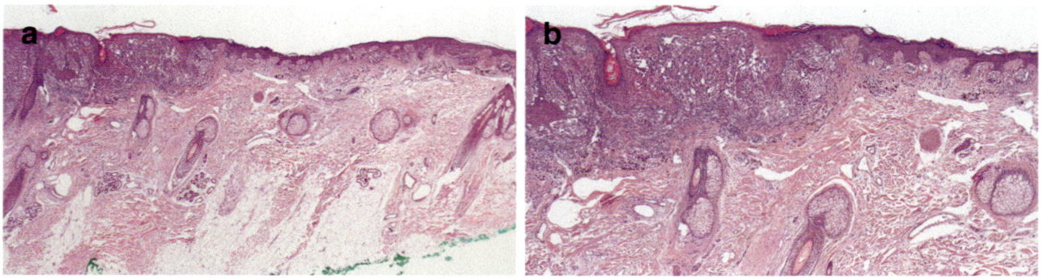

Fig. 3.4 (**a**) Superficial spreading melanoma: histopathologic findings—Low-power view demonstrates an asymmetric, poorly circumscribed, broad, atypical compound melanocytic proliferation (H&E, 20×). (**b**) There is confluent lentiginous spread, prominent nesting, and focal pagetoid upward migration of the atypical melanocytes. There is mild solar elastosis (cumulative solar damage grade I) (H&E, 40×)

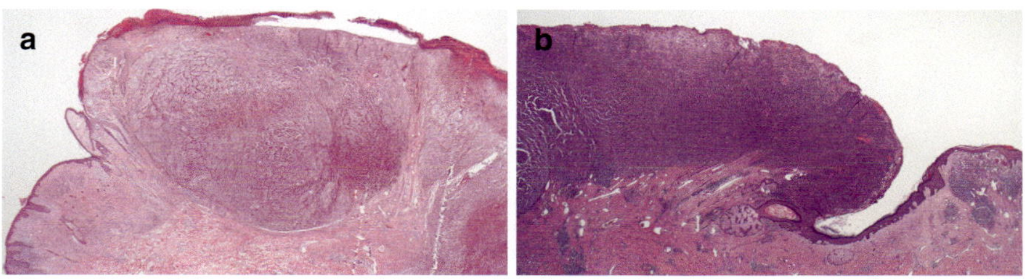

Fig. 3.5 (**a**) Low-power view of an ulcerated expansile nodule adjacent to an associated intradermal melanocytic nevus on the left side (H&E, 10×). (**b**) Another example of an ulcerated expansile nodule with a skip area of regression on the right of the nodule and lymphocytic infiltrate at the base of the nodules (H&E, 10×)

or perineural invasion, satellitosis, and associated melanocytic nevus are present (Fig. 3.5). The significant architectural findings in SSM include asymmetry (one half of the lesion appears different from the other half), poor circumscription (the edges of the lesion do not start with a nest and end with a nest, rather have single scattered atypical melanocytes at the edge), large size (>6 mm; often >10 mm), confluent spread (or contiguous proliferation/fusion of nests characterized by contiguous cell bodies of melanocytes that are touching each other), and pagetoid scatter (or buckshot scatter termed due to its appearance reminiscent of Paget disease of the nipple in which breast cancer cells scatter into the epidermis) (Fig. 3.6) [68]. Pagetoid upward migration of melanocytes was found in approximately one-third of SSM, and hence, although helpful in diagnosis, lack of pagetoid scatter shouldn't preclude the diagnosis [70]. The architectural findings are best appreciated at scanning magnification. SSM typically demonstrates irregular epidermal thickness, along with band-like lymphocytic infiltrate and fibroplasia in the papillary dermis [71]. The lack of maturation with vertical dermal descent of melanoma cells is also helpful in diagnosis. In some cases, there are biphenotypic or multiple phenotypes of atypical cells and expansile growth or "puffy shirt appearance" (Fig. 3.7) [72]. The melanoma cells might "consume" or replace the lowermost layers of epidermis,

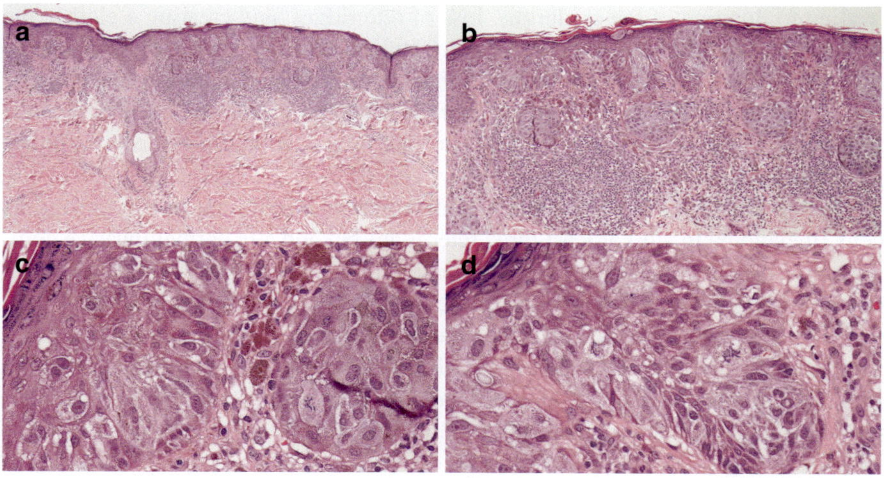

Fig. 3.6 (**a**) Prominent pagetoid upward migration of the atypical melanocytes (Buckshot scatter) (H&E, 40×). (**b**) There is a brisk lymphocytic response with melanophages in the underlying stroma (H&E, 100×). (**c**) Higher magnification demonstrating enlarged atypical melanocytes with abundant amphophilic cytoplasm, dusty melanin pigment, irregular round to oval nucleus, opened up chromatin, and prominent eosinophilic nucleoli (H&E, 400×). (**d**) There are interspersed numerous mitosis in the intraepidermal melanocytes (H&E, 400×)

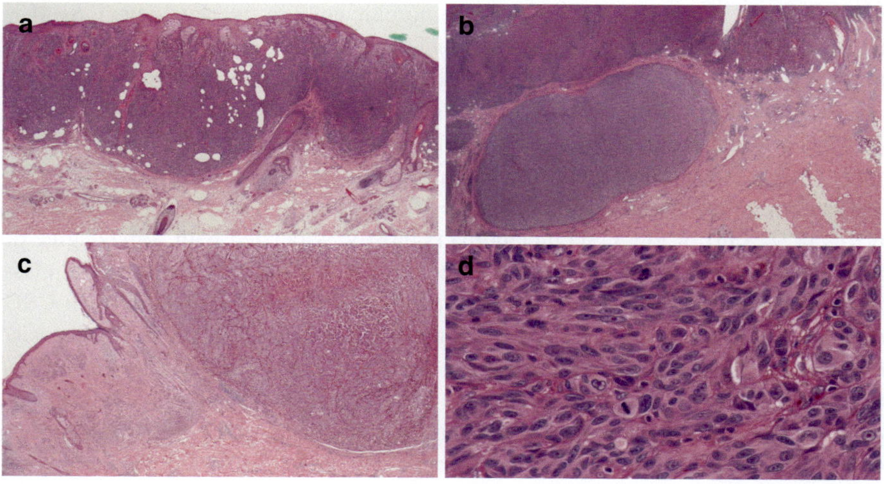

Fig. 3.7 (**a**) Expansile nodules of atypical melanocytes ("puffy shirt" appearance) (H&E, 20×). (**b**) Expansile nodule separately lying in the dermis (H&E, 10×). (**c**) Associated nevus on the left with maturation pattern with dermal descent in contrast to melanoma on the right with no maturation (H&E, 20×). (**d**) Higher magnification of the expansile nodule demonstrating typical and atypical mitosis (H&E, 400×)

leading to thinning of the epidermis, loss of rete ridges, and creating a cleft in the dermal-epidermal junction, giving rise to "zipper effect" or "consumption of the epidermis." [73–76] Consumption of the epidermis is present in approximately 40% of cases of SSM [77]. In some cases, there is follicular or adnexal extension of the melanoma cells, which percolates down the hair follicle epithelium or eccrine ducts, respectively [78].

Histologically, SSM demonstrates intraepidermal proliferation of melanoma cells (melanoma in situ) at least three rete ridges beyond any dermal invasive component of melanoma cells (in contrast to nodular melanoma with an intraepidermal component of less than three rete ridges beyond the dermal component). The dermal invasive component may be an expansile nest, a solid mass, or rarely fascicular arrangement. The cytologically atypical melanocytes are enlarged, epithelioid round to polygonal cells, with mild anisocytosis, increased eosinophilic to amphophilic cytoplasm, dusty melanin pigment, enlarged oval to irregular nuclei, anisokaryosis, irregularly clumped or dense chromatin, and variably conspicuous to prominent nucleoli. Less frequently, the cells may be spindle-shaped or nevoid, without evidence of maturation with dermal descent. There is mostly uniform atypia defined as cytologic atypia involving more than 50% of the lesional cells. The nuclear features of cytologic atypia include enlarged nuclei in comparison to basal keratinocytes, irregularity of nuclear membrane, hyperchromasia, irregularly clumped chromatin, and amphophilic to eosinophilic macronucleoli [6]. The melanoma cells are uniformly or monotonously pleomorphic (indicating the same neoplastic clone), in contrast to random pleomorphic cells in dysplastic nevi. SSM is associated with nevus, either conventional (common or banal) or dysplastic, in approximately one-third to half of cases [43, 79–81]. The associated nevus is generally easily recognizable as a separate population of cells that are demonstrating features of maturation with dermal descent (diminution of nest, cell size, and pigment with dermal descent and acquiring spindle-shape and separation of cells in the lower dermis) as in conventional nevus, or less cytologic atypia as in dysplastic nevus [82]. SSM or low-CSD melanoma is mostly associated with some degree of solar elastosis in the surrounding skin, generally low to moderate (individual elastotic fibers are still identifiable), in contrast to severe solar elastosis in high-CSD melanomas (individual elastotic fibers are not recognizable). Mild solar elastosis/CSD (grade I) is characterized by single elastotic fibers visible at 20× magnification; moderate solar elastosis/CSD (grade II) by presence of fascicles or bunches of elastotic fibers; in contrast to severe solar elastosis/CSD (grade III), seen in high CSD melanomas, by homogeneous amorphous aggregates or nodules of grayish elastotic material, not identifiable as separate individual elastotic fibrils [83, 84]. Of note, rarely melanomas with features characteristic of SSM such as extensive pagetoid scatter and nested proliferation of large epithelioid melanocytes with dusty cytoplasmic melanin can be seen in association with severe or grade III solar elastosis and should be classified as SSM or low CSD melanoma.

Breslow thickness or primary tumor thickness, considered to be one of the dominant independent prognostic factors of SSM, is measured from the upper edge of the granular layer of the epidermis of the overlying skin or the upper edge of the base of the ulcer, if the lesion is ulcerated over the entire dermal component to the deepest point of tumor invasion, either the deepest isolated cell or the deepest edge of a single mass [85]. Traditionally, it is measured with the help of a calibrated ocular micrometer with calibrations perpendicular to the surface of adjacent normal skin at 10× magnification of the objective lens. Recently, it can be measured on whole slide scanned images as per the software specifications. If the tumor is transected at the deep margin of the specimen, then the Breslow depth is indicated as "at least." The Clark level or anatomic level of invasion, another independent predictor of outcome, is categorized as I–V depending on whether the tumor is intraepidermal only (melanoma in situ), is present in the papillary dermis, fills and expands the papillary dermis, invades into the reticular dermis, or invades subcutis, respectively [3, 86].

Ulceration, another major independent predictor of outcome, is defined as a full-thickness epidermal defect including loss of stratum corneum and basement membrane with definitive evidence of reactive changes, including fibrin deposition, neutrophilic aggregate, or granulation tissue (excluding prior biopsy-related change or sectioning artifact) [86, 87]. Several studies have emphasized the significance of measuring the ulceration (maximum diameter or as a percentage of the maximum diameter of the dermal invasive component) in better predicting outcome [87, 88].

Mitotic rate in the dermal component of melanoma is another strong independent prognostic factor and is expressed as the number of mitoses per mm^2 in the dermal component of the tumor. First, the "hotspot" or "area with most mitotic figures" should be identified, and then the mitosis is counted in that high-power field (HPF; 40× magnification of objective lens) plus adjacent HPFs equivalent to 1 mm^2 for that microscope (generally 4.5–5 HPF) [89]. There might be some atypical mitosis, including multipolar spindles (tripolar, tetrapolar, or multipolar), rod-like structures, dispersed mitosis, polar asymmetry, anaphase bridge, and ring mitosis.

Radial growth phase (RGP) or nontumorigenic horizontal growth phase is typical of most SSM or low CSD melanoma. It signifies the early developmental phase of melanoma, following its origin from melanocytes at the dermal-epidermal junction. Histologically, RGP is characterized by a proliferation of melanoma cells in the epidermis, with or without neoplastic melanocytes in the superficial papillary dermis, either as single cells or small clusters of cells without any dermal mitosis or formation of an expansile mass/tumor nodule. Therefore, RGP includes melanoma in situ (melanoma cells confined to the epidermis) and microinvasive melanoma (melanoma cells involving superficial papillary dermis) [90, 91]. RGP is associated with excellent survival [92]. RGP is followed by the tumorigenic vertical growth phase (VGP), which is defined as the presence of a nodule/nest/cluster of melanoma cells in the dermis that is larger than the largest nest/cluster of cells in the epidermis, or the presence of any dermal mitosis [6]. This tumor nodule formation signifies that the net direction of growth of melanoma is vertically perpendicular to that in RGP, further indicating the evolution of a clone capable of expansile growth [93].

Regression, partial or complete, is a common feature in SSM that signifies immunologic rejection and is of diagnostic and prognostic importance [94]. Histologically, regression appears as an area where melanoma cells have been replaced by variably dense infiltrate comprising of lymphocytes and melanophages, along with attenuation of the epidermis (thinning and loss of rete ridges), dermal fibrosis, and increased number of thick-walled and dilated blood vessels [95, 96]. Generally, the area of regression has invasive melanoma or melanoma in situ on one or both sides, indicating the "footprint" of melanoma that dwindled. Partial regression is found in approximately one-third of melanomas [97–100]. Other characteristic stromal changes associated with SSM include diffuse fibroplasia, with a plaque-like/band-like lymphocytic infiltrate and scattered melanophages [95]. Tumor-infiltrating lymphocyte (TIL) is another important prognostic factor that is inversely related to outcome. It is classified as "brisk" if the lymphocytes completely cover the base of the invasive melanoma component, otherwise termed "non-brisk." It is termed "not identified or absent" if there are no lymphocytes within the tumor.

"Large nested melanoma," an uncommon variant of SSM or low-CSD melanoma, is characterized by large, irregular junctional nests with nests predominating over pagetoid pattern and nests mostly surrounded by a cuff of epidermal keratinocytes. Like classic SSM, the nested melanoma may be associated with a benign nevus [69, 101]. Infrequently, SSM demonstrates a predominant lentiginous pattern, with confluent proliferation of single atypical melanocytes along the dermal-epidermal junction with minimal pagetoid scatter and rare nests. Another rare variant, "verrucous melanoma," is characterized by marked acanthosis, verrucous hyperplasia and hyperkeratosis, sometimes extensive pseudoepitheliomatous hyperplasia mimicking squamous cell carcinoma, proliferation of eccrine ducts, and elongated rete ridges [38, 102–104].

Electron microscopy, although not commonly used, has helped characterize ultrastructurally SSM [105, 106]. Stage II melanosomes, considered a hallmark of melanoma, are largely spheroid in SSM in contrast to ellipsoid in lentigo maligna melanoma and normal melanocytes [107, 108]. These melanosomes are abundant in the large pagetoid melanoma cells, and the melanization is often incomplete within the melanosomes [109].

Immunohistochemistry

Immunohistochemical stains that confirm the tumor cells to be of melanocytic origin include cytoplasmic staining with tyrosinase, HMB45, and Melan-A; both cytoplasmic and nuclear staining with S100; and nuclear staining with SOX10 and MITF. Markers that are helpful in differentiation from nevus include HMB45 (maturation marker), Ki-67 (proliferation marker), p16 (cell cycle arrest marker), and PRAME (PReferentially expressed Antigen in MElanoma). HMB45 demonstrates vertical gradient or diminution of staining with maturation in nevus, and patchy or random staining with no predictability from left to right or top to bottom in melanoma (Fig. 3.8) [110–112]. The dual Ki-67/Melan-A stain is very helpful in identifying proliferative melanocytes in heavily inflamed lesions. Melanomas usually

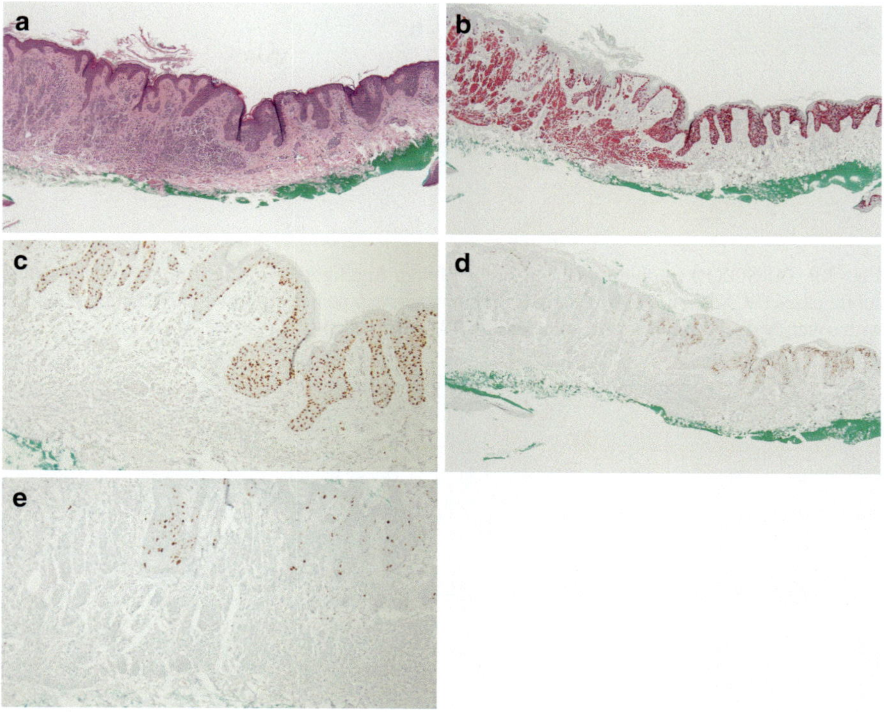

Fig. 3.8 (**a**) Superficial spreading melanoma with associated intradermal melanocytic nevus on the left (H&E, 40×). (**b**) Immunohistochemical staining with Melan-A highlights the melanoma cells as well as intradermal melanocytic nevus cells (Melan-A, 40×). (**c**) PRAME immunostain highlights the nuclei of the melanoma cells and is negative in the intradermal melanocytic nevus cells (PRAME, 100×). (**d**) HMB45 immunostain stains the melanoma cells and demonstrates a maturation pattern in the intradermal melanocytic nevus cells (HMB45, 40×). (**e**) Ki-67 immunostain stains some melanoma cells and basal keratinocytes and is negative in the intradermal melanocytic nevus cells (Ki-67, 100×)

demonstrate a Ki-67 proliferation rate of more than 20%, in contrast to less than 10% in the Spitz nevus, less than 5% in dysplastic nevus, and less than 1% in the conventional melanocytic nevus [113]. Melanomas often demonstrate loss of staining for p16, in contrast to checkerboard or mosaic staining in the nevus [114–116]. PRAME immunostaining is often positive (defined as nuclear immunoreactivity in 75–100% of melanoma cells) in SSM and negative in conventional or dysplastic nevus (<75% staining in melanocytes) (Fig. 3.9) [117, 118]. Other immunohistochemical markers revealing molecular alteration, such as BRAF, beta-catenin, BAP1, ALK, and NTRK1, are helpful in the differentiation of specific lesions and SSM. BRAF immunostain can help differentiate SSM from Spitzoid lesions, as the BRAF V600E mutation is uncommon in Spitzoid lesions. The dual D2–40/Melan-A or D2–40/SOX10 immunohistochemical stain, highlighting lymphatic endothelial cells and melanoma cells, can be used to confirm equivocal lymphovascular invasion (Fig. 3.10).

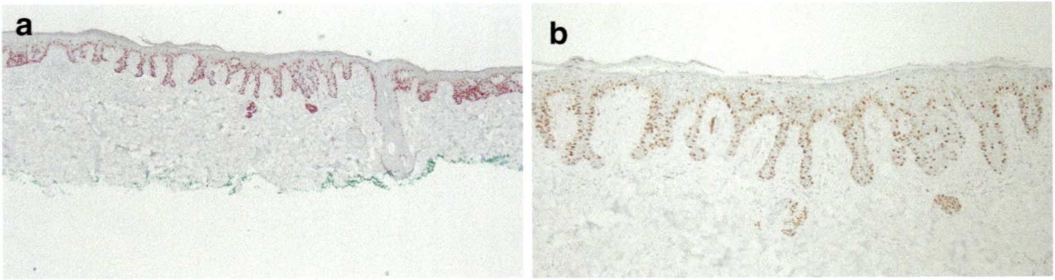

Fig. 3.9 (**a**) SOX10 immunostain can be helpful in highlighting the melanoma cells in some subtle cases (SOX10, 40×). (**b**) PRAME immunostain can be helpful in the differential diagnosis with severely dysplastic nevus in some cases (PRAME, 100×)

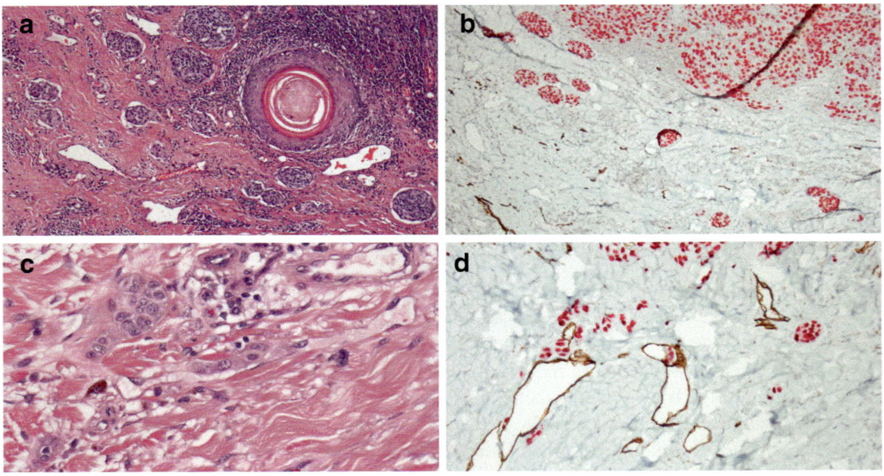

Fig. 3.10 (**a**) Superficial spreading melanoma with focus suspicious of lymphovascular invasion (H&E, 100×). (**b**) Immunohistochemical staining with dual D2–40 (brown cytoplasmic)/SOX10 (red nuclear) highlights the melanoma cell nests, but there are no D2–40-positive lymphatic/endothelial cells around these nests (not true lymphovascular invasion) (D2–40/SOX10, 100×). (**c**) Another case with a focus suspicious for lymphovascular invasion (H&E, 400×). (**d**) Dual D2–40 (brown cytoplasmic) /SOX10 (red nuclear) highlights the melanoma cells within the D2–40 positive lymphatic/endothelial vessel (true lymphovascular invasion) (D2–40/SOX10, 200×)

Differential Diagnosis

Dysplastic Nevus

The distinction of early SSM and severely dysplastic nevus is very challenging; however, it is encountered very commonly in day-to-day practice, and it is very important to distinguish them as most dysplastic nevi are stable and will never transform to melanoma or even involute over time (annual risk of transformation as low as 0.005%) [119, 120]. Dysplastic nevus is generally smaller in size (>4 mm and rarely >10 mm), somewhat symmetrical and circumscribed as compared to SSM, which is large (mostly >6 mm, often >10 mm), asymmetric, and poorly circumscribed (Table 3.1). There are uniformly elongated, delicate rete ridges without any significant epidermal changes in dysplastic nevus. In contrast, there is irregular acanthosis of epidermis, with thinning or consumption, sometimes ulceration, and effaced rete ridges in SSM. In dysplastic nevus, relatively uniform nests predominate over single cells in the epidermis, and there is little or no pagetoid spread, in contrast to SSM, in which there is predominance of intraepidermal single cells with confluent spread, prominent pagetoid scatter even at the edges, and irregular nests. If features of trauma or irritation are present, such as parakeratosis, pigment in the stratum corneum, subepidermal fibrosis, and/or hemorrhage, then focal suprabasilar/pagetoid upward migration of the melanocytes restricted to such a focus should be discounted. The pagetoid spread, if present, in dysplastic nevus is focal and only limited to the lower layers of the epidermis, in contrast to SSM, in which there is extensive pagetoid scatter, even at the edge of the lesion and very high-level, going as high as stratum corneum. In the dermis, the dysplastic nevus has a patchy lymphocytic infiltrate and regression is absent; however, caution should be exercised not to confuse the concentric and lamellar fibroplasia mixed with inflammation and melanophages as regression. SSM demonstrates brisk lymphocytic infiltrate in a bandlike arrangement, diffusely covering the base of the invasive tumor in most cases, and is commonly associated with partial or complete regression. The dermal melanocytic component is mostly nested in dysplastic nevus and demonstrates maturation, in contrast to the expansile pattern of melanoma cells in the dermis without any evidence of maturation in SSM. There is often mitosis in the dermal melanocytes in SSM, and one-third of SSM has intraepidermal mitosis. In contrast, dysplastic nevus almost never has mitoses in the epidermis or dermis. There is uniform severe cytologic atypia in SSM, in contrast to dysplastic nevus, in which most of the cells are not atypical, and only some cells demonstrate random atypia (Table 3.1). In equivocal cases, immunohistochemical staining for PRAME, p16, and/or Ki-67 (or dual Melan-A/Ki-67) or, rarely, in even more challenging cases, molecular testing such as a 5-probe FISH assay (interrogating gain of *RREB1*, *MYC*, *CCND1*, and homozygous deletion of *CDKN2A*) or NGS might be helpful [121]. In such cases, dermoscopic information and clinical findings might also be helpful in supporting one diagnosis over the other.

Special Site Nevi/Nevi of Special Sites

Nevus of special sites, occurring on the anogenital region, axillae, umbilicus, breast, scalp, and ears, may pose a diagnostic challenge. These nevi may have one or more architectural features of dysplastic nevus or even melanoma. In addition, these nevi may have superimposed features of trauma/irritation, halo-type regression, and age-related changes. These nevi generally demonstrate maturation with descent into the deeper dermis and are devoid of mitoses, necrosis, or significant host response

Table 3.1 Findings helpful in differentiating superficial spreading melanoma from dysplastic nevus

Histologic features	Dysplastic nevus	Superficial spreading melanoma (SSM)
Size	Small (>4 mm; rarely >10 mm)	Large (mostly >6 mm; often >10 mm)
Symmetry	Symmetric	Asymmetric
Circumscription	Relatively well circumscribed	Poorly circumscribed
Epidermis	No significant change	Irregular thickening with effaced rete ridges
Consumption	Absent	Present
Ulceration	Absent	Present
Nests	Uniform	Irregular
Nests vs single cells	Predominantly nested	Predominantly single cells
Pagetoid spread	Absent	Prominent
Confluent spread	Absent	Present
Lymphocytic infiltrate	Patchy	Brisk
Regression	Absent	Present
Dermal melanocytes	Mostly nested	Expansile
Maturation	Present	Absent
Mitosis	Absent	Present (mostly in epidermis, often in the dermis)
Cytologic atypia	Patchy, random	Uniform severe atypia
PRAME immunostain	Mostly negative or patchy	Mostly positive
Ki-67 proliferation rate	<5%	usually >20%

(lymphocytic infiltrate and fibrosis). When a nevus is from these sites and demonstrates some atypical features, one should be careful before overcalling them. Immunohistochemical staining for PRAME and dermoscopic findings may be helpful in distinguishing from SSM [122, 123].

Recurrent Nevus/Persistent Nevus/Traumatized Nevus

Recurrent nevus might need to be distinguished from SSM in some cases. These nevi demonstrate an atypical junctional and often superficial dermal melanocytic proliferation overlying and strictly confined to the area of dermal scar. The atypical cells do not extend laterally beyond the scar, and there is generally a residual banal nevus beneath the scar. Although there can be lentiginous spread and pagetoid scatter in the atrophic epidermis with effacement of the rete ridges, generally the cytologic atypia is not severe and uniform. The clinical history recurrent nevus/persistent nevus/traumatized nevus of trauma or a previous biopsy-proven nevus at the same site is helpful [124].

Pagetoid Spitz Nevus

Spitz nevus, especially pagetoid Spitz nevus, might be diagnostically challenging to differentiate from melanoma in situ, superficial spreading type. Generally, Pagetoid Spitz nevus comprises predominantly single cells with Spitzoid cytologic features, including large epithelioid cells having abundant amphophilic cytoplasm devoid of pigment mostly, large nuclei with evenly dispersed chromatin, and prominent eosinophilic nucleoli. Mostly, these nevi are small (<4 mm) in size, symmetrical, and with sharply defined borders. The cells are evenly distributed in the lower half of the epidermis and lack severe cytologic atypia. Most of the cases display epidermal hyperplasia and have Kamino bodies [125, 126]. They are mostly seen as a pigmented macule on the extremities of young females [127]. In contrast, SSM with or without spitzoid features are large and asymmetrical and demonstrate poor circumscription with single cells at one or both advancing edges, sometimes with pagetoid cells at the edge. There is prominent pagetoid scatter, consumption of the epidermis, and severe cytologic atypia [128]. In challenging cases, such as SSM with nevoid morphology and sharp borders, immunohistochemical stains with BRAF can be helpful if it is positive, as most of the Spitz nevi are negative for BRAF. Also, ancillary studies, such as FISH or cytogenetic studies, may be helpful [129, 130]. Dermoscopic findings and clinical information are also helpful in establishing a diagnosis [131].

Other Melanoma Subtypes

Although not very important from a management point of view, the distinction can sometimes be challenging. Lentigo maligna melanoma or high-CSD melanoma demonstrates lentiginous or basal proliferation of atypical melanocytes with minimal nesting or pagetoid scatter, thinned epidermis with loss of rete ridges, and severe solar elastosis. Nodular melanoma demonstrates predominantly dermal nodules with focal overlying epidermal involvement, and by definition, the intraepidermal in situ component extends less than three rete ridges beyond any dermal invasive component.

Prognosis

The prognosis of SSM is not significantly different from that of most other subtypes of low-CSD melanoma, other than acral-lentiginous melanoma [132]. The prognosis of SSM may be affected by the primary anatomic site [133]. The most powerful predictors of survival in SSM are tumor thickness (Breslow thickness) and ulceration. Other predictive factors include microsatellite, TILs, mitosis, and lymphovascular invasion. Molecular biomarkers of prognostic significance will be discussed in Chap. 12.

Molecular Findings

SSM or low-CSD melanoma is mostly associated with *BRAF* p.V600E mutation, the earliest driver oncogenic mutation identified in over 50% of cases [10, 134–136]. This mutation results in an amino acid substitution at position 600 from valine (V) to glutamic acid (E) [137]. It is the most common alteration that activates the mitogen-activated protein (MAP) kinase pathway in melanoma. Most SSM have a mutually exclusive driver oncogenic mutation of the *BRAF*, and less often *NRAS* or other alterations. SSM with prominent nesting and pagetoid scatter of melanoma cells are more likely to be associated with an activating *BRAF* mutation than other melanoma subtypes [17, 136, 138]. The probability of *BRAF* mutation in no or low-CSD melanomas is significantly higher in individuals younger than 50 years [139]. *BRAF* mutation rate is significantly higher in melanomas in intermittently sun-damaged skin rather than chronically sun-damaged skin and when melanomas are associated with a precursor nevus [140]. The detection of *BRAF* mutation can be helpful in differentiating Spitzoid lesions from SSM, as *BRAF* mutation is significantly higher in SSM as compared to Spitzoid lesions. Most banal nevi (up to 82%) also harbor the same *BRAF V600E* mutation [140–143].

Interestingly, most of the banal nevi only harbors single mutation, such as *BRAF V600E* and no other additional oncogenic alterations in contrast to melanoma, and their risk of progression to melanoma is estimated to be as low as 1 in 200,000 [119]. Therefore, these molecularly clonal lesions are considered "benign." [142, 143] These stable benign neoplasms harboring single driver oncogenic alterations are still called melanocytic nevus, although traditionally the term "nevus" was used for hamartomas.

The burden of point mutation increases with the progression of the neoplasm, from benign nevus through intermediate lesions (melanocytoma or dysplastic nevus) to melanoma [144]. A strong UV mutation signature is detectable at all these stages [140]. SSM or low-CSD melanoma harbors a high mutation burden with strong UV radiation signatures, confirming its epidemiologic link to sun exposure [134, 145–147]. These canonical point mutations are mostly cytosine transitioning to thymidine (C > T) at dipyrimidine sites, which is characteristic of UV radiation-induced mutation [134]. SSM is associated with multiple DNA copy number changes and aberrations, mostly in chromosomal arms or entire chromosomes. In fact, melanomas have the highest tumor mutation burden compared to any cancer in humans, which is the basis for immunotherapy in these cases [148]. SSM or low-CSD melanoma harbors a mutation burden of approximately 15 mutations per megabase [149]. Some of the SSM and rarely benign nevus are also associated with microsatellite instability, which is more common in children compared to adult melanoma [150–155].

The progression or melanomagenesis from a normal melanocyte to the development of invasive malignant melanoma and metastasis, with progressive accumulation of mutations and other genetic or epigenetic alterations (so-called hits), related to mutagenic effects on nucleic acid of sun exposure or other UV radiation, can be modeled to put it in a simplified way as:

Normal melanocyte → benign nevus → moderate or low-grade dysplasia → severe or high-grade dysplasia or melanocytoma → melanoma in situ → invasive melanoma → metastatic melanoma.

Although there are gaps in our knowledge of molecular progression, the alterations or "hits" can be related to these lesions in a simplified way as follows:

Normal melanocyte (no alteration) → benign nevus (*BRAF* V600E or rarely *NRAS*) → moderate or low-grade dysplasia → severe or high-grade dysplasia or melanocytoma (*BRAF* V600E or rarely *NRAS* + *TERT* promoter mutation) → melanoma in situ → invasive melanoma (*BRAF* V600E or rarely *NRAS* + *TERT* promoter mutation + *CDKN2A* loss + SWI/SNF) → metastatic melanoma (*BRAF* V600E or rarely *NRAS* + *TERT* promoter mutation + *CDKN2A* loss + SWI/SNF + *TP53* mutation and/or *PTEN*) [147, 156–158].

The initiating event or hit that leads to fully evolved SSM involves the MAP kinase pathway. The MAP kinase signaling is transmitted as follows: *RAS* → *RAF* → *MEK* → *ERK* [159]. Transmission of signal through this pathway allows the cell to progress through the cell cycle and regulates apoptosis. The RAF (rapidly accelerated fibrosarcoma) family of serine/threonine protein kinases includes *BRAF* (V-Raf Murine Sarcoma Viral Oncogene Homolog B1, located on chr 7; 7q34) that phosphorylates MEK when activated, activating the MAP kinase cascade and leading to cell proliferation and survival [160–163]. *BRAF* is the most common oncogene somatically mutated in SSM, with *BRAF* p.V600E mutation occurring in over 50% of cases and in 82% of benign acquired nevus [134, 141, 164, 165]. The single hit of *BRAF* mutation in the absence of any other oncogenic alteration leads to benign nevus formation, the proliferation of which is kept in check by tumor suppressor mechanisms such as oncogene-induced and replicative senescence, after some cell divisions, hence not progressing further [166–168]. However, when one of these partially transformed melanocytes acquires additional molecular "hit," such as *TERT* promoter mutation, that somehow nullifies the oncogene-induced senescence or other mechanisms that restrict uncontrolled proliferation of nevus, then it progresses further. *TERT* promoter mutation leads to increased telomerase expression, which in turn allows cells to avoid replicative senescence due to critical telomere shortening and thus resulting in immortalization of the cell [169–171]. The clonal expansion of these genetically intermediate lesions with more than one driver oncogenic alteration increases the risk of additional alterations, such as *CDKN2A* inactivation by loss or mutation, *PTEN* alteration, and SWI/SNF or *TP53* mutation, leading to transformation to melanoma [140, 172].

TERT (telomerase reverse transcriptase; 5p15) promoter mutation is found in the majority of SSM or low-CSD melanoma and is rare in nevus as well as nevus associated with low-CSD melanoma [173–175]. Again, it is found more commonly in metastatic melanoma than in primary melanoma [169]. *TERT* promoter mutation as well as copy-number gains is associated with worse prognosis in SSM [176, 177]. *PTEN* (phosphatase and tensin homolog: 10q23) inactivation by deletion or mutation, that leads to the activation of PI3K/AKT/mTOR pathway which in turn leads to cell proliferation and survival, is found in advanced primary SSM and also rarely (8%) in nevus [172, 178–181]. Inactivation of *CDKN2A* (cyclin-dependent kinase N2A; 9p21) that encodes tumor suppressor proteins p16 INK4A and p14, by loss or mutation, is also very common in SSM or low-CSD melanoma, and biallelic inactivation of *CDKN2A* is only found in invasive melanoma [144, 182–186]. p16 inhibits CDK4/6, releasing E2F from Rb, which in turn transitions the cells from G1 → S phase, initiating cell cycle. Loss of p16 leads to unchecked CDK4/6 and hence uncontrolled cell division and proliferation. Absence of p14, which inhibits MDM2 from degrading the tumor suppressor protein p53, leads to absence of p53, hindering apoptosis and hence leading to proliferation. *TP53* mutation occurs in advanced primary melanomas. Copy-number alterations are initially seen in intermediate and in situ lesions and keep on accumulating as the lesions progress to invasive melanoma and metastatic melanoma [144, 186]. Chromosomal abnormalities involving mostly losses at chromosomes 6q, 9, 10, and 20 and gains of chromosomes 1q, 6p, 7, 8q, 17q, and 20q are also common in SSM [187]. *CDKN2A/CDK4/Rb* pathway is also very commonly associated with germline alterations, leading to familial SSM [188, 189]. Germline mutations of the *TERT* promoter are also associated with familial melanoma susceptibility [188]. Approximately 10% of melanomas are known to be familial or hereditary with either a strong family history or/and established germline alteration.

The molecular techniques used to detect alterations for diagnostic evaluation and management of SSM include fluorescence in situ hybridization (FISH), comparative genomic hybridization (CGH), gene expression profiling (GEP) by qualitative reverse transcription polymerase chain reaction (qRT-PCR), and mutation or alteration analysis by various methods, including Sanger sequencing, pyrosequencing, allele-specific polymerase chain reaction (PCR), TaqMan RT-PCR, PCR with mass spectroscopy, and next-generation sequencing (NGS). Recently, the most frequently used techniques are FISH and NGS. Tape-stripping to extract cells from the surface of atypical, pigmented lesions for GEP (two-gene GEP evaluating *PRAME* and *LINC00518* mutation or three-gene GEP evaluating *PRAME*, *LINC00518*, and *TERT* promoter mutation) or toluidine blue cytology is used by some centers [190–194].

References

1. Horn-Ross PL, Holly EA, Brown SR, Aston DA. Temporal trends in the incidence of cutaneous malignant melanoma among Caucasians in the San Francisco-Oakland MSA. Cancer Causes Control. 1991;2(5):299–305. https://doi.org/10.1007/bf00051669.
2. Clark WH Jr, Elder DE, Van Horn M. The biologic forms of malignant melanoma. Hum Pathol. 1986;17(5):443–50. https://doi.org/10.1016/s0046-8177(86)80032-6.
3. Clark WH Jr, From L, Bernardino EA, Mihm MC. The histogenesis and biologic behavior of primary human malignant melanomas of the skin. Cancer Res. 1969;29(3):705–27.
4. McGovern VJ. The classification of melanoma and its relationship with prognosis. Pathology. 1970;2(2):85–98. https://doi.org/10.3109/00313027009077330.

5. Elder DE, Barnhill RL, Bastian BC, et al. Melanocytic tumour classification, and the pathway concept of melanoma pathogenesis. In: Elder DE, Massi D, Scolyer RA, Willemze R, editors. WHO classification of skin tumours, vol. 11. 4th ed. Lyon: Tumours, FIWHOCo.
6. Elder DE, Bastian BC, Cree IA, Massi D, Scolyer RA. The 2018 World Health Organization classification of cutaneous, mucosal, and uveal melanoma: detailed analysis of 9 distinct subtypes defined by their evolutionary pathway. Arch Pathol Lab Med. 2020;144(4):500–22. https://doi.org/10.5858/arpa.2019-0561-RA.
7. Sagebiel RW. Histopathology of borderline and early malignant melanomas. Am J Surg Pathol. 1979;3(6):543–52. https://doi.org/10.1097/00000478-197912000-00007.
8. Bay C, Kejs AM, Storm HH, Engholm G. Incidence and survival in patients with cutaneous melanoma by morphology, anatomical site and TNM stage: a Danish population-based register study 1989-2011. Cancer Epidemiol. 2015;39(1):1–7. https://doi.org/10.1016/j.canep.2014.10.010.
9. Lachiewicz AM, Berwick M, Wiggins CL, Thomas NE. Epidemiologic support for melanoma heterogeneity using the surveillance, epidemiology, and end results program. J Invest Dermatol. 2008;128(5):1340–2. https://doi.org/10.1038/jid.2008.18.
10. Maldonado JL, Fridlyand J, Patel H, et al. Determinants of BRAF mutations in primary melanomas. J Natl Cancer Inst. 2003;95(24):1878–90. https://doi.org/10.1093/jnci/djg123.
11. Arnold M, Singh D, Laversanne M, et al. Global burden of cutaneous melanoma in 2020 and projections to 2040. JAMA Dermatol. 2022;158(5):495–503. https://doi.org/10.1001/jamadermatol.2022.0160.
12. Sung H, Ferlay J, Siegel RL, et al. Global cancer statistics 2020: GLOBOCAN estimates of incidence and mortality worldwide for 36 cancers in 185 countries. CA Cancer J Clin. 2021;71(3):209–49. https://doi.org/10.3322/caac.21660.
13. NCIScsfmots. https://seer.cancer.gov/statfacts/html/melan.html.
14. Lancaster HO, Nelson J. Sunlight as a cause of melanoma; a clinical survey. Med J Aust. 1957;44(14):452–6.
15. Holman CD, Mulroney CD, Armstrong BK. Epidemiology of pre-invasive and invasive malignant melanoma in Western Australia. Int J Cancer. 1980;25(3):317–23. https://doi.org/10.1002/ijc.2910250303.
16. Arnold M, de Vries E, Whiteman DC, et al. Global burden of cutaneous melanoma attributable to ultraviolet radiation in 2012. Int J Cancer. 2018;143(6):1305–14. https://doi.org/10.1002/ijc.31527.
17. Curtin JA, Fridlyand J, Kageshita T, et al. Distinct sets of genetic alterations in melanoma. N Engl J Med. 2005;353(20):2135–47. https://doi.org/10.1056/NEJMoa050092.
18. Elder DE. Skin cancer. Melanoma and other specific nonmelanoma skin cancers. Cancer. 1995;75(1 Suppl):245–56. https://doi.org/10.1002/1097-0142(19950101)75:1+<245::aid-cncr2820751310>3.0.co;2-7.
19. Burbidge TE, Bastian BC, Guo D, et al. Association of Indoor Tanning Exposure with age at melanoma diagnosis and BRAF V600E mutations. J Natl Cancer Inst. 2019;111(11):1228–31. https://doi.org/10.1093/jnci/djz048.
20. Naldi L, Lorenzo Imberti G, Parazzini F, Gallus S, La Vecchia C. Pigmentary traits, modalities of sun reaction, history of sunburns, and melanocytic nevi as risk factors for cutaneous malignant melanoma in the Italian population: results of a collaborative case-control study. Cancer. 2000;88(12):2703–10. https://doi.org/10.1002/1097-0142(20000615)88:12<2703::aid-cncr8>3.0.co;2-q.
21. Gandini S, Sera F, Cattaruzza MS, et al. Meta-analysis of risk factors for cutaneous melanoma: I. Common and atypical naevi. Eur J Cancer. 2005;41(1):28–44. https://doi.org/10.1016/j.ejca.2004.10.015.
22. Tucker MA, Halpern A, Holly EA, et al. Clinically recognized dysplastic nevi. A central risk factor for cutaneous melanoma. JAMA. 1997;277(18):1439–44.
23. Arumi-Uria M, McNutt NS, Finnerty B. Grading of atypia in nevi: correlation with melanoma risk. Mod Pathol. 2003;16(8):764–71. https://doi.org/10.1097/01.Mp.0000082394.91761.E5.

24. Xiong MY, Rabkin MS, Piepkorn MW, et al. Diameter of dysplastic nevi is a more robust biomarker of increased melanoma risk than degree of histologic dysplasia: a case-control study. J Am Acad Dermatol. 2014;71(6):1257–1258.e1254. https://doi.org/10.1016/j.jaad.2014.07.030.
25. Shors AR, Kim S, White E, et al. Dysplastic naevi with moderate to severe histological dysplasia: a risk factor for melanoma. Br J Dermatol. 2006;155(5):988–93. https://doi.org/10.1111/j.1365-2133.2006.07466.x.
26. Law MH, Macgregor S, Hayward NK. Melanoma genetics: recent findings take us beyond well-traveled pathways. J Invest Dermatol. 2012;132(7):1763–74. https://doi.org/10.1038/jid.2012.75.
27. Greene MH, Clark WH Jr, Tucker MA, Kraemer KH, Elder DE, Fraser MC. High risk of malignant melanoma in melanoma-prone families with dysplastic nevi. Ann Intern Med. 1985;102(4):458–65. https://doi.org/10.7326/0003-4819-102-4-458.
28. Rigel DS, Friedman RJ, Kopf AW, Polsky D. ABCDE—an evolving concept in the early detection of melanoma. Arch Dermatol. 2005;141(8):1032–4. https://doi.org/10.1001/archderm.141.8.1032.
29. Guibert P, Mollat F, Ligen M, Dreno B. Melanoma screening: report of a survey in occupational medicine. Arch Dermatol. 2000;136(2):199–202. https://doi.org/10.1001/archderm.136.2.199.
30. Friedman RJ, Rigel DS, Kopf AW. Early detection of malignant melanoma: the role of physician examination and self-examination of the skin. CA Cancer J Clin. 1985;35(3):130–51. https://doi.org/10.3322/canjclin.35.3.130.
31. Abbasi NR, Shaw HM, Rigel DS, et al. Early diagnosis of cutaneous melanoma: revisiting the ABCD criteria. JAMA. 2004;292(22):2771–6. https://doi.org/10.1001/jama.292.22.2771.
32. Robinson JK, Turrisi R. Skills training to learn discrimination of ABCDE criteria by those at risk of developing melanoma. Arch Dermatol. 2006;142(4):447–52. https://doi.org/10.1001/archderm.142.4.447.
33. Bystryn JC. A confusing message will not improve the detection of melanoma. Arch Dermatol. 2007;143(6):806; author reply 806–807. https://doi.org/10.1001/archderm.143.6.806-a.
34. Fox GN. ABCD-EFG for diagnosis of melanoma. Clin Exp Dermatol. 2005;30(6):707. https://doi.org/10.1111/j.1365-2230.2005.01857.x.
35. Piepkorn M, Odland PB. Quality of care in the diagnosis of melanoma and related melanocytic lesions. Arch Dermatol. 1997;133(11):1393–6.
36. Koch SE, Henneberry JM. Clinically subtle primary cutaneous melanoma. J Am Acad Dermatol. 1999;40(2 Pt 1):252–4. https://doi.org/10.1016/s0190-9622(99)70198-2.
37. Askari SK, Schram SE, Wenner RA, et al. Evaluation of prospectively collected presenting signs/symptoms of biopsy-proven melanoma, basal cell carcinoma, squamous cell carcinoma, and seborrheic keratosis in an elderly male population. J Am Acad Dermatol. 2007;56(5):739–47. https://doi.org/10.1016/j.jaad.2006.11.032.
38. Steiner A, Konrad K, Pehamberger H, Wolff K. Verrucous malignant melanoma. Arch Dermatol. 1988;124(10):1534–7.
39. Sober AJ, Fitzpatrick TB, Mihm MC Jr. Primary melanoma of the skin: recognition and management. J Am Acad Dermatol. 1980;2(3):179–97. https://doi.org/10.1016/s0190-9622(80)80001-6.
40. Borges SZ, Bakos L, Cartell A, Wagner M, Agostini A, Lersch E. Distribution of clinical-pathological types of cutaneous melanomas and mortality rate in the region of Passo Fundo, RS, Brazil. Int J Dermatol. 2007;46(7):679–86. https://doi.org/10.1111/j.1365-4632.2007.03037.x.
41. Bulliard JL, Ess S, Bordoni A, Konzelmann I, Levi F. Left-sided excess in the laterality of cutaneous melanoma. Arch Dermatol. 2008;144(4):556–8. https://doi.org/10.1001/archderm.144.4.556.
42. Brewster DH, de Vries E. Left-sided excess in the laterality of cutaneous melanoma. Arch Dermatol. 2008;144(9):1235. https://doi.org/10.1001/archderm.144.9.1235-a.

43. Shitara D, Nascimento MM, Puig S, et al. Nevus-associated melanomas: clinicopathologic features. Am J Clin Pathol. 2014;142(4):485–91. https://doi.org/10.1309/ajcp4l5cjgktjvdd.
44. Scope A, Dusza SW, Halpern AC, et al. The "ugly duckling" sign: agreement between observers. Arch Dermatol. 2008;144(1):58–64. https://doi.org/10.1001/archdermatol.2007.15.
45. Ladewig G, Reinhold U, Thirkill CE, Kerber A, Tilgen W, Pföhler C. Incidence of antiretinal antibodies in melanoma: screening of 77 serum samples from 51 patients with American joint committee on cancer stage I-IV. Br J Dermatol. 2005;152(5):931–8. https://doi.org/10.1111/j.1365-2133.2005.06480.x.
46. Pföhler C, Haus A, Palmowski A, et al. Melanoma-associated retinopathy: high frequency of subclinical findings in patients with melanoma. Br J Dermatol. 2003;149(1):74–8. https://doi.org/10.1046/j.1365-2133.2003.05377.x.
47. Wagner RF Jr, Nathanson L. Paraneoplastic syndromes, tumor markers, and other unusual features of malignant melanoma. J Am Acad Dermatol. 1986;14(2 Pt 1):249–56. https://doi.org/10.1016/s0190-9622(86)70029-7.
48. Argenziano G, Catricalà C, Ardigo M, et al. Seven-point checklist of dermoscopy revisited. Br J Dermatol. 2011;164(4):785–90. https://doi.org/10.1111/j.1365-2133.2010.10194.x.
49. Gereli MC, Onsun N, Atilganoglu U, Demirkesen C. Comparison of two dermoscopic techniques in the diagnosis of clinically atypical pigmented skin lesions and melanoma: seven-point and three-point checklists. Int J Dermatol. 2010;49(1):33–8. https://doi.org/10.1111/j.1365-4632.2009.04152.x.
50. Kittler H, Marghoob AA, Argenziano G, et al. Standardization of terminology in dermoscopy/dermatoscopy: results of the third consensus conference of the International Society of Dermoscopy. J Am Acad Dermatol. 2016;74(6):1093–106. https://doi.org/10.1016/j.jaad.2015.12.038.
51. Maskalane J, Salijuma E, Lallas K, et al. Distribution of the dermoscopic features of melanoma of trunk and extremities according to the anatomic sublocation. J Am Acad Dermatol. 2021;84(6):1717–9. https://doi.org/10.1016/j.jaad.2020.08.058.
52. Rosendahl C, Tschandl P, Cameron A, Kittler H. Diagnostic accuracy of dermatoscopy for melanocytic and nonmelanocytic pigmented lesions. J Am Acad Dermatol. 2011;64(6):1068–73. https://doi.org/10.1016/j.jaad.2010.03.039.
53. Verzi AE, Quan VL, Walton KE, et al. The diagnostic value and histologic correlate of distinct patterns of shiny white streaks for the diagnosis of melanoma: a retrospective, case-control study. J Am Acad Dermatol. 2018;78(5):913–9. https://doi.org/10.1016/j.jaad.2017.11.021.
54. Ascierto PA, Palmieri G, Celentano E, et al. Sensitivity and specificity of epiluminescence microscopy: evaluation on a sample of 2731 excised cutaneous pigmented lesions. The melanoma cooperative study. Br J Dermatol. 2000;142(5):893–8. https://doi.org/10.1046/j.1365-2133.2000.03468.x.
55. Andreassi L, Perotti R, Rubegni P, et al. Digital dermoscopy analysis for the differentiation of atypical nevi and early melanoma: a new quantitative semiology. Arch Dermatol. 1999;135(12):1459–65. https://doi.org/10.1001/archderm.135.12.1459.
56. Menzies SW. Surface microscopy of pigmented skin tumours. Australas J Dermatol. 1997;38(Suppl 1):S40–3. https://doi.org/10.1111/j.1440-0960.1997.tb01008.x.
57. Argenziano G, Fabbrocini G, Carli P, De Giorgi V, Delfino M. Epiluminescence microscopy: criteria of cutaneous melanoma progression. J Am Acad Dermatol. 1997;37(1):68–74. https://doi.org/10.1016/s0190-9622(97)70213-5.
58. Braun RP, Meier M, Pelloni F, et al. Teledermatoscopy in Switzerland: a preliminary evaluation. J Am Acad Dermatol. 2000;42(5 Pt 1):770–5. https://doi.org/10.1067/mjd.2000.103977.
59. Carli P, Massi D, de Giorgi V, Giannotti B. Clinically and dermoscopically featureless melanoma: when prevention fails. J Am Acad Dermatol. 2002;46(6):957–9. https://doi.org/10.1067/mjd.2002.120569.
60. Stante M, Carli P, Massi D, de Giorgi V. Dermoscopic features of naevus-associated melanoma. Clin Exp Dermatol. 2003;28(5):476–80. https://doi.org/10.1046/j.1365-2230.2003.01332.x.

61. Zalaudek I, Argenziano G, Ferrara G, et al. Clinically equivocal melanocytic skin lesions with features of regression: a dermoscopic-pathological study. Br J Dermatol. 2004;150(1):64–71. https://doi.org/10.1111/j.1365-2133.2004.05657.x.
62. Braun RP, Gaide O, Oliviero M, et al. The significance of multiple blue-grey dots (granularity) for the dermoscopic diagnosis of melanoma. Br J Dermatol. 2007;157(5):907–13. https://doi.org/10.1111/j.1365-2133.2007.08145.x.
63. Pezzini C, Kaleci S, Chester J, Farnetani F, Longo C, Pellacani G. Reflectance confocal microscopy diagnostic accuracy for malignant melanoma in different clinical settings: systematic review and meta-analysis. J Eur Acad Dermatol Venereol. 2020;34(10):2268–79. https://doi.org/10.1111/jdv.16248.
64. Suppa M, Palmisano G, Tognetti L, et al. Line-field confocal optical coherence tomography in melanocytic and non-melanocytic skin tumors. Ital J Dermatol Venerol. 2023;158(3):180–9. https://doi.org/10.23736/s2784-8671.23.07639-9.
65. Schneider SL, Kohli I, Hamzavi IH, Council ML, Rossi AM, Ozog DM. Emerging imaging technologies in dermatology: part II: applications and limitations. J Am Acad Dermatol. 2019;80(4):1121–31. https://doi.org/10.1016/j.jaad.2018.11.043.
66. Schneider SL, Kohli I, Hamzavi IH, Council ML, Rossi AM, Ozog DM. Emerging imaging technologies in dermatology: part I: basic principles. J Am Acad Dermatol. 2019;80(4):1114–20. https://doi.org/10.1016/j.jaad.2018.11.042.
67. Fink C, Haenssle HA. Non-invasive tools for the diagnosis of cutaneous melanoma. Skin Res Technol. 2017;23(3):261–71. https://doi.org/10.1111/srt.12350.
68. Price NM, Rywlin AM, Ackerman AB. Histologic criteria for the diagnosis of superficial spreading malignant melanoma: formulated on the basis of proven metastatic lesions. Cancer. 1976;38(6):2434–41. https://doi.org/10.1002/1097-0142(197612)38:6<2434::aid-cncr2820380631>3.0.co;2-n.
69. Kutzner H, Metzler G, Argenyi Z, et al. Histological and genetic evidence for a variant of superficial spreading melanoma composed predominantly of large nests. Mod Pathol. 2012;25(6):838–45. https://doi.org/10.1038/modpathol.2012.35.
70. Fallowfield ME, Cook MG. Pagetoid infiltration in primary cutaneous melanoma. Histopathology. 1992;20(5):417–20. https://doi.org/10.1111/j.1365-2559.1992.tb01012.x.
71. Bono A, Bartoli C, Moglia D, et al. Small melanomas: a clinical study on 270 consecutive cases of cutaneous melanoma. Melanoma Res. 1999;9(6):583–6.
72. Moyer AB, Diwan AH. Puffy shirt appearance: cell crowding at low magnification may represent nevoid melanoma. J Cutan Pathol. 2019;46(11):805–9. https://doi.org/10.1111/cup.13531.
73. Bandino JP, Kazlouskaya V, Ergin Ş, et al. Epidermal consumption in benign and malignant melanocytic neoplasms. J Cutan Pathol. 2015;42(12):937–43. https://doi.org/10.1111/cup.12545.
74. Urso C. Cleft formation and consumption of the epidermis in cutaneous melanocytic lesions. Hum Pathol. 2006;37(2):246; author reply 247. https://doi.org/10.1016/j.humpath.2005.08.027.
75. Braun-Falco M, Friedrichson E, Ring J. Subepidermal cleft formation as a diagnostic marker for cutaneous malignant melanoma. Hum Pathol. 2005;36(4):412–5. https://doi.org/10.1016/j.humpath.2005.02.005.
76. Cramer SF. Consumption of the epidermis—what is its place in the spectrum of aberrant melanocyte-keratinocyte interactions? Am J Dermatopathol. 2008;30(2):200–3. https://doi.org/10.1097/DAD.0b013e318164ede6.
77. Walters RF, Groben PA, Busam K, et al. Consumption of the epidermis: a criterion in the differential diagnosis of melanoma and dysplastic nevi that is associated with increasing breslow depth and ulceration. Am J Dermatopathol. 2007;29(6):527–33. https://doi.org/10.1097/DAD.0b013e318156e0a7.
78. Elder DE. Pathology of melanoma. Surg Oncol Clin N Am. 2015;24(2):229–37. https://doi.org/10.1016/j.soc.2014.12.002.

79. Sagebiel RW. Melanocytic nevi in histologic association with primary cutaneous melanoma of superficial spreading and nodular types: effect of tumor thickness. J Invest Dermatol. 1993;100(3):322s–5s. https://doi.org/10.1111/1523-1747.ep12470218.
80. Stolz W, Schmoeckel C, Landthaler M, Braun-Falco O. Association of early malignant melanoma with nevocytic nevi. Cancer. 1989;63(3):550–5. https://doi.org/10.1002/1097-0142(19890201)63:3<550::aid-cncr2820630325>3.0.co;2-a.
81. Gruber SB, Barnhill RL, Stenn KS, Roush GC. Nevomelanocytic proliferations in association with cutaneous malignant melanoma: a multivariate analysis. J Am Acad Dermatol. 1989;21(4 Pt 1):773–80. https://doi.org/10.1016/s0190-9622(89)70253-x.
82. Harley S, Walsh N. A new look at nevus-associated melanomas. Am J Dermatopathol. 1996;18(2):137–41. https://doi.org/10.1097/00000372-199604000-00005.
83. Lee EY, Williamson R, Watt P, Hughes MC, Green AC, Whiteman DC. Sun exposure and host phenotype as predictors of cutaneous melanoma associated with neval remnants or dermal elastosis. Int J Cancer. 2006;119(3):636–42. https://doi.org/10.1002/ijc.21907.
84. Landi MT, Bauer J, Pfeiffer RM, et al. MC1R germline variants confer risk for BRAF-mutant melanoma. Science. 2006;313(5786):521–2. https://doi.org/10.1126/science.1127515.
85. Breslow A. Thickness, cross-sectional areas and depth of invasion in the prognosis of cutaneous melanoma. Ann Surg. 1970;172(5):902–8. https://doi.org/10.1097/00000658-197011000-00017.
86. Gershenwald JE, Scolyer R Hess KR, et al. Melanoma of the skin, In: Amin MB, Edge SB, Greene FL, et al., editors. AJCC cancer staging manual. 8th ed. New York: Springer; 2017.
87. Gershenwald JE, Scolyer RA, Hess KR, et al. Melanoma staging: evidence-based changes in the American joint committee on cancer eighth edition cancer staging manual. CA Cancer J Clin. 2017;67(6):472–92. https://doi.org/10.3322/caac.21409.
88. In 't Hout FE, Haydu LE, Murali R, Bonenkamp JJ, Thompson JF, Scolyer RA. Prognostic importance of the extent of ulceration in patients with clinically localized cutaneous melanoma. Ann Surg. 2012;255(6):1165–70. https://doi.org/10.1097/SLA.0b013e31824c4b0b.
89. Scolyer RA, Shaw HM, Thompson JF, et al. Interobserver reproducibility of histopathologic prognostic variables in primary cutaneous melanomas. Am J Surg Pathol. 2003;27(12):1571–6. https://doi.org/10.1097/00000478-200312000-00011.
90. English DR, Heenan PJ, Holman CD, et al. Melanoma in Western Australia in 1980-81: incidence and characteristics of histological types. Pathology. 1987;19(4):383–92. https://doi.org/10.3109/00313028709103888.
91. Durnick A, Stolz W, Landthaler M, Vogt T. Lentigo maligna and lentigo maligna melanoma in young adults. Dermatologic Surg. 2004;30(5):813–6. https://doi.org/10.1111/j.1524-4725.2004.30222.x.
92. Gillgren P, Månsson-Brahme E, Frisell J, Johansson H, Larsson O, Ringborg U. Epidemiological characteristics of cutaneous malignant melanoma of the head and neck—a population-based study. Acta Oncol. 1999;38(8):1069–74. https://doi.org/10.1080/028418699432383.
93. Clark WH Jr, Elder DE, Dt G, et al. Model predicting survival in stage I melanoma based on tumor progression. J Natl Cancer Inst. 1989;81(24):1893–904. https://doi.org/10.1093/jnci/81.24.1893.
94. McGovern VJ. Spontaneous regression of melanoma. Pathology. 1975;7(2):91–9. https://doi.org/10.3109/00313027509092702.
95. Clark WH Jr, Tucker MA, Goldstein AM. Parenchymal-stromal interactions in neoplasia. Theoretical considerations and observations in melanocytic neoplasia. Acta Oncol. 1995;34(6):749–57. https://doi.org/10.3109/02841869509127182.
96. Clark WH Jr, Tucker MA. Problems with lesions related to the development of malignant melanoma: common nevi, dysplastic nevi, malignant melanoma in situ, and radial growth phase malignant melanoma. Hum Pathol. 1998;29(1):8–14. https://doi.org/10.1016/s0046-8177(98)90384-7.

97. Blessing K, McLaren KM. Histological regression in primary cutaneous melanoma: recognition, prevalence and significance. Histopathology. 1992;20(4):315–22. https://doi.org/10.1111/j.1365-2559.1992.tb00988.x.
98. Trau H, Rigel DS, Harris MN, et al. Metastases of thin melanomas. Cancer. 1983;51(3):553–6. https://doi.org/10.1002/1097-0142(19830201)51:3<553::aid-cncr2820510332>3.0.co;2-t.
99. McGovern VJ, Shaw HM, Milton GW. Prognosis in patients with thin malignant melanoma: influence of regression. Histopathology. 1983;7(5):673–80. https://doi.org/10.1111/j.1365-2559.1983.tb02279.x.
100. Trau H, Kopf AW, Rigel DS, et al. Regression in malignant melanoma. J Am Acad Dermatol. 1983;8(3):363–8. https://doi.org/10.1016/s0190-9622(83)70040-x.
101. Leecy TN, McQuillan P, Harvey NT, et al. Large nested melanoma: a clinicopathological, morphometric and cytogenetic study of 12 cases. Pathology. 2020;52(4):431–8. https://doi.org/10.1016/j.pathol.2020.02.006.
102. Kamino H, Tam ST, Alvarez L. Malignant melanoma with pseudocarcinomatous hyperplasia—an entity that can simulate squamous cell carcinoma. A light-microscopic and immunohistochemical study of four cases. Am J Dermatopathol. 1990;12(5):446–51. https://doi.org/10.1097/00000372-199010000-00003.
103. Reis-Filho JS, Gasparetto EL, Schmitt FC, Fillus-Neto J. Pseudoepitheliomatous hyperplasia in cutaneous malignant melanoma: a rare and misleading feature. J Cutan Pathol. 2001;28(9):496–7. https://doi.org/10.1034/j.1600-0560.2001.028009496.x.
104. Hanly AJ, Jorda M, Elgart GW. Cutaneous malignant melanoma associated with extensive pseudoepitheliomatous hyperplasia. Report of a case and discussion of the origin of pseudoepitheliomatous hyperplasia. J Cutan Pathol. 2000;27(3):153–6. https://doi.org/10.1034/j.1600-0560.2000.027003153.x.
105. Wellings SR, Siegel BV. Electron microscopy of human malignant melanoma. J Natl Cancer Inst. 1960;24:437–61.
106. Hunter JA, Zaynoun S, Paterson WD, Bleehen SS, Mackie R, Cochran AJ. Cellular fine structure in the invasive nodules of different histogenetic types of malignant melanoma. Br J Dermatol. 1978;98(3):255–72. https://doi.org/10.1111/j.1365-2133.1978.tb06152.x.
107. Mishima Y. Melanocytic and nevocytic malignant melanomas. Cellular and subcellular differentiation. Cancer. 1967;20(5):632–49. https://doi.org/10.1002/1097-0142(1967)20:5<632::aid-cncr2820200510>3.0.co;2-7.
108. Bhuta S. Electron microscopy in the evaluation of melanocytic tumors. Semin Diagn Pathol. 1993;10(1):92–101.
109. Clark WH Jr, Ainsworth AM, Bernardino EA, Yang CH, Mihm CM Jr, Reed RJ. The developmental biology of primary human malignant melanomas. Semin Oncol. 1975;2(2):83–103.
110. Prieto VG, Shea CR. Immunohistochemistry of melanocytic proliferations. Arch Pathol Lab Med. 2011;135(7):853–9. https://doi.org/10.5858/2009-0717-rar.1.
111. Gown AM, Vogel AM, Hoak D, Gough F, McNutt MA. Monoclonal antibodies specific for melanocytic tumors distinguish subpopulations of melanocytes. Am J Pathol. 1986;123(2):195–203.
112. Colombari R, Bonetti F, Zamboni G, et al. Distribution of melanoma specific antibody (HMB-45) in benign and malignant melanocytic tumours. An immunohistochemical study on paraffin sections. Virchows Arch A Pathol Anat Histopathol. 1988;413(1):17–24. https://doi.org/10.1007/bf00844277.
113. Rudolph P, Lappe T, Schubert C, Schmidt D, Parwaresch RM, Christophers E. Diagnostic assessment of two novel proliferation-specific antigens in benign and malignant melanocytic lesions. Am J Pathol. 1995;147(6):1615–25.
114. Reed JA, Loganzo F Jr, Shea CR, et al. Loss of expression of the p16/cyclin-dependent kinase inhibitor 2 tumor suppressor gene in melanocytic lesions correlates with invasive stage of tumor progression. Cancer Res. 1995;55(13):2713–8.
115. Mihic-Probst D, Saremaslani P, Komminoth P, Heitz PU. Immunostaining for the tumour suppressor gene p16 product is a useful marker to differentiate melanoma metastasis

from lymph-node nevus. Virchows Arch. 2003;443(6):745–51. https://doi.org/10.1007/s00428-003-0897-9.
116. Chinchanikar SS, Fraga GR. Ancillary immunohistochemistry testing for loss of p16 in melanoma: a systematic review and meta-analysis of diagnostic accuracy studies. J Cutan Pathol. 2024;51(12):971–9. https://doi.org/10.1111/cup.14717.
117. Lezcano C, Jungbluth AA, Nehal KS, Hollmann TJ, Busam KJ. PRAME expression in melanocytic Tumors. Am J Surg Pathol. 2018;42(11):1456–65. https://doi.org/10.1097/pas.0000000000001134.
118. Lezcano C, Jungbluth AA, Busam KJ. Immunohistochemistry for PRAME in dermatopathology. Am J Dermatopathol. 2023;45(11):733–47. https://doi.org/10.1097/dad.0000000000002440.
119. Tsao H, Bevona C, Goggins W, Quinn T. The transformation rate of moles (melanocytic nevi) into cutaneous melanoma: a population-based estimate. Arch Dermatol. 2003;139(3):282–8. https://doi.org/10.1001/archderm.139.3.282.
120. Halpern AC, Guerry DP IV, Elder DE, Trock B, Synnestvedt M, Humphreys T. Natural history of dysplastic nevi. J Am Acad Dermatol. 1993;29(1):51–7. https://doi.org/10.1016/0190-9622(93)70151-i.
121. Gerami P, Li G, Pouryazdanparast P, et al. A highly specific and discriminatory FISH assay for distinguishing between benign and malignant melanocytic neoplasms. Am J Surg Pathol. 2012;36(6):808–17. https://doi.org/10.1097/PAS.0b013e31824b1efd.
122. Larre Borges A, Zalaudek I, Longo C, et al. Melanocytic nevi with special features: clinical-dermoscopic and reflectance confocal microscopic-findings. J Eur Acad Dermatol Venereol. 2014;28(7):833–45. https://doi.org/10.1111/jdv.12291.
123. Merkel EA, Martini MC, Amin SM, Lee CY, Gerami P. Evaluation of dermoscopic features for distinguishing melanoma from special site nevi of the breast. J Am Acad Dermatol. 2016;75(2):364–70. https://doi.org/10.1016/j.jaad.2016.04.006.
124. Brenn T. Pitfalls in the evaluation of melanocytic lesions. Histopathology. 2012;60(5):690–705. https://doi.org/10.1111/j.1365-2559.2011.04042.x.
125. Fernandez AP, Billings SD, Bergfeld WF, Ko JS, Piliang MP. Pagetoid spitz nevi: clinicopathologic characterization of a series of 12 cases. J Cutan Pathol. 2016;43(11):932–9. https://doi.org/10.1111/cup.12774.
126. Han MH, Koh KJ, Choi JH, Sung KJ, Moon KC, Koh JK. Pagetoid spitz nevus: a variant of spitz nevus. Int J Dermatol. 2000;39(7):555–7. https://doi.org/10.1046/j.1365-4362.2000.00819-4.x.
127. Busam KJ, Barnhill RL. Pagetoid spitz nevus. Intraepidermal spitz tumor with prominent pagetoid spread. Am J Surg Pathol. 1995;19(9):1061–7.
128. Connors RC, Chalet MD, Ackerman AB. Benign juvenile melanoma (spitz nevus) vs. superficial spreading malignant melanoma: criteria for histologic differentiation. J Dermatol Surg. 1975;1(2):14–5. https://doi.org/10.1111/j.1524-4725.1975.tb00064.x.
129. Gerami P, Barnhill RL, Beilfuss BA, LeBoit P, Schneider P, Guitart J. Superficial melanocytic neoplasms with pagetoid melanocytosis: a study of interobserver concordance and correlation with FISH. Am J Surg Pathol. 2010;34(6):816–21. https://doi.org/10.1097/PAS.0b013e3181dd1e72.
130. Gerami P, Wass A, Mafee M, Fang Y, Pulitzer MP, Busam KJ. Fluorescence in situ hybridization for distinguishing nevoid melanomas from mitotically active nevi. Am J Surg Pathol. 2009;33(12):1783–8. https://doi.org/10.1097/PAS.0b013e3181ba6db6.
131. Lallas A, Apalla Z, Ioannides D, et al. Update on dermoscopy of spitz/Reed naevi and management guidelines by the international Dermoscopy society. Br J Dermatol. 2017;177(3):645–55. https://doi.org/10.1111/bjd.15339.
132. Gumaste PV, Fleming NH, Silva I, et al. Analysis of recurrence patterns in acral versus non-acral melanoma: should histologic subtype influence treatment guidelines? J Natl Compr Cancer Netw. 2014;12(12):1706–12. https://doi.org/10.6004/jnccn.2014.0172.

133. Balch CM, Soong SJ, Gershenwald JE, et al. Prognostic factors analysis of 17,600 melanoma patients: validation of the American joint committee on cancer melanoma staging system. J Clin Oncol. 2001;19(16):3622–34. https://doi.org/10.1200/jco.2001.19.16.3622.
134. Cancer Genome Atlas Network. Genomic classification of cutaneous melanoma. Cell. 2015;161(7):1681–96. https://doi.org/10.1016/j.cell.2015.05.044.
135. Krauthammer M, Kong Y, Ha BH, et al. Exome sequencing identifies recurrent somatic RAC1 mutations in melanoma. Nat Genet. 2012;44(9):1006–14. https://doi.org/10.1038/ng.2359.
136. Viros A, Fridlyand J, Bauer J, et al. Improving melanoma classification by integrating genetic and morphologic features. PLoS Med. 2008;5(6):e120. https://doi.org/10.1371/journal.pmed.0050120.
137. Richtig G, Hoeller C, Kashofer K, et al. Beyond the BRAF(V)(600E) hotspot: biology and clinical implications of rare BRAF gene mutations in melanoma patients. Br J Dermatol. 2017;177(4):936–44. https://doi.org/10.1111/bjd.15436.
138. Broekaert SM, Roy R, Okamoto I, et al. Genetic and morphologic features for melanoma classification. Pigment Cell Melanoma Res. 2010;23(6):763–70. https://doi.org/10.1111/j.1755-148X.2010.00778.x.
139. Long GV, Menzies AM, Nagrial AM, et al. Prognostic and clinicopathologic associations of oncogenic BRAF in metastatic melanoma. J Clin Oncol. 2011;29(10):1239–46. https://doi.org/10.1200/jco.2010.32.4327.
140. Shain AH, Yeh I, Kovalyshyn I, et al. The genetic evolution of melanoma from precursor lesions. N Engl J Med. 2015;373(20):1926–36. https://doi.org/10.1056/NEJMoa1502583.
141. Pollock PM, Harper UL, Hansen KS, et al. High frequency of BRAF mutations in nevi. Nat Genet. 2003;33(1):19–20. https://doi.org/10.1038/ng1054.
142. Yeh I, von Deimling A, Bastian BC. Clonal BRAF mutations in melanocytic nevi and initiating role of BRAF in melanocytic neoplasia. J Natl Cancer Inst. 2013;105(12):917–9. https://doi.org/10.1093/jnci/djt119.
143. Saroufim M, Habib R, Karram S, et al. BRAF analysis on a spectrum of melanocytic neoplasms: an epidemiological study across differing UV regions. Am J Dermatopathol. 2014;36(1):68–73. https://doi.org/10.1097/DAD.0b013e318293f355.
144. Zeng H, Jorapur A, Shain AH, et al. Bi-allelic loss of CDKN2A initiates melanoma invasion via BRN2 activation. Cancer Cell. 2018;34(1):56–68.e59. https://doi.org/10.1016/j.ccell.2018.05.014.
145. Pleasance ED, Cheetham RK, Stephens PJ, et al. A comprehensive catalogue of somatic mutations from a human cancer genome. Nature. 2010;463(7278):191–6. https://doi.org/10.1038/nature08658.
146. Hayward NK, Wilmott JS, Waddell N, et al. Whole-genome landscapes of major melanoma subtypes. Nature. 2017;545(7653):175–80. https://doi.org/10.1038/nature22071.
147. Lu X, Zhang Q, Wang Y, et al. Molecular classification and subtype-specific characterization of skin cutaneous melanoma by aggregating multiple genomic platform data. J Cancer Res Clin Oncol. 2018;144(9):1635–47. https://doi.org/10.1007/s00432-018-2684-7.
148. Chalmers ZR, Connelly CF, Fabrizio D, et al. Analysis of 100,000 human cancer genomes reveals the landscape of tumor mutational burden. Genome Med. 2017;9(1):34. https://doi.org/10.1186/s13073-017-0424-2.
149. Krauthammer M, Kong Y, Bacchiocchi A, et al. Exome sequencing identifies recurrent mutations in NF1 and RASopathy genes in sun-exposed melanomas. Nat Genet. 2015;47(9):996–1002. https://doi.org/10.1038/ng.3361.
150. Hussein MR, Roggero E, Sudilovsky EC, Tuthill RJ, Wood GS, Sudilovsky O. Alterations of mismatch repair protein expression in benign melanocytic nevi, melanocytic dysplastic nevi, and cutaneous malignant melanomas. Am J Dermatopathol. 2001;23(4):308–14. https://doi.org/10.1097/00000372-200108000-00006.
151. Hussein MR, Sun M, Tuthill RJ, et al. Comprehensive analysis of 112 melanocytic skin lesions demonstrates microsatellite instability in melanomas and dysplastic nevi, but not in

benign nevi. J Cutan Pathol. 2001;28(7):343–50. https://doi.org/10.1034/j.1600-0560.2001.280702.x.
152. Ponti G, Losi L, Pellacani G, et al. Malignant melanoma in patients with hereditary non-polyposis colorectal cancer. Br J Dermatol. 2008;159(1):162–8. https://doi.org/10.1111/j.1365-2133.2008.08575.x.
153. Korabiowska M, Cordon-Cardo C, Jaenckel F, Stachura J, Fischer G, Brinck U. Application of in situ hybridization probes for MLH-1 and MSH-2 in tissue microarrays of paraffin-embedded malignant melanomas: correlation with immunohistochemistry and tumor stage. Hum Pathol. 2004;35(12):1543–8. https://doi.org/10.1016/j.humpath.2004.09.016.
154. Kroiss MM, Vogt TM, Schlegel J, Landthaler M, Stolz W. Microsatellite instability in malignant melanomas. Acta Derm Venereol. 2001;81(4):242–5. https://doi.org/10.1080/00015550152572840.
155. Uribe P, Wistuba II, Solar A, Balestrini C, Perez-Cotapos ML, Gonzalez S. Comparative analysis of loss of heterozygosity and microsatellite instability in adult and pediatric melanoma. Am J Dermatopathol. 2005;27(4):279–85. https://doi.org/10.1097/01.dad.0000171599.40562.7c.
156. IARC. WHO. WHO classification of tumours series. 5th ed, vol. 12. Available from: https://tumourclassification.iarc.who.int/chapters/64.
157. Zaidi MR, Day CP, Merlino G. From UVs to metastases: modeling melanoma initiation and progression in the mouse. J Invest Dermatol. 2008;128(10):2381–91. https://doi.org/10.1038/jid.2008.177.
158. Bastian BC. The molecular pathology of melanoma: an integrated taxonomy of melanocytic neoplasia. Annu Rev Pathol. 2014;9:239–71. https://doi.org/10.1146/annurev-pathol-012513-104658.
159. Davies MA, Samuels Y. Analysis of the genome to personalize therapy for melanoma. Oncogene. 2010;29(41):5545–55. https://doi.org/10.1038/onc.2010.323.
160. Stephens RM, Sithanandam G, Copeland TD, Kaplan DR, Rapp UR, Morrison DK. 95-kilodalton B-Raf serine/threonine kinase: identification of the protein and its major autophosphorylation site. Mol Cell Biol. 1992;12(9):3733–42. https://doi.org/10.1128/mcb.12.9.3733-3742.1992.
161. Hillier LW, Fulton RS, Fulton LA, et al. The DNA sequence of human chromosome 7. Nature. 2003;424(6945):157–64. https://doi.org/10.1038/nature01782.
162. Sithanandam G, Kolch W, Duh FM, Rapp UR. Complete coding sequence of a human B-raf cDNA and detection of B-raf protein kinase with isozyme specific antibodies. Oncogene. 1990;5(12):1775–80.
163. Chang L, Karin M. Mammalian MAP kinase signalling cascades. Nature. 2001;410(6824):37–40. https://doi.org/10.1038/35065000.
164. Davies H, Bignell GR, Cox C, et al. Mutations of the BRAF gene in human cancer. Nature. 2002;417(6892):949–54. https://doi.org/10.1038/nature00766.
165. Dhomen N, Marais R. BRAF signaling and targeted therapies in melanoma. Hematol Oncol Clin North Am. 2009;23(3):529–45, ix. https://doi.org/10.1016/j.hoc.2009.04.001.
166. Michaloglou C, Vredeveld LC, Soengas MS, et al. BRAFE600-associated senescence-like cell cycle arrest of human naevi. Nature. 2005;436(7051):720–4. https://doi.org/10.1038/nature03890.
167. Wajapeyee N, Serra RW, Zhu X, Mahalingam M, Green MR. Oncogenic BRAF induces senescence and apoptosis through pathways mediated by the secreted protein IGFBP7. Cell. 2008;132(3):363–74. https://doi.org/10.1016/j.cell.2007.12.032.
168. Tsao H, Chin L, Garraway LA, Fisher DE. Melanoma: from mutations to medicine. Genes Dev. 2012;26(11):1131–55. https://doi.org/10.1101/gad.191999.112.
169. Huang FW, Hodis E, Xu MJ, Kryukov GV, Chin L, Garraway LA. Highly recurrent TERT promoter mutations in human melanoma. Science. 2013;339(6122):957–9. https://doi.org/10.1126/science.1229259.

170. Kirkpatrick KL, Mokbel K. The significance of human telomerase reverse transcriptase (hTERT) in cancer. Eur J Surg Oncol. 2001;27(8):754–60. https://doi.org/10.1053/ejso.2001.1151.
171. Szostak JW. Telomerase: the beginning of the ends. Nature. 1989;337(6205):303–4. https://doi.org/10.1038/337303a0.
172. Dankort D, Curley DP, Cartlidge RA, et al. Braf(V600E) cooperates with Pten loss to induce metastatic melanoma. Nat Genet. 2009;41(5):544–52. https://doi.org/10.1038/ng.356.
173. Horn S, Figl A, Rachakonda PS, et al. TERT promoter mutations in familial and sporadic melanoma. Science. 2013;339(6122):959–61. https://doi.org/10.1126/science.1230062.
174. Hosler GA, Davoli T, Mender I, et al. A primary melanoma and its asynchronous metastasis highlight the role of BRAF, CDKN2A, and TERT. J Cutan Pathol. 2015;42(2):108–17. https://doi.org/10.1111/cup.12444.
175. Thomas NE, Edmiston SN, Tsai YS, et al. Utility of TERT promoter mutations for cutaneous primary melanoma diagnosis. Am J Dermatopathol. 2019;41(4):264–72. https://doi.org/10.1097/dad.0000000000001259.
176. Griewank KG, Murali R, Puig-Butille JA, et al. TERT promoter mutation status as an independent prognostic factor in cutaneous melanoma. J Natl Cancer Inst. 2014;106(9):dju246. https://doi.org/10.1093/jnci/dju246.
177. Motaparthi K, Kim J, Andea AA, et al. TERT and TERT promoter in melanocytic neoplasms: current concepts in pathogenesis, diagnosis, and prognosis. J Cutan Pathol. 2020;47(8):710–9. https://doi.org/10.1111/cup.13691.
178. Tsao H, Mihm MC Jr, Sheehan C. PTEN expression in normal skin, acquired melanocytic nevi, and cutaneous melanoma. J Am Acad Dermatol. 2003;49(5):865–72. https://doi.org/10.1016/s0190-9622(03)02473-3.
179. Tsao H, Zhang X, Fowlkes K, Haluska FG. Relative reciprocity of NRAS and PTEN/MMAC1 alterations in cutaneous melanoma cell lines. Cancer Res. 2000;60(7):1800–4.
180. Zhou XP, Gimm O, Hampel H, Niemann T, Walker MJ, Eng C. Epigenetic PTEN silencing in malignant melanomas without PTEN mutation. Am J Pathol. 2000;157(4):1123–8. https://doi.org/10.1016/s0002-9440(10)64627-5.
181. Wu H, Goel V, Haluska FG. PTEN signaling pathways in melanoma. Oncogene. 2003;22(20):3113–22. https://doi.org/10.1038/sj.onc.1206451.
182. Kamb A, Gruis NA, Weaver-Feldhaus J, et al. A cell cycle regulator potentially involved in genesis of many tumor types. Science. 1994;264(5157):436–40. https://doi.org/10.1126/science.8153634.
183. Guan KL, Jenkins CW, Li Y, et al. Growth suppression by p18, a p16INK4/MTS1- and p14INK4B/MTS2-related CDK6 inhibitor, correlates with wild-type pRb function. Genes Dev. 1994;8(24):2939–52. https://doi.org/10.1101/gad.8.24.2939.
184. Udayakumar D, Tsao H. Melanoma genetics: an update on risk-associated genes. Hematol Oncol Clin North Am. 2009;23(3):415–29, vii. https://doi.org/10.1016/j.hoc.2009.03.011.
185. Greenwald HS, Friedman EB, Osman I. Superficial spreading and nodular melanoma are distinct biological entities: a challenge to the linear progression model. Melanoma Res. 2012;22(1):1–8. https://doi.org/10.1097/CMR.0b013e32834e6aa0.
186. Shain AH, Joseph NM, Yu R, et al. Genomic and transcriptomic analysis reveals incremental disruption of key Signaling pathways during melanoma evolution. Cancer Cell. 2018;34(1):45–55.e44. https://doi.org/10.1016/j.ccell.2018.06.005.
187. Bastian BC, Olshen AB, LeBoit PE, Pinkel D. Classifying melanocytic tumors based on DNA copy number changes. Am J Pathol. 2003;163(5):1765–70. https://doi.org/10.1016/s0002-9440(10)63536-5.
188. Potrony M, Badenas C, Aguilera P, et al. Update in genetic susceptibility in melanoma. Ann Transl Med. 2015;3(15):210. https://doi.org/10.3978/j.issn.2305-5839.2015.08.11.
189. Leachman SA, Carucci J, Kohlmann W, et al. Selection criteria for genetic assessment of patients with familial melanoma. J Am Acad Dermatol. 2009;61(4):677.e671–14. https://doi.org/10.1016/j.jaad.2009.03.016.

190. Wachsman W, Morhenn V, Palmer T, et al. Noninvasive genomic detection of melanoma. Br J Dermatol. 2011;164(4):797–806. https://doi.org/10.1111/j.1365-2133.2011.10239.x.
191. Ferris LK, Jansen B, Ho J, et al. Utility of a noninvasive 2-gene molecular assay for cutaneous melanoma and effect on the decision to biopsy. JAMA Dermatol. 2017;153(7):675–80. https://doi.org/10.1001/jamadermatol.2017.0473.
192. Bass J, Hill H, Jaworsky C. Significant discordance in DermTech test results when paired with histopathology: caveat emptor. J Am Acad Dermatol. 2023;89(5):1039–41. https://doi.org/10.1016/j.jaad.2023.07.1022.
193. Ludzik J, Lee C, Witkowski A. Potential limitations in the clinical adoption of 3-GEP pigmented lesion assay for melanoma triage by dermatologists and advanced practice practitioners. Cureus. 2022;14(11):e31914. https://doi.org/10.7759/cureus.31914.
194. Berardi P, Arcangeli F. The tape stripping toluidine blue (TSTB) method in the diagnosis of malignant melanoma: an investigator-blind study. Melanoma Res. 1992;2(2):93–9. https://doi.org/10.1097/00008390-199207000-00003.

Chapter 4
Lentigo Maligna

Shaymaa Hegazy and Doina Ivan

Introduction

Lentigo maligna (LM) is a subtype of melanoma that arises in chronically sun-exposed skin. LM was initially described in 1894 by Sir John Hutchinson, and the term "Hutchinson melanotic freckle" was used for a while [1, 2]. Dubreuilh in 1894, and respectively in 1912, proposed the terms "malignant lentigo of elderly people" and "melanosis circumscripta precancerosa," as a slowly enlarging pigmented macular lesion with variegated black-brown color and irregular outline, most commonly seen on the face [3]. In 1967, Clark coined the term lentigo maligna [4].

The term lentigo maligna melanoma (LMM) was historically used when invasion of the melanoma within the dermis was noted, while the term lentigo maligna (LM) was reserved for melanoma in situ. However, currently, the term lentigo maligna (LM) is used for both invasive and in situ melanoma of this morphologic type. LM is typically associated with chronic sun exposure or a high cumulative sun damage (CSD). Microscopically, LM is characterized by a lentiginous and confluent growth pattern of melanocytes in a background of marked solar elastosis. A stepwise accumulation of genetic abnormalities leads to proliferation of melanocytes, initially involving only epidermis (referred to as "radial growth phase" or "non-tumorigenic growth phase") and later on invading dermis ("vertical growth phase" or "tumorigenic growth phase") [5, 6].

S. Hegazy · D. Ivan (✉)
UT MD Anderson Cancer Center, Houston, TX, USA
e-mail: DSIvan@mdanderson.org

V. G. Prieto, C. A. Torres-Cabala (eds.), *Precision Molecular Pathology of Melanocytic Lesions*, Molecular Pathology Library,
https://doi.org/10.1007/978-3-032-18222-7_4

Incidence

LM represents approximately 5–15% of total cases of melanoma and 10–26% of melanomas on the head and neck. They constitute the third most frequent subtype of melanoma, preceded by superficial spreading melanoma (SSM) and nodular melanoma (NM).

Worldwide, the incidence of melanoma is highest in Australia, where LM is reported at an annual rate of 1.3 new cases per 100,000 inhabitants. In the USA, the incidence of LM is most significant in Hawaii and lowest in the northern states. This distribution correlates with prolonged, possibly occupational, sun exposure. LM is most frequently diagnosed in patients with fair skin (prone to sunburn), who also have red hair and blue eyes. In the last few decades, the incidence of LM has significantly increased; for example, a study performed in Minnesota showed an increased incidence from 2.2 to 13.7 cases per 100,000 person-years between 1970–1989 and 2004–2007 [7].

Age

The patients diagnosed with LM are typically older than those with superficial spreading melanoma/low-CSD melanoma or nodular melanoma. The mean age at diagnosis ranges from approximately 65–73 years, and it is rarely seen before the fourth decade of life [8]. Given its predilection for chronically sun-exposed areas, LM is often associated with the presence of solar lentigo and actinic changes and has a lower incidence of associated melanocytic naevi [9, 10].

Gender

A slight male preponderance has been reported in LM, with a male-to-female ratio of approximately 1.7:1 [11]. However, a melanoma study on a Spanish population observed a higher frequency of invasive melanomas, including LMM, in female patients. This suggests that regional variations may influence the gender distribution of LMM [12].

Site

LM most commonly affects chronically sun-exposed skin of the head and neck region, with a predilection for the face, nose (in particular, ala and tip of the nose), and cheeks. Less frequently, LM arises on extremities, especially in women [13]. In men, ears (in particular, the ear lobule) and bald scalp are frequent sites of involvement, likely because of increased sun exposure resulting from the absence of hair coverage [12].

Clinical Features

In general, melanoma is often suspected when a patient presents with a new pigmented patch or plaque (Fig. 4.1). It may also be considered when an existing mole shows changes in size, shape, or color, particularly if it meets the clinical ABCDE criteria (asymmetry, border irregularity, color variation, diameter greater than 6 mm, and evolution/change of lesion) used for melanoma diagnosis. LM often develops de novo, without a preexisting melanocytic lesion. LM commonly debuts as a variably pigmented area on chronically sun-exposed skin, frequently exhibiting irregular contour and variegation of the pigmentation (Fig. 4.2) [14].

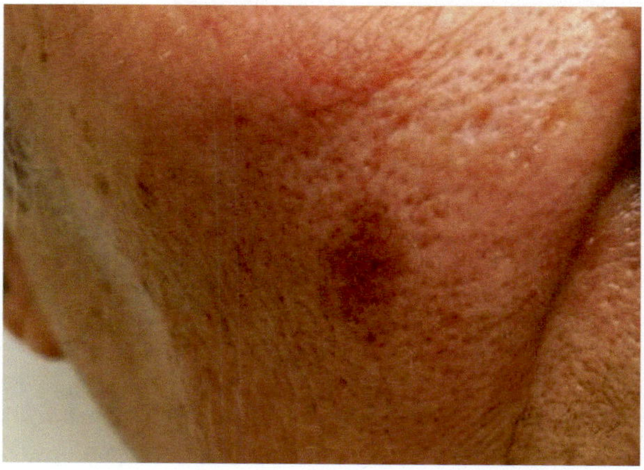

Fig. 4.1 Lentigo maligna, a pigmented, irregular patch on the malar cheek

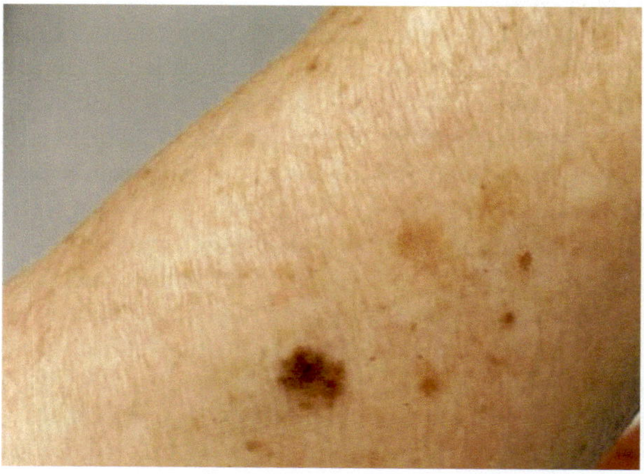

Fig. 4.2 Lentigo maligna, pigmented patch on the forearm with irregular borders and variegation in color

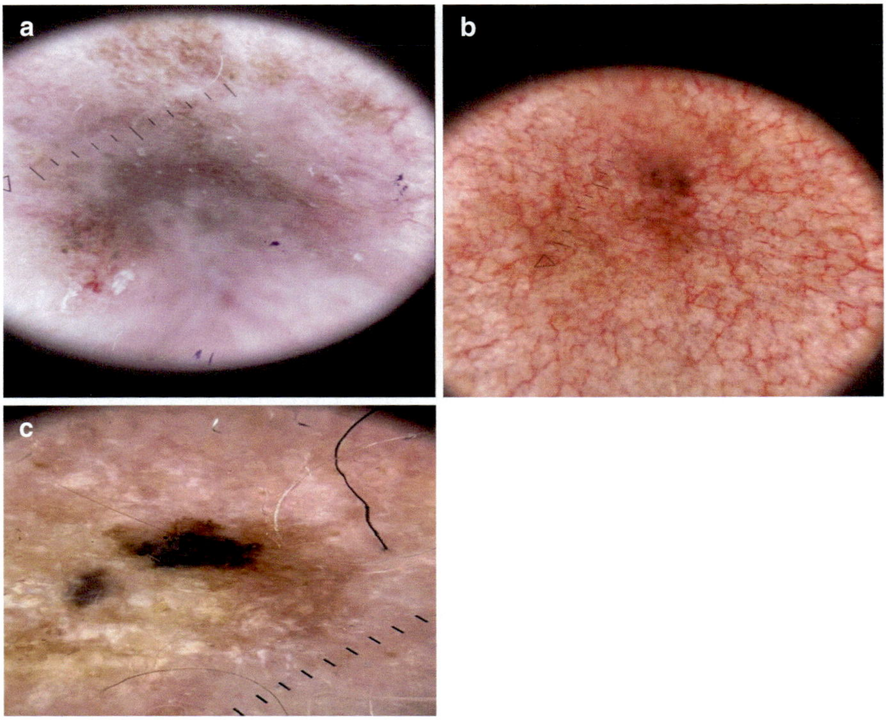

Fig. 4.3 (**a**, **b**) Dermoscopically, lentigo maligna shows an annular-granular pattern, asymmetric pigmented follicular openings, dark rhomboidal structures, gray dots, and increased vasculature network. (**c**) Dermoscopically, invasive lentigo maligna melanoma shows an asymmetric pigmented nodule, pigmented follicular openings, gray dots, and homogenous areas

Dermoscopically, LM is characterized by features such as an annular-granular pattern, asymmetric pigmented follicular openings, dark rhomboidal structures, occasionally homogeneous areas, gray dots, and increased vasculature network [15] (Fig. 4.3a–c).

In early LM, clinical and dermoscopic features may be subtle and can overlap with those of benign lesions. To improve diagnostic accuracy, a dermoscopic "inverse approach" has been proposed, which emphasizes the absence of characteristic prevalent patterns seen in pigmented actinic keratoses and solar lentigo/early flat pigmented seborrheic keratoses. Application of the "inverse approach" has enhanced the sensitivity for diagnosing LM, raising it from 51.5% to 83.6%, thereby demonstrating its value as a diagnostic aid [16]. In some cases, LM can present as amelanotic lesions, often as an erythematous patch [17].

LM may remain on the in situ stage for extended periods of time, ranging from 5 to 20 years, before progressing to invasive disease. However, cases of rapid progression within months have also been reported [18, 19]. The exact rate at which LM progresses from in situ to an invasive lesion (LMM) remains poorly defined. One retrospective study estimated a 5% lifetime risk for invasion for a person given a lentigo maligna diagnosis at the age of 45, while a recent Australian prospective study reported a 3.5% annual progression rate, with an average progression time of 28.3 years, indicating that LM can become invasive, despite a reportedly relatively low risk [20]. Once dermal involvement occurs, lentigo maligna has the same prognosis as other types of invasive melanomas when adjusted for Breslow thickness.

Distinguishing LM from its invasive counterpart on a clinical basis remains challenging, particularly in patients with a history of prior treatments such as cryotherapy, which can alter lesion appearance. The presence of a dermal nodule or thickened plaque is strongly associated with invasive disease; however, early invasive LM may lack overt clinical signs, limiting the reliability of physical examination alone. The risk for progression of LM appears to be proportional to the size of the lesion. Given these clinical diagnostic limitations, a low threshold for performing a biopsy of pigmented lesions in chronically sun-exposed areas is recommended to ensure accurate diagnosis and timely intervention [20].

Histologic Features

While complete excisional biopsy remains the gold standard for evaluating pigmented lesions, it is not always feasible, particularly when dealing with large lesions in cosmetically sensitive areas such as the face or when the clinical diagnosis is uncertain. In such cases, multiple punch biopsies are often performed, as they allow sampling from different areas of the lesion. These punch biopsies should extend into the subcutaneous adipose tissue to ensure adequate histopathologic evaluation.

Superficial techniques, such as shave biopsy, scissors excision, or curettage, are discouraged for melanocytic lesions, as they may preclude accurate histopathologic assessment of tumor thickness, which is essential for staging. Notably, the choice of biopsy technique does not appear to impact patient survival or metastasis rates in melanoma cases [21].

The lesion should be grossly examined and documented, describing its size, pattern, and distribution of pigmentation, involvement of surgical margins by pigment, and the presence of any scarring suggestive of prior biopsy or features of regression. It is advisable to ink all specimens (including shave biopsies) to assess whether the lesion extends to the tissue edges.

On histologic examination, LM is characterized by intraepidermal proliferation of cytologically atypical melanocytes (single cells or small nests), present along the basal layer. The growth pattern is predominantly lentiginous, and occasional pagetoid spread of atypical melanocytes may also be observed. The hallmark of LM is the contiguous, confluent growth pattern of the melanocytic proliferation, often with extension into follicular structures, arising in skin with significant solar elastosis and actinic changes [6, 21]. It is important to note that sometimes these changes are very subtle, and a high index of suspicion is recommended when examining skin with extensive solar damage.

Histologically, the atypical melanocytes may exhibit a variety of cytologic features, including epithelioid, spindled, and pleomorphic forms. These cells are typically hyperchromatic and may demonstrate cytoplasmic retraction. Occasionally, large multinucleated melanocytes, referred to as "starburst cells," may be observed [22].

Typically, in classic lentigo maligna, the epidermis is atrophic, with loss of the normal rete ridge architecture (Fig. 4.4a). In areas where numerous confluent atypical melanocytes are present along the dermoepidermal junction or extend into the adnexal structures (Fig. 4.4b), separation of the epidermis from the underlying dermis may occur, a phenomenon described as "epidermal consumption." Additional histologic features often include fibrosis of the papillary dermis, scattered melanophages, a lymphocytic host response, and, in some cases, findings consistent with regression are noted, such as dermal fibrosis, melanophage accumulation, and reduced melanocytic density (Fig. 4.4c).

When the atypical melanocytes invade the dermis, the diagnosis of invasive LM (or LMM) is made. The invasive component is indistinguishable from other types of invasive melanoma; however, the intraepidermal component helps in the differential diagnosis. LM can also be associated in up to 25% of cases with desmoplastic melanoma, which is a melanoma variant characterized by scattered spindled melanocytes in a dense collagenous stroma, which is also linked with chronic sun exposure [23].

A less common histologic variant is the small cell (nevoid) type of lentigo maligna, which may resemble a benign or a dysplastic nevus and can pose significant diagnostic difficulty [24].

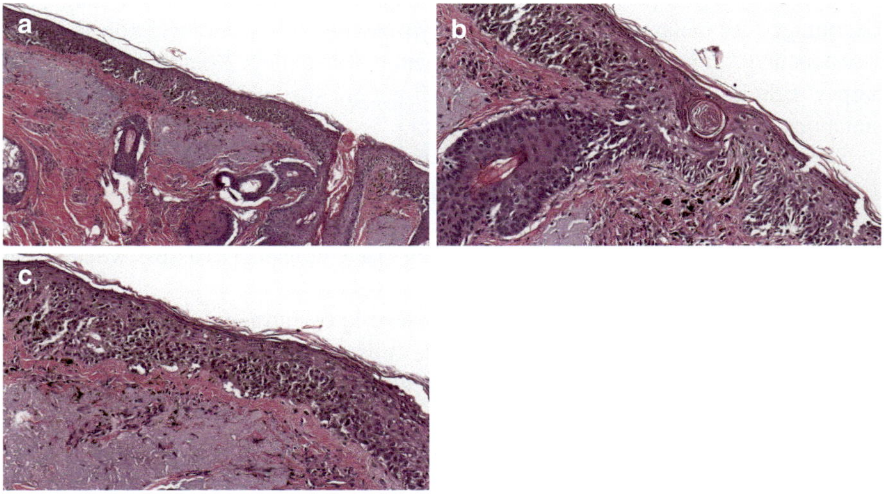

Fig. 4.4 (**a**) Shave biopsy of skin showing a junctional melanocytic proliferation with confluent growth pattern and epidermal flattening and loss of rete ridges (H&E, 40×). (**b**) Melanoma in situ, lentigo maligna type, with adnexal extension (H&E, 200×). (**c**) Lentigo maligna in situ with pagetoid upward migration and dermal regression (H&E, 200×)

Differential Diagnosis

The differential diagnosis of LM includes melanocytic hyperplasia in a background of actinic damage, where the melanocytes may be increased in number, occasionally may exhibit cytologic atypia but lack the confluent growth pattern seen in LM. Pigmented actinic keratosis or benign lichenoid keratoses may be clinically or histologically included in the differential diagnosis of LM, but they lack the melanocytic proliferation. [25] In some instances, immunohistochemical studies may be performed to help with the differential diagnosis.

Dysplastic nevi, particularly those exhibiting marked architectural disorder, can be mistaken for LM. However, in elderly patients with extensive actinic damage and evidence of focal confluent growth of junctional melanocytes, LM is the more likely diagnosis. Given that dysplastic nevi are uncommon in chronically sun-damaged skin of older individuals, this diagnosis should be made cautiously, with careful consideration of the potential for a nevoid variant of LM, which can closely mimic dysplastic nevi both clinically and histologically [24].

Immunohistochemical Studies

Junctional melanocytes with cytologic atypia may be frequently noted in chronic sun-damaged skin, and melanocytic hyperplasia may be seen in such cases. Moreover, in lesions of pigmented actinic keratosis, scattered junctional atypical melanocytes may be present. The accurate evaluation of the density of the atypical melanocytes is essential in distinguishing LM from melanocytic hyperplasia or pigmented actinic keratosis [26]. For the diagnosis of melanoma in situ, lentigo maligna type, immunohistochemical studies with melanocytic markers highlight the confluent growth pattern of atypical intraepithelial melanocytes, with pagetoid upward migration and extension within the adnexal structures (Fig. 4.5a, b). In contrast, in skin with actinic damage, melanocytic hyperplasia may be noted; there are scattered atypical melanocytes, relatively increased in number, but not having a confluent growth pattern as seen in lentigo maligna [27]. It is not uncommon for the histologic evaluation of such lesions on H&E sections alone to be very difficult.

Immunohistochemical studies can be used for the differential diagnosis in such a setting. While MART-1 reliably labels melanocytes, the extensive dendritic staining by MART-1 may mimic a confluent growth of melanocytes, potentially leading to overdiagnosis, unless the number of labeled cell bodies is carefully evaluated [27, 28]. Another potential diagnostic pitfall involves interpreting dermal cells that express MART1, since MART1 also labels melanophages, and they should not be mistaken for invasive melanoma [29]. Using MART1 with a red chromogen may facilitate the distinction of melanocytes and aid in the correct diagnosis.

To improve specificity, HMB45 may be used, since it is not showing a significant labeling of the melanocytes' dendritic processes or of the melanophages [28]. In

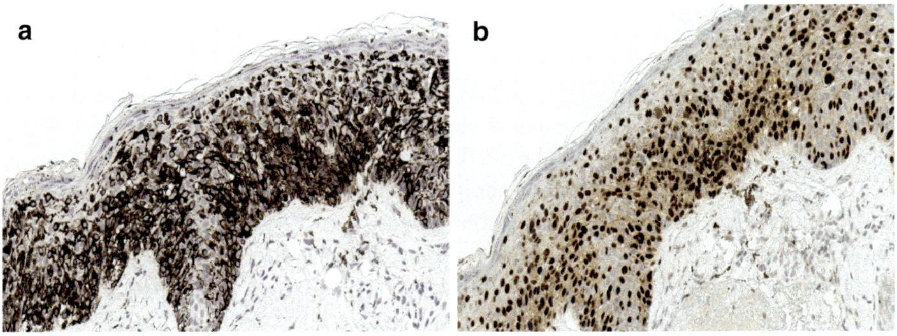

Fig. 4.5 (**a**) Pan-melanoma cocktail (tyrosinase and MART1) immunohistochemical study highlights an extensive and confluent intraepidermal melanocytic proliferation, with pagetoid upward migration and extension within the adnexal structures, while (**b**) PRAME immunohistochemical study labels the majority of the melanocytes (>75% of cells) (400x)

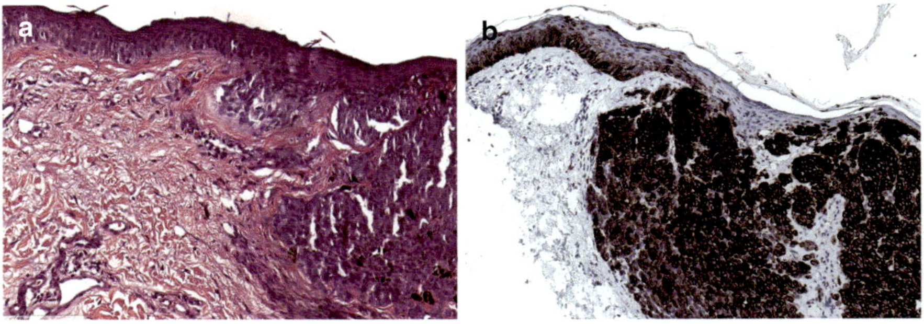

Fig. 4.6 (**a**) A punch biopsy of skin demonstrating invasive lentigo maligna (H&E, 200×). (**b**) HMB45 immunohistochemical study highlights the atypical melanocytes in both the epidermis and dermis, without evidence of maturation (200x)

addition, in invasive melanoma, HMB45 demonstrates patchy labeling of the dermal melanocytes, without evidence of maturation, therefore supporting the differential diagnosis from invasive LM from benign nevi or dysplastic nevi (Fig. 4.6a, b).

Another useful immunohistochemical marker is SOX10, a nuclear marker that is easier to interpret, allowing for a better quantitative appreciation of the melanocytic proliferation [28]. In addition, SOX10 will highlight dermal melanocytes in cases in which desmoplastic melanoma is associated with LM. MiTF1 is another nuclear marker that may be used in such cases. The sensitivity of MiTF1 can be as high as 80%; however, it declines to approximately 55% in cases of desmoplastic melanoma [30]. Despite its usefulness, the specificity of MiTF1 is limited, as it may also label non-melanocytic cells such as macrophages and fibroblasts.

The pan-melanoma antibody cocktail (comprising HMB45, tyrosinase, and MART1) (Fig. 4.5a) has demonstrated greater sensitivity (up to 98%) compared to individual markers in the diagnosis of complex in situ lesions such as LM and LMM or detecting micrometastasis [31, 32].

The dual immunohistochemical study using MART1/Ki67 enables an easier assessment of a melanocyte-specific proliferation index, which is crucial for differentiating challenging nevoid melanoma from dysplastic nevi [33]. Other dual immunohistochemical studies, such as MiTF/D2-40 or SOX10/D2-40, are used in evaluating the presence or absence of lymphovascular invasion.

PRAME (Preferentially Expressed Antigen in Melanoma) is a nuclear immunohistochemical marker that demonstrates high diagnostic accuracy in melanoma in general and PM in particular, with a reported sensitivity of 93.5% and specificity of 94.7% (Fig. 4.5b). It is particularly valuable for evaluating surgical margins and distinguishing LM from benign melanocytic hyperplasia. It is crucial to be aware that PRAME expression may be absent in some confirmed cases of LM. Conversely, diffuse nuclear positivity can be observed in a subset of dysplastic nevi, especially those arising in sun-damaged skin, exhibiting marked architectural and cytologic atypia. Studies have documented diffuse PRAME expression in approximately 5–13% of dysplastic nevi, underscoring that lack of PRAME staining does not exclude malignancy, while its presence does not definitively confirm melanoma [34].

Molecular Studies

Approximately 10% of melanomas are thought to have a hereditary component. A first-degree relative of a patient with melanoma has an estimated 8- to 12-fold increased risk of melanoma [35]. One of the principal susceptibility loci is located on chromosome 9p21, which harbors the *CDKN2A* (also known as MTS1) tumor suppressor gene [36]. Another gene implicated in familial melanoma is *CDK4*, with germline mutations identified in some melanoma-prone kindreds [37].

In LMM, comparative genomic hybridization (CGH) studies have more frequently demonstrated chromosomal losses involving chromosome 13, with less frequent losses on chromosome 10 [38]. Moreover, a link between DNA repair deficiency and a high frequency of *TP53* mutations in LMM arising in patients with xeroderma pigmentosum, supporting the contribution of genomic instability to melanoma pathogenesis in this context [39].

Since LMM is a high-CSD melanoma, it exhibits a distinct genetic signature. Curtin and his colleagues identified *KIT* aberrations (mutations, gene gain, or amplifications) in 28% of chronically sun-damaged melanomas (LM/LMM) [40]. Bastian and colleagues reported additional mutations or amplifications in *KIT* downstream effectors (*PTPN11* and *GAB2*) in a subset of CSD melanomas [41].

LMM has a lower frequency of BRAF V600E mutations compared with other melanomas, especially those related to intermittent sun exposure; instead, when *BRAF* mutation is present, it is often non-V600E [42]. LMM frequently carries other MAPK pathway mutations, such as NF1 inactivating mutations (30%) and *NRAS* activating mutations [43]. Also, inactivating mutations of *ARID2* and *TERT* promoter mutations have been identified in LMM [44]. LMM is characterized by a very high mutation burden and ultraviolet radiation signature [45].

References

1. Hutchinson J. Lentigo-melanosis: a further report. Arch Surg. 1894;5:253–6.
2. Cohen LM. Lentigo maligna and lentigo maligna melanoma. J Am Acad Dermatol. 1995;33(6):923–36; quiz 937–40.
3. Dudreulih MW. Lentigo malin des veillards. Ann Dermatol Syphilis. 1984;5:1092–9.
4. Clark WH Jr. A classification of malignant melanoma. Advances in the biology of the skin, vol. 8. New York: Pergamon Press; 1967. p. 621.
5. Holman CD, Armstrong BK. Cutaneous malignant melanoma and indicators of total accumulated exposure to the sun: an analysis separating histogenetic types. J Natl Cancer Inst. 1984;73(1):75–82.
6. Koh HK, Kligler BE, Lew RA. Sunlight and cutaneous malignant melanoma: evidence for and against causation. Photochem Photobiol. 1990;51(6):765–79.
7. Mirzoyev SA, Knudson RM, Reed KB, Hou JL, Lohse CM, Frohm ML, Brewer JD, Otley CC, Roenigk RK. Incidence of lentigo maligna in Olmsted County, Minnesota, 1970 to 2007. J Am Acad Dermatol. 2014;70(3):443–8.
8. Cox NH, Aitchison TC, Sirel JM, MacKie RM. Comparison between lentigo maligna melanoma and other histogenetic types of malignant melanoma of the head and neck. Scottish Melanoma Group. Br J Cancer. 1996;73(7):940–4. https://doi.org/10.1038/bjc.1996.168.
9. Whiteman DC, Watt P, Purdie DM, Hughes MC, Hayward NK, Green AC. Melanocytic nevi, solar keratoses, and divergent pathways to cutaneous melanoma. J Natl Cancer Inst. 2003;95(11):806–12. https://doi.org/10.1093/jnci/95.11.806. PMID: 12783935.
10. Lee EY, Williamson R, Watt P, Hughes MC, Green AC, Whiteman DC. Sun exposure and host phenotype as predictors of cutaneous melanoma associated with neval remnants or dermal elastosis. Int J Cancer. 2006;119(3):636–42. https://doi.org/10.1002/ijc.21907. PMID: 16572428.
11. Punchihewa N, Wee E, Kelly JW, Mclean C, Mar VJ, Pan Y. The anatomical distribution of lentiginous melanoma (lentigo maligna and lentigo maligna melanoma): differences according to sex. Australas J Dermatol. 2023;64(3):e277–80. https://doi.org/10.1111/ajd.14058.
12. Castro E, Souza B, Morais Silva DH, Valente NYS, Kakizaki P, Luce MCA, Bandeira LG. Cutaneous melanoma: a retrospective study of 18 years. Are there gender differences? An Bras Dermatol. 2021;96(5):619–23. https://doi.org/10.1016/j.abd.2020.08.022.
13. Elder DE. Skin cancer. Melanoma and other specific nonmelanoma skin cancers. Cancer. 1995;75(1 Suppl):245–56. https://doi.org/10.1002/1097-0142(19950101)75:1+<245::aid-cncr2820751310>3.0.co;2-7. PMID: 8000999.
14. Friedman RJ, Rigel DS, Kopf AW. Early detection of malignant melanoma: the role of physician examination and self-examination of the skin. CA Cancer J Clin. 1985;35(3):130–51. https://doi.org/10.3322/canjclin.35.3.130.
15. Stante M, Giorgi V, Stanganelli I, Alfaioli B, Carli P. Dermoscopy for early detection of facial lentigo maligna. Br J Dermatol. 2005;152(2):361–4. https://doi.org/10.1111/j.1365-2133.2004.06328.
16. Lallas A, Paschou E, Manoli SM, Papageorgiou C, Spyridis I, Liopyris K, Bobos M, Moutsoudis A, Lazaridou E, Apalla Z. Dermatoscopy of melanoma according to type, anatomic site and stage. Ital J Dermatol Venerol. 2021;156(3):274–88. https://doi.org/10.23736/S2784-8671.20.06784-X. Epub 2020 Dec 14. PMID: 33314891.
17. Borkovic SP, Schwartz RA. Amelanotic lentigo maligna melanoma manifesting as a dermatitis like plaque. Arch Dermatol. 1983;119(5):423–5.
18. Odom RB, James WD, Berger TG. Melanocytic nevi and neoplasms. In: Odom RB, James WD, Berger TG, editors. Andrew's diseases of the skin. ed 9 ed. Philadelphia: WB Saunders Co; 2000. p. 869–92.
19. Bevona C, Fewkes J, Liu V, Sober AJ. Prolonged evolution of a lentigo maligna. J Am Acad Dermatol. 2004;51(5):830–5. https://doi.org/10.1016/j.jaad.2002.09.002.

20. Menzies SW, Liyanarachchi S, Coates E, Smith A, Cooke-Yarborough C, Lo S, Armstrong B, Scolyer RA, Guitera P. Estimated risk of progression of lentigo maligna to lentigo maligna melanoma. Melanoma Res. 2020;30(2):193–7. https://doi.org/10.1097/CMR.0000000000000619.
21. Swetter SM, Tsao H, Bichakjian CK, Curiel-Lewandrowski C, Elder DE, Gershenwald JE, Guild V, Grant-Kels JM, Halpern AC, Johnson TM, Sober AJ, Thompson JA, Wisco OJ, Wyatt S, Hu S, Lamina T. Guidelines of care for the management of primary cutaneous melanoma. J Am Acad Dermatol. 2019;80(1):208–50. https://doi.org/10.1016/j.jaad.2018.08.055.
22. Busam KJ. Dermatopathology. 2nd ed. Philadelphia: Elsevier; 2010.
23. Walters RF, Groben PA, Busam K, Millikan RC, Rabinovitz H, Cognetta A, Mihm MC Jr, Prieto VG, Googe PB, King R, Moore DT, Woosley JT, Thomas NE. Consumption of the epidermis: a criterion in the differential diagnosis of melanoma and dysplastic nevi that is associated with increasing Breslow depth and ulceration. Am J Dermatopathol. 2007;29(6):527–33.
24. Kossard S, Wilkinson B. Small cell (naevoid) melanoma: a clinicopathologic study of 131 cases. Australas J Dermatol. 1997;38(Suppl 1):S54–8. https://doi.org/10.1111/j.1440-0960.1997.tb01011.x. PMID: 10994474.
25. Reinehr CPH, Bakos RM. Actinic keratoses: review of clinical, dermoscopic, and therapeutic aspects. An Bras Dermatol. 2019;94(6):637–57. https://doi.org/10.1016/j.abd.2019.10.004.
26. Kelly GL, Berlingeri-Ramos AC, Taylor CR, McCalmont TH. Distinction of melanoma in situ from solar lentigo on sun-damaged skin using morphometrics and MITF immunohistochemistry. Am J Dermatopathol. 2012;34(4):344–50. https://doi.org/10.1097/DAD.0b013e318244b3a1.
27. Prieto VG, Shea CR. Use of immunohistochemistry in melanocytic lesions. J Cutan Pathol. 2008;35:1–10.
28. Prieto V, Shea CR, Suster J. Immunohistochemistry of melanocytic proliferations. Am J Dermatopathol. 2011;33(14):A–Z.
29. Danga ME, Yaar R, Bhawan J. Melan-A positive dermal cells in malignant melanoma in situ. J Cutan Pathol. 2015;42(6):388–93. https://doi.org/10.1111/cup.12473.
30. Granter SR, Weilbaecher KN, Quigley C, Fletcher CD, Fisher DE. Microphthalmia transcription factor: not a sensitive or specific marker for the diagnosis of desmoplastic melanoma and spindle cell (non-desmoplastic) melanoma. Am J Dermatopathol. 2001;23(3):185–9.
31. Orchard G. Evaluation of melanocytic neoplasms: application of a pan-melanoma antibody cocktail. Br J Biomed Sci. 2002;59(4):196–202. https://doi.org/10.1080/09674845.2002.11783659.
32. Shidham VB, Qi D, Rao RN, Acker SM, Chang CC, Kampalath B, Dawson G, Machhi JK, Komorowski RA. Improved immunohistochemical evaluation of micrometastases in sentinel lymph nodes of cutaneous melanoma with 'MCW melanoma cocktail',a mixture of monoclonal antibodies to MART-1, Melan-A, and tyrosinase. BMC Cancer. 2003;3:15. Published 2003 May 7. https://doi.org/10.1186/1471-2407-3-15.
33. Nielsen PS, Spaun E, Riber-Hansen R, Steiniche T. Immunohistochemical double stains against Ki-67/MART-1 and HMB-45/MITF: promising diagnostic tools in melanocytic lesions. Am J Dermatopathol. 2011;33(4):361–70.
34. Lezcano C, Jungbluth AA, Nehal KS, Hollmann TJ, Busam KJ. PRAME expression in melanocytic tumors. Am J Surg Pathol. 2018;42(11):1456–65. https://doi.org/10.1097/PAS.0000000000001134.
35. Bishop DT, Demenais F, Goldstein AM, Bergman W, Newton Bishop JA, Bressac-de Paillerets B, Chompret A, Ghiorzo P, Gruis NA, Hansson J, Harland M, Hayward NK, Holland EA, Mann GJ, Mantelli M, Nancarrow D, Platz A, Tucker MA. Geographical variation in the penetrance of CDKN2A mutations for melanoma. J Natl Cancer Inst. 2002;94(12):894–903. https://doi.org/10.1093/jnci/94.12.894.
36. Kamb A, Gruis NA, Weaver-Feldhaus J, Liu Q, Harshman K, Tavtigian SV, Stockert E, Day RS III, Johnson BE, Skolnick MH. A cell cycle regulator potentially involved in genesis of many tumor types. Science. 1994;264(5157):436–40. https://doi.org/10.1126/science.8153634.

37. Zuo L, Weger J, Yang Q, Goldstein M, Tucker A, Walker J, Hayward N, Dracopoli C. Germline mutations in the p16INK4a binding domain of CDK4 in familial melanoma. Nat Genet. 1996;12(1):97–9. https://doi.org/10.1038/ng0196-97.
38. Bastian BC, LeBoit PE, Hamm H, Bröcker EB, Pinkel D. Chromosomal gains and losses in primary cutaneous melanomas detected by comparative genomic hybridization. Cancer Res. 1998;58(10):2170–5. PMID: 9605761.
39. D'Errico M, Teson M, Calcagnile A, Degan P, Lemma T, Fronza G, Dogliotti E. Differential expression of key genes in DNA repair pathways in melanoma: a study on xeroderma pigmentosum melanomas. J Invest Dermatol. 2000;115(2):246–53. https://doi.org/10.1046/j.1523-1747.2000.00033.x.
40. Curtin JA, Busam K, Pinkel D, Bastian BC. Somatic activation of KIT in distinct subtypes of melanoma. J Clin Oncol. 2006;24(26):4340–6. https://doi.org/10.1200/JCO.2006.06.2984.
41. Bastian BC. The molecular pathology of melanoma: an integrated taxonomy of melanocytic neoplasia. Annu Rev Pathol. 2014;9:239–71. https://doi.org/10.1146/annurev-pathol-012513-104658.
42. Thomas NE, Edmiston SN, Alexander A, Groben PA, Parrish E, Kricker A, Busam K, Marghoob AA, Panageas KS, Begg CB, Halpern AC. Number of nevi and early-life ambient UV exposure are associated with BRAF-mutant melanoma. Cancer Epidemiol Biomarkers Prev. 2007;16(5):991–7. https://doi.org/10.1158/1055-9965.EPI-06-1071.
43. Loras A, Gil-Barrachina M, Marqués-Torrejón MÁ, Perez-Pastor G, Martinez-Cadenas C. UV-induced somatic mutations driving clonal evolution in healthy skin, nevus, and cutaneous melanoma. Life (Basel). 2022;12(9):1339. Published 2022 Aug 29. https://doi.org/10.3390/life12091339.
44. Bobos M. Histopathologic classification and prognostic factors of melanoma: a 2021 update. Ital J Dermatol Venerol. 2021;156:300–21. https://doi.org/10.23736/S2784-8671.21.06958-3.
45. Hayward NK, Wilmott JS, Waddell N, Johansson PA, Field MA, Nones K, Patch A-M, Kakavand H, Alexandrov LB, Burke H, Jakrot V, Kazakoff SH, Holmes O, Pupo GM, Jung J, Kefford RF, Gómez-López G, Pessoa Rodrigues C, Menzies AM, Ferguson PM, Thompson JF, Saw RPM, López-Bigas N, Thorne H, Corbin J, Gruis NA, McArthur GA, Lo S, Hirst M, Stratford EW, Dutton-Regester K, Scolyer RA, Grimmond SM. Whole-genome landscapes of major melanoma subtypes. Nature. 2017;545(7653):175–80. https://doi.org/10.1038/nature22071.

Chapter 5
Acral Melanoma

Kaitlin Vanderbeck and Carlos A. Torres-Cabala

Introduction

Acral melanoma (AM) refers to melanomas that occur on the glabrous (hairless) or volar skin of palms, soles, and digits [1]. Subungual melanoma (SUM) may be considered a variant of acral melanoma. Subungual melanoma affects nail apparatus, specifically nail bed or matrix [2, 3]. Histopathologically, acral melanoma can demonstrate several subtypes, including acral-lentiginous melanoma (ALM), superficial spreading melanoma (SSM or low-CSD melanoma), nodular melanoma (NM), and desmoplastic melanoma [1]. Weight-bearing regions are most often affected. Acral melanoma is more commonly found on the soles of the feet/ heel compared to the palms, while subungual melanomas are more often seen on fingernails rather than toenails [1, 2, 4, 5]. Typically, great toe and thumb are the most commonly affected digits [6, 7]. It appears that regional differences in melanocytes (likely related to a positional identity of oncogenes) may account for the development of acral melanoma through *CRKL* amplification and subsequent activation of the HOX13-IGF axis, potentially explaining why melanocytes found at acral sites are susceptible to certain oncogenic insults, in contrast to melanocytes other anatomical locations [8].

K. Vanderbeck
Department of Pathology and Molecular Medicine, Kingston Health Sciences Centre, Queen's University, Kingston, ON, Canada

C. A. Torres-Cabala (✉)
Departments of Pathology, Dermatology, and Translational Molecular Pathology, The University of Texas MD Anderson Cancer Center, Houston, TX, USA
e-mail: ctcabala@mdanderson.org

V. G. Prieto, C. A. Torres-Cabala (eds.), *Precision Molecular Pathology of Melanocytic Lesions*, Molecular Pathology Library,
https://doi.org/10.1007/978-3-032-18222-7_5

Clinical Features

Acral melanoma is relatively rare in Caucasian populations, compared to melanomas arising in association with ultraviolet (UV) damage. In contrast, acral melanoma is the most common type of melanoma seen in Asian, Hispanic, and African populations, comprising more than 50% of cutaneous melanomas in East Asian countries [9–12]. Subungual melanoma accounts for approximately 30% of acral melanomas [13, 14]. The overall age-adjusted incidence of acral melanoma is 1.8 per million person-years [11]. The occurrence of acral melanoma increases with age, with a mean age of onset of 63 years [1, 11, 15, 16].

Subungual melanomas represent 0.7–3.5% of all melanomas reported globally [3]. Subungual melanomas comprise 75% of all melanomas seen in African patients, 25% in Chinese patients, and 10% in Japanese patients [3, 17]. Subungual melanomas typically occur in the seventh decade in male patients and the sixth decade in female patients [3, 6, 7].

Acral Melanoma

The most common histological subtype of acral melanoma is acral lentiginous melanoma [1]. Clinically, these lesions often start as pigmented macules that progressively develop into invasive melanoma over several months or years, with a mean time to diagnosis of 1 year [18]. Acral melanomas are often advanced at diagnosis because hyperkeratotic epidermis may cover the lesion, possibly leading to clinical misdiagnosis [19] (Fig. 5.1).

Subungual Melanoma

Subungual melanomas typically present as a longitudinal discoloration of the nail, known as longitudinal melanonychia, and may progress to involve adjacent skin. This latter finding is referred to as Hutchinson sign [20–23]. As with acral melanomas, there is often a delay in diagnosis as lesions are sometimes attributed to local factors such as trauma. Up to 73% of cases are AJCC stage II/III at diagnosis and 79% of cases are considered Clark level IV or V. The acral lentiginous subtype is the most common subtype of subungual melanoma reported (66%). Sentinel lymph node metastases are seen in 24% of cases [24].

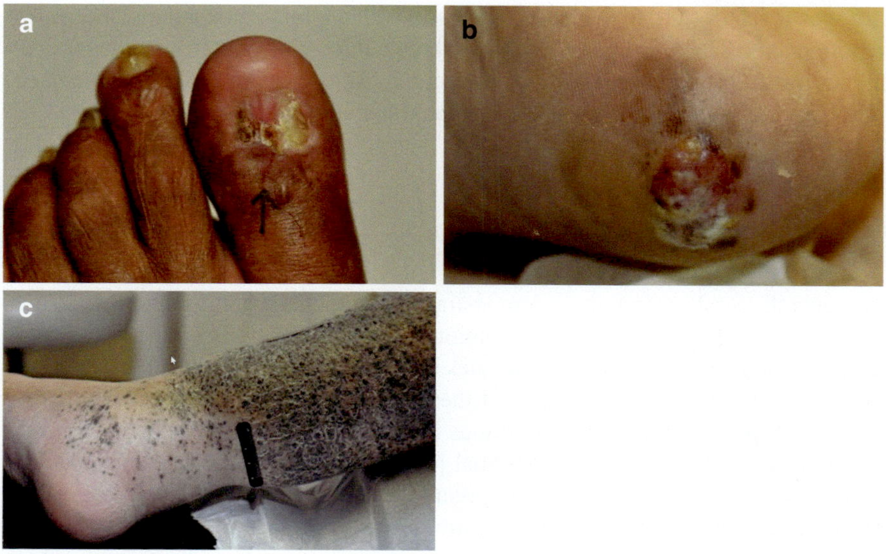

Fig. 5.1 Clinical characteristics of acral melanoma. (**a**) Melanoma in situ. The clinical appearance of acral and subungual melanoma in situ can be subtle, especially in dark-skinned individuals. (**b**) Acral melanoma of the heel. In addition to peripheral melanoma in situ there is invasive melanoma with ulceration. (**c**) In transit metastasis of acral melanoma. In some cases, innumerable deposits of melanoma are present

Dermoscopy

On dermoscopy, acral melanomas may demonstrate a characteristic "parallel ridge pattern" where the pigmentation aligns with the ridges of skin markings. Lesions may also display irregular pigmentation with variable coloration [25]. In addition to the Hutchinson sign, subungual melanomas may demonstrate longitudinal, irregular lines, triangular bands, increased vascularity, and ulceration [2, 25–27].

Prognosis

The prognosis of acral and subungual melanomas is significantly influenced by several factors, including Breslow thickness, ulceration, increased mitotic rate, and presence of microsatellites [28, 29]. Metastasis to sentinel lymph nodes is the most important predictor of recurrence [30]. It appears that acral melanoma (in particular acral lentiginous subtype) is inherently more aggressive than other types of melanoma, a finding also seen in pT1 thin melanomas [31]. For both acral melanoma and subungual melanoma, poor prognosis is likely related to late presentation/detection [3, 32]. Although a subungual location is sometimes regarded as indicative of aggressive behavior, it seems that this clinical presentation is not an independent prognostic factor [33]. Indeed, the 5-year survival rate for subungual melanoma was reported to be 87.1% in one study, with subungual location conferring a better overall survival (OS) compared to acral melanoma [32]. Acral and subungual melanomas demonstrate a poorer survival rate than other subtypes of melanoma.

Histopathology

In general, acral melanomas demonstrate prominent acanthosis of epidermis. Elongation of the rete ridges is a common feature, and there is typically cytologic atypia and pleomorphism of melanocytes with an increased nuclear-to-cytoplasmic ratio. It is important to recognize that these features may be subtle in some cases. Some subtypes, such as acral lentiginous melanoma, show increased confluence of melanocytes along the dermo-epidermal junction. Pagetoid scatter of melanocytes is also characteristic; however, interpretation of pagetoid scatter of melanocytes must be made with caution as this feature may also be seen in reactive or traumatized skin, particularly in weight-bearing areas. Epidermal consumption, which involves the attenuation of basal or suprabasal layers of epidermis with loss of rete ridges, is also a common finding, particularly in advanced cases [34, 35]. In early lesions, there may be proliferation of solitary atypical melanocytes within the epidermis, including rete ridges [36].

Acral lentiginous melanoma (ALM) is the most common subtype, followed by superficial spreading melanoma (SSM) and nodular melanoma (NM) [37–39]. Up to 66% of subungual melanomas are of the acral lentiginous subtype [3]. ALM in situ demonstrates an increase in the number and confluence of melanocytes at the base of the epidermis. Melanocytes demonstrate variable cytologic atypia with hyperchromatic nuclei and prominent dendrites. As the melanoma progresses, the vertical growth phase is observed with significant invasion into dermis. The superficial spreading melanoma subtype demonstrates similar histologic features, except melanocytes appear largely in nests, particularly along the dermo-epidermal junction. The in situ component will extend at least three rete pegs past the intradermal component in this subtype; otherwise, it would correspond to a nodular subtype. Nodular melanomas tend to exhibit a more prominent, if not solely intradermal component than the other subtypes. Of note, invasive melanocytes with a spindled phenotype are more likely to harbor *NF1* mutations, while an epithelioid phenotype is often associated with *BRAF* mutations [40].

In early subungual melanomas, there is a mild proliferation of atypical melanocytes with hyperchromatic nuclei, increased nuclear-to-cytoplasmic ratio, and elongated dendrites [41–43]. There is often abundant melanin deposition in the nail plate. The atypical melanocytic proliferation may be seen within nail bed and matrix, with an increased number and confluence of junctional melanocytes. Pagetoid scatter may also be seen. As the melanoma progresses, features like ALM are observed, including a vertical growth phase. Importantly, lymphocyte-predominant inflammation can help distinguish melanoma from other conditions, such as melanonychia [3]. The presence of melanocytes or remnants thereof (e.g., melanin pigment) in the nail plate may also indicate the presence of an underlying melanoma [44]. Increased melanocyte density may also help with diagnosis. It has been reported that melanocyte density in Caucasian patients is between 6.5 and 7.7 cells per millimeter within the basal layer, with a melanocyte density of 40 per millimeter or greater being concerning for melanoma in situ [44–46].

Immunohistochemistry

Lesional cells express conventional melanocytic markers, including SOX10, S100, MelanA/MART-1, and MITF. HMB45 labeling can be useful for identifying melanoma cells, as it typically highlights epidermal and intradermal melanocytes throughout the lesion in melanoma. In contrast, acral nevi lose HMB45 expression with increasing depth within the dermal component of the lesion ("maturation pattern"). Of note, HMB45 may be focal in amelanotic acral melanoma. Importantly, MelanA/MART-1 and HMB45 may stain pigment and, in so doing may lead to overestimation of the number of melanocytes [44]. These immunostains may also highlight long melanocyte dendrites further contributing to diagnostic confusion [47, 48]. Other markers, including PRAME, tend to be positive in melanoma and negative in nevi [49–52]. Cyclin D1 positivity is supportive of melanoma [1, 53]. Complete loss of expression of p16 may indicate homozygous loss of *CDKN2A* and be supportive of melanoma [54]. LEF1 staining pattern may be of utility in the distinction between benign acral nevi and acral melanoma. Benign melanocytic nevi typically show LEF1 "maturation pattern", with stronger nuclear staining in superficial (junctional and superficial dermal) melanocytes that gradually decreases with depth. This pattern of expression is not typically seen in acral melanoma [55]. TERT positivity by immunohistochemistry appears to be more frequent in acral lentiginous melanoma but not associated with prognosis or specific for *TERT* gene amplification [56, 57]. Nuclear localization of *YAP1* has been reported to be more frequent in acral melanoma and to correlate with proliferative activity and propensity for invasion[58].

It is important to note that certain markers may be negative in cases with desmoplastic features, in which S100 and SOX10 are still expected to be positive. Other immunohistochemical markers might be used to evaluate mutational status of certain genes, such as *BRAF V600E* and *NRAS Q61R*, which are usually negative, especially in the acral lentiginous type [54]. Interestingly, it appears that a heterogeneous expression of *BRAF V600E* may be more common in acral melanomas seen in patients from Japan and Latin America; this might be in relation to intratumor heterogeneity (authors' personal observation and [59]). Biomarkers potentially used to guide certain immune checkpoint inhibitor therapies, like PD-L1, are variably expressed in acral melanoma. A subset of cases requires dual immunostains, such as PD-L1/SOX10, for a more accurate evaluation of PD-L1 expression due to a possible heavy melanin content [60]. Apoptosis-related proteins like BLC2, MCL1, and BIM are frequently expressed in acral melanoma, perhaps indicating a potential role for apoptosis-directed therapies [61] (Fig. 5.2).

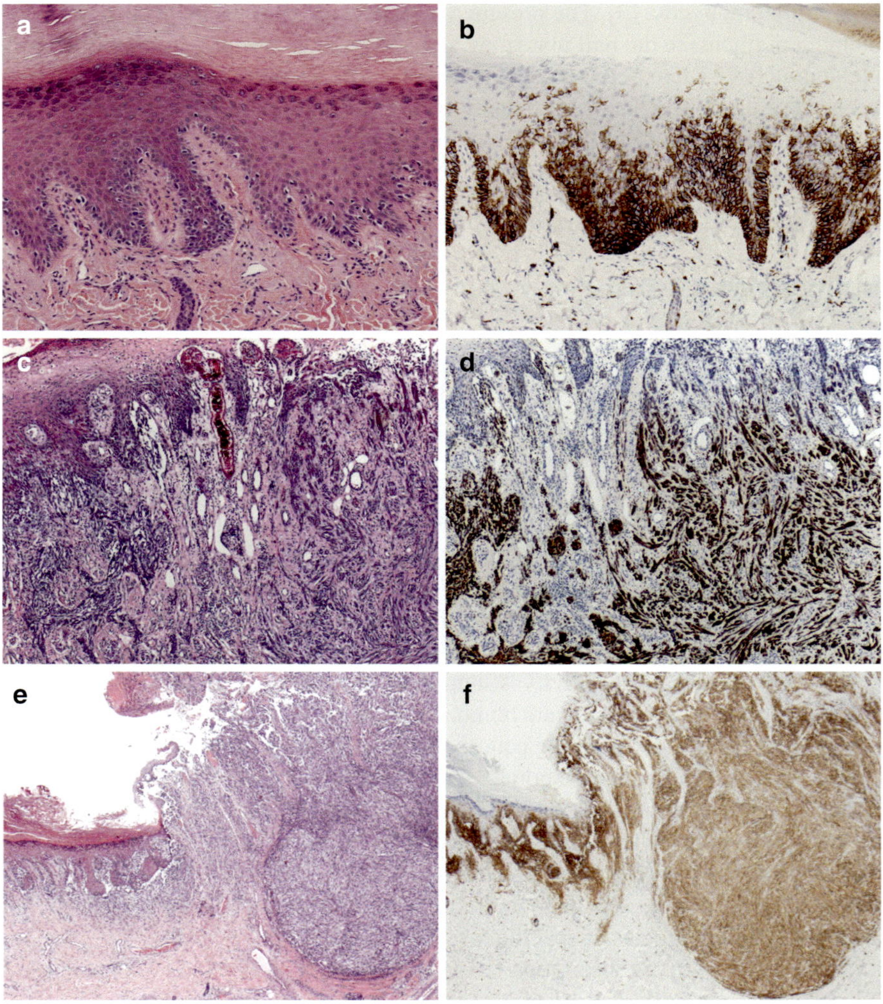

Fig. 5.2 Histopathological features of acral melanoma. (**a**) Acral lentiginous melanoma in situ. Notice the proliferation of single melanocytes with focal confluence. Pagetoid upward migration is not obviously seen in these H&E sections (H&E, ×200). (**b**) The same lesion evaluated for HMB45 by immunohistochemistry reveals long dendrites and more evident pagetoid scatter (×200). (**c**) The invasive component of this acral melanoma displays spindle cell morphology (H&E, ×100). (**d**) Melanomas with spindle cell morphology are many times negative for melanocytic markers such as Melan-A/MART1 or HMB45. In this case, expression of S100 by immunohistochemistry supports the melanocytic nature of the tumor (×100). (**e**) In situ and adjacent invasive acral lentiginous melanoma, with ulceration. (H&E, ×40). (**f**) This tumor with epithelioid morphology is positive for Melan-A/MART-1 by immunohistochemistry (×40)

Molecular Findings

Acral Melanoma

The etiology and pathophysiology of acral melanoma are multifactorial, with trauma and physical stress possibly contributing to its development [13]. Family history and UV-radiation exposure are thought to play a minimal role in tumorigenesis [28, 62]. Signature 7 (ultraviolet, UV), characterized by UV-induced C > T or CC > TT transitions, has been detected as a nonzero signature in up to 40% of acral melanomas, supporting a small role of UV radiation in the pathogenesis in some cases [63]. By analysis of single microscopic tumor nests, it has been reported that acral melanomas show extensive intratumor genomic heterogeneity, even in early stages [64]. Also, invasiveness appears to be associated with subclonal diversification, increased epithelial-mesenchymal transition, and increased CD163+macrophages expressing APOE [65].

Acral melanomas tend to have a low tumor mutational burden relative to other melanoma subtypes and are more frequently associated with other aberrations, such as gene amplifications, deletions, and chromosomal rearrangements, leading to genomic instability [1, 66–68]. Some of the frequently reported gene amplifications include loci associated with *CCND1* (early in the genesis of acral melanoma, in melanoma in situ, and in phenotypically normal melanocytes as "field effect"), *CDK4*, *hTERT*, *PAK1*, *GAB2*, *EP300*, *YAP1*, *MDM2*, *MYC*, *CRKL*, and *KIT* [1, 20, 67, 69–74]. *TERT* gene amplification might be involved in progression of acral melanoma to metastasis and also be present in some non-acral melanomas [55]. Targeting amplified genes such as *MYC* or *CRKL* has been postulated as a therapeutic option for these patients [75]. Overexpression of *ERBB2* mRNA has been reported in acral melanoma, suggesting a potential therapeutic target [63, 76]. *PTEN* and *CDKN2a* deletions have been documented in approximately 25% of cases [1, 68]. Gene fusions appear to be rare; a report of a case harboring a fusion involving *RAF1* has been documented [77].

This being stated, acral melanomas are mostly "triple negative" (*BRAF*, *NRAS*, *KIT* negative), with gene amplifications as the primary driver [1, 74]. However, there are some cases with mutations in genes related to the mitogen-activating protein kinase pathway (MAPK-pathway), including *BRAF*, *NRAS*, and *NF1* [1]. Mutations in the *KIT* gene are detected in acral melanoma in about 12–40% of cases, perhaps slightly less frequently than in mucosal melanomas [1, 68, 78, 79]. Expression of KIT by immunohistochemistry does not correlate with *KIT* mutations, although it can be used as a negative predictor of a mutation if absent [79]. *BRAF* mutations are more common in superficial spreading melanomas affecting acral sites and may be associated with a pre-existing nevus [2, 39, 40, 71]. *BRAF V600E* mutations are more commonly reported in patients with European ancestry, with fewer mutations within the MAPK pathway exhibited in Korean patients [1, 39, 40, 80]. Inactivation of *NF1* and its cooperating factor *SPRED1* is present in around 10% of cases [20]. Cyclin D1 protein expression, characterized either via

Fig. 5.3 Acral melanoma demonstrating amplification of *TERT* by fluorescence in situ hybridization (FISH). This is a relatively common event in acral melanoma. (FISH, red probe covering *TERT* at 5p15; green probe as control, covering 5q31)

molecular studies or immunohistochemistry, is associated with increased *CCDN1* copy number in acral melanoma [1, 53]. Amplifications of genes like *CCND1* and *CDK4* are relatively common and associated with poor prognosis [66, 67, 73, 81]. By DNA methylation analysis, hypermethylation of epigenetic markers such as *HHEX*, *NELFB*, *IFITM1*, and *SIK3* was linked to histopathological and clinical features associated with worse prognosis [82] (Fig. 5.3).

Tumor-infiltrating lymphocytes in acral melanoma are reported to be relatively low, and lower levels are associated with poor outcome [83]. Tumor microenvironment characterization of acral melanomas has disclosed fewer effector CD8+T cells and NK cells, and near-complete absence of γδ T cells, in contrast to non-acral cutaneous melanomas, suggesting a suppressed-immune microenvironment [84]. Novel immune checkpoints, such as ADORA2, TIGIT, and VISTA, have been identified in acral melanoma [84].

Subungual Melanoma

Specific to subungual melanomas, *SPRED1* rearrangements are more frequently observed than in other melanoma subtypes [1, 2, 70].

Subungual melanomas are more likely than acral melanoma to demonstrate a UV-radiation related mutational signature [32, 71]. Similar to other acral melanomas, trauma and melanocyte activation are suspected contributors to its pathogenesis [3]. Somatic mutations, including *KIT*, *CDK4*, *GNAQ*, *NF1*, *BRAF*, *NRAS*, *SMAD4*, *ERBB2*, *TP53*, and *TERTp* mutations, have been documented in subungual melanomas [32, 68, 70–73, 85–88]. However, notably, many subungual melanomas fail to demonstrate mutations in *BRAF* (*BRAFV600E*), *NRAS*, or *NF1*. Instead, they often demonstrate mutations involving *GNAQ R183* and *KIT* in most cases, with a minority of cases exhibiting *RAS* and *BRAF* mutations [19, 32]. Subungual melanomas tend to demonstrate single nucleotide variations (SNVs) more frequently than copy number alterations (CNAs), the latter of which are more commonly seen in acral melanoma [19, 32]. *CDK4/CCND1* amplifications are reportedly more common in subungual melanoma than in acral melanoma [72]. Because of all these peculiarities in its molecular profile, some authors have postulated that subungual melanoma should be regarded as a melanoma subtype distinct from acral melanoma [72] (Fig. 5.3).

Key genetic alterations in both acral melanoma and subungual melanoma are summarized in Table 5.1 and Fig. 5.4.

Table 5.1 Molecular findings in acral and subungual melanomas

Alteration type	Genes involved	Frequency	Notes
Acral melanoma[a]			
Oncogenic mutations	*BRAF*	15–21%	Mutually exclusive with *NRAS* [1, 2, 20, 32, 39, 41, 67–69] *BRAF p.V600E* mutations more common in patients with European ancestry [1, 39, 80] Fewer *BRAF* mutations in Korean patients [1, 40, 80]
	NRAS	15–28%	Mutually exclusive with *BRAF* [1, 2, 20, 32, 39, 41, 67–69] Fewer NRAS mutations in Korean patients [1, 40, 80]
	KIT	12–40%	Can co-occur with *NF1* mutations [1, 2, 20, 32, 39, 41, 67–69, 71, 73, 78, 79] Fewer *KIT* mutations in Korean patients [1, 40, 80]
	NF1	11–23%	May co-occur with *KIT* mutations [1, 2, 20, 32, 39, 41, 67–69, 71, 73] Inactivation of *NF1* and *SPRED1* present in 10% of cases [20]
	"Signature 7" (UV-induced)	Up to 40%	C > T or CC > TT transitions [63]
Structural rearrangements	*BRAF, NTRK3, ALK, PRKCA*	Approximately 7%	[20]

(continued)

Table 5.1 (continued)

Alteration type	Genes involved	Frequency	Notes
Amplifications	*CCND1, CDK4, hTERT, PAK1, GAB2, EP300, YAP1, MDM2, MYC, CRKL, KIT, ERBB2*	Frequent	[1, 19, 20, 67, 69–72, 74] *TERT* gene amplifications may be involved in progression to metastasis [55] *MYC* and *CRKL* amplifications may be therapeutic targets [75] Amplifications of *CCND1* and *CDK4* are relatively common and associated with poor prognosis [66, 67, 73, 81] Overexpression of *ERBB2* mRNA has been described in AM and may be a therapeutic target [63, 76]
Deletions	*PTEN, CDKN2A*	Up to 25%	[1, 68] CDKN2A loss more common in AM than in SUM [72]
Fusions	*RAF1*	Rare	[77]
DNA hypermethylation	*HHEX, NELFB, IFITM1, SIK3*	—	Associated with worse prognosis [82]
Subungual melanoma[b]			
Structural rearrangement	*SPRED1*	—	[1, 2, 70–72, 86]
MAPK pathway mutations	*KIT, GNAQ, NF1, BRAF, NRAS, CDK4, TERTp, SMAD4, ERBB2, TP53*	—	Mutations in *KIT* with *GNAQ* (*especially R183*) prevalent [1, 19, 20, 32, 68, 70–72, 85, 86]
Amplifications	*CDK4, CCND1*, CNAs, SNVs	—	SNVs are more common than CNAs (more common in acral melanoma) [32, 68] CDK4/CCND1 amplifications more common in SUM than in AM [72]
Deletions	*PTEN, CDKN2A*	Possible, but not well characterized	[1, 68] Less frequent in SUM compared to AM [72]

[a]Acral melanomas generally exhibit a lower mutational burden and are often "triple negative" (*BRAF, NRAS, KIT*)
[b]Subungual melanomas are more likely to exhibit a UV-radiation induced mutagenic signature than acral melanoma occurring on volar surfaces

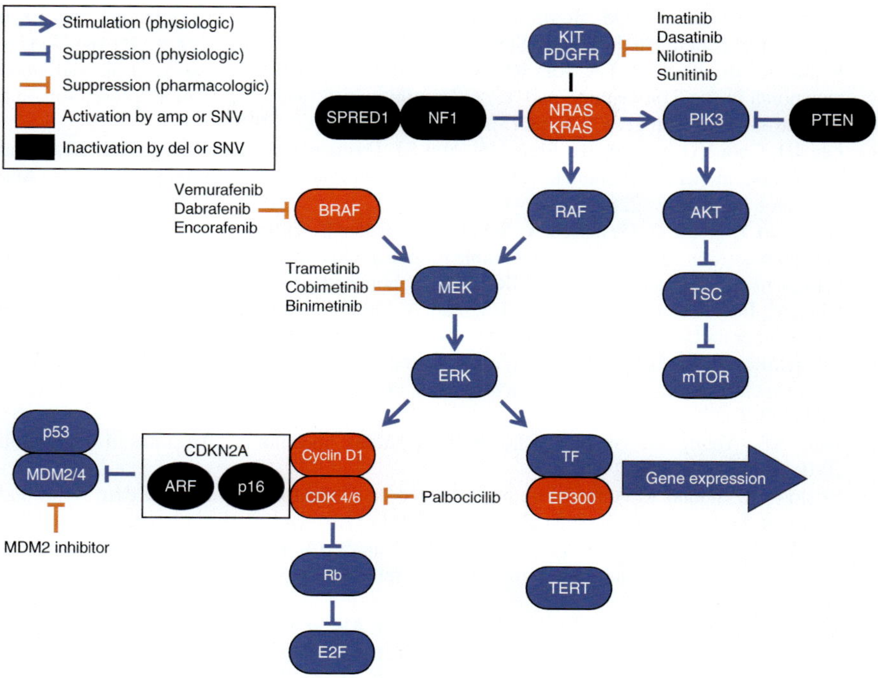

Fig. 5.4 Summary of molecular alterations in acral melanoma

References

1. World Health Organization (WHO). In: Massi D, Scolyer R, Willemze R, editors. Classification of skin tumours. 5th ed. Lyon: International Agency for Research on Cancer; 2023.
2. Ahn SY, Bae GE, Park SY, Yeo MK. Differences in the clinical and molecular profiles of subungual melanoma and acral melanoma in Asian patients. Cancers (Basel). 2023;15(17):4417.
3. Mole RJ. Subungual melanoma. Treasure Island: StatPearls Publishing; 2023. Available from: https://www.ncbi.nlm.nih.gov/books/NBK482480/.
4. Minagawa A, Omodaka T, Okuyama R. Melanomas and mechanical stress points on the plantar surface of the foot. N Engl J Med. 2016;374(24):2404–6.
5. Nguyen JT, Bakri K, Nguyen EC, Johnson CH, Moran SL. Surgical management of subungual melanoma: mayo clinic experience of 124 cases. Ann Plast Surg. 2013;71(4):346–54.
6. Decker A, Connolly KL, Lee EH, Busam KJ, Nehal KS. Frequency of subungual melanoma in longitudinal melanonychia: a single-center experience. Dermatologic Surg. 2017;43(6):798–804.
7. Ingkaninanda P, Visessiri Y, Rutnin S. Clinicopathological features and prognostic factors of malignant melanoma: a retrospective analysis of Thai patients in Ramathibodi hospital. J Med Assoc Thail. 2015;98(8):820–7.
8. Weiss JM, Hunter MV, Cruz NM, Baggiolini A, Tagore M, Ma Y, et al. Anatomic position determines oncogenic specificity in melanoma. Nature. 2022;604(7905):354–61.
9. Chang JW. Acral melanoma: a unique disease in Asia. JAMA Dermatol. 2013;149(11):1272–3.
10. Wang Y, Zhao Y, Ma S. Racial differences in six major subtypes of melanoma: descriptive epidemiology. BMC Cancer. 2016;16(1):691.

11. Bradford PT, Goldstein AM, McMaster ML, Tucker MA. Acral lentiginous melanoma: incidence and survival patterns in the United States, 1986–2005. Arch Dermatol. 2009;145(4):427–34.
12. Markovic SN, Erickson LA, Rao RD, Weenig RH, Pockaj BA, Bardia A, et al. Malignant melanoma in the 21st century, part 1: epidemiology, risk factors, screening, prevention, and diagnosis. Mayo Clin Proc. 2007;82(3):364–80.
13. Lee JH, Choi YD, Hwang JH, Shin MH, Yun SJ. Frequency of trauma, physical stress, and occupation in acral melanoma: analysis of 313 acral melanoma patients in Korea. Ann Dermatol. 2021;33(3):228–36.
14. Teramoto Y, Keim U, Gesierich A, Schuler G, Fiedler E, Tüting T, et al. Acral lentiginous melanoma: a skin cancer with unfavourable prognostic features. A study of the German central malignant melanoma registry (CMMR) in 2050 patients. Br J Dermatol. 2018;178(2):443–51.
15. Wada M, Ito T, Tsuji G, Nakahara T, Hagihara A, Furue M, et al. Acral lentiginous melanoma versus other melanoma: a single-center analysis in Japan. J Dermatol. 2017;44(8):932–8.
16. Kuchelmeister C, Schaumburg-Lever G, Garbe C. Acral cutaneous melanoma in caucasians: clinical features, histopathology and prognosis in 112 patients. Br J Dermatol. 2000;143(2):275–80.
17. Thai KE, Young R, Sinclair RD. Nail apparatus melanoma. Australas J Dermatol. 2001;42(2):71–81; quiz 2–3.
18. Bristow IR, Acland K. Acral lentiginous melanoma of the foot and ankle: a case series and review of the literature. J Foot Ankle Res. 2008;1(1):11.
19. Haugh AM, Zhang B, Quan VL, Garfield EM, Bubley JA, Kudalkar E, et al. Distinct patterns of acral melanoma based on site and relative sun exposure. J Invest Dermatol. 2018;138(2):384–93.
20. Yeh I, Jorgenson E, Shen L, Xu M, North JP, Shain AH, et al. Targeted genomic profiling of acral melanoma. J Natl Cancer Inst. 2019;111(10):1068–77.
21. Ren M, Ren J, Cai X, Shen XX, Kong JC, Dai B, et al. Clinicopathological, immunohistochemical and fluorescence in-situ hybridisation features of early subungual melanoma: an analysis of 65 cases. Histopathology. 2021;78(5):717–26.
22. Lee WJ, Lee JH, Won CH, Chang SE, Choi JH, Moon KC, et al. Nail apparatus melanoma: a comparative, clinicoprognostic study of the initial clinical and morphological characteristics of 49 patients. J Am Acad Dermatol. 2015;73(2):213–20.
23. Yun SJ, Kim SJ. Images in clinical medicine. Hutchinson's nail sign. N Engl J Med. 2011;364(18):e38.
24. Tan KB, Moncrieff M, Thompson JF, McCarthy SW, Shaw HM, Quinn MJ, et al. Subungual melanoma: a study of 124 cases highlighting features of early lesions, potential pitfalls in diagnosis, and guidelines for histologic reporting. Am J Surg Pathol. 2007;31(12):1902–12.
25. Saida T, Koga H, Uhara H. Key points in dermoscopic differentiation between early acral melanoma and acral nevus. J Dermatol. 2011;38(1):25–34.
26. Soon SL, Solomon AR Jr, Papadopoulos D, Murray DR, McAlpine B, Washington CV. Acral lentiginous melanoma mimicking benign disease: the Emory experience. J Am Acad Dermatol. 2003;48(2):183–8.
27. Mun JH, Kim GW, Jwa SW, Song M, Kim HS, Ko HC, et al. Dermoscopy of subungual haemorrhage: its usefulness in differential diagnosis from nail-unit melanoma. Br J Dermatol. 2013;168(6):1224–9.
28. Liang WS, Hendricks W, Kiefer J, Schmidt J, Sekar S, Carpten J, et al. Integrated genomic analyses reveal frequent TERT aberrations in acral melanoma. Genome Res. 2017;27(4):524–32.
29. Phan A, Touzet S, Dalle S, Ronger-Savlé S, Balme B, Thomas L. Acral lentiginous melanoma: histopathological prognostic features of 121 cases. Br J Dermatol. 2007;157(2):311–8.
30. Egger ME, McMasters KM, Callender GG, Quillo AR, Martin RC 2nd, Stromberg AJ, et al. Unique prognostic factors in acral lentiginous melanoma. Am J Surg. 2012;204(6):874–9; discussion 9–80.

31. Mejbel HA, Torres-Cabala CA, Milton DR, Ivan D, Feldmeyer L, Namikawa K, et al. Prognostic significance of acral lentiginous histologic type in T1 melanoma. Mod Pathol. 2021;34(3):572–83.
32. Blessing K, Kernohan NM, Park KG. Subungual malignant melanoma: clinicopathological features of 100 cases. Histopathology. 1991;19(5):425–9.
33. Mejbel HA, Torres-Cabala CA, Milton DR, Ivan D, Nagarajan P, Curry JL, et al. Prognostic significance of subungual anatomic site in acral lentiginous melanoma. Arch Pathol Lab Med. 2021;145(8):943–52.
34. Gumaste PV, Fleming NH, Silva I, Shapiro RL, Berman RS, Zhong J, et al. Analysis of recurrence patterns in acral versus nonacral melanoma: should histologic subtype influence treatment guidelines? J Natl Compr Cancer Netw. 2014;12(12):1706–12.
35. Ohata C, Nakai C, Kasugai T, Katayama I. Consumption of the epidermis in acral lentiginous melanoma. J Cutan Pathol. 2012;39(6):577–81.
36. Ishihara Y, Saida T, Miyazaki A, Koga H, Taniguchi A, Tsuchida T, et al. Early acral melanoma in situ: correlation between the parallel ridge pattern on dermoscopy and microscopic features. Am J Dermatopathol. 2006;28(1):21–7.
37. Jung HJ, Kweon SS, Lee JB, Lee SC, Yun SJ. A clinicopathologic analysis of 177 acral melanomas in Koreans: relevance of spreading pattern and physical stress. JAMA Dermatol. 2013;149(11):1281–8.
38. Lv J, Dai B, Kong Y, Shen X, Kong J. Acral melanoma in Chinese: a clinicopathological and prognostic study of 142 cases. Sci Rep. 2016;6:31432.
39. Carrera C, Gual A, Díaz A, Puig-Butillé JA, Noguès S, Vilalta A, et al. Prognostic role of the histological subtype of melanoma on the hands and feet in Caucasians. Melanoma Res. 2017;27(4):315–20.
40. Moon KR, Choi YD, Kim JM, Jin S, Shin MH, Shim HJ, et al. Genetic alterations in primary acral melanoma and acral melanocytic nevus in Korea: common mutated genes show distinct cytomorphological features. J Invest Dermatol. 2018;138(4):933–45.
41. Teixido C, Castillo P, Martinez-Vila C, Arance A, Alos L. Molecular markers and targets in melanoma. Cells. 2021;10(9):2320.
42. Izumi M, Ohara K, Hoashi T, Nakayama H, Chiu CS, Nagai T, et al. Subungual melanoma: histological examination of 50 cases from early stage to bone invasion. J Dermatol. 2008;35(11):695–703.
43. Park SW, Jang KT, Lee JH, Park JH, Kwon GY, Mun GH, et al. Scattered atypical melanocytes with hyperchromatic nuclei in the nail matrix: diagnostic clue for early subungual melanoma in situ. J Cutan Pathol. 2016;43(1):41–52.
44. Jiang AJ, Abbott JJ, Higgins HW, Elenitsas R, Rubin AI. Clinicohistopathologic challenges and traps in the diagnosis of nail unit melanoma. J Cutan Pathol. 2023;50(6):580–90.
45. Amin B, Nehal KS, Jungbluth AA, Zaidi B, Brady MS, Coit DC, et al. Histologic distinction between subungual lentigo and melanoma. Am J Surg Pathol. 2008;32(6):835–43.
46. Tosti A, Cameli N, Piraccini BM, Fanti PA, Ortonne JP. Characterization of nail matrix melanocytes with anti-PEP1, anti-PEP8, TMH-1, and HMB-45 antibodies. J Am Acad Dermatol. 1994;31(2 Pt 1):193–6.
47. Kim YC, Lee MG, Choe SW, Lee MC, Chung HG, Cho SH. Acral lentiginous melanoma: an immunohistochemical study of 20 cases. Int J Dermatol. 2003;42(2):123–9.
48. Choi YD, Chun SM, Jin SA, Lee JB, Yun SJ. Amelanotic acral melanomas: clinicopathological, BRAF mutation, and KIT aberration analyses. J Am Acad Dermatol. 2013;69(5):700–7.
49. Hu J, Cai X, Lv JJ, Wan XC, Zeng XY, Feng ML, et al. Preferentially expressed antigen in melanoma immunohistochemistry as an adjunct for differential diagnosis in acral lentiginous melanoma and acral nevi. Hum Pathol. 2022;120:9–17.
50. McBride JD, McAfee JL, Piliang M, Bergfeld WF, Fernandez AP, Ronen S, et al. Preferentially expressed antigen in melanoma and p16 expression in acral melanocytic neoplasms. J Cutan Pathol. 2022;49(3):220–30.

51. Lezcano C, Jungbluth AA, Nehal KS, Hollmann TJ, Busam KJ. PRAME expression in melanocytic tumors. Am J Surg Pathol. 2018;42(11):1456–65.
52. Rothrock AT, Torres-Cabala CA, Milton DR, Cho WC, Nagarajan P, Vanderbeck K, et al. Diagnostic utility of PRAME expression by immunohistochemistry in subungual and non-subungual acral melanocytic lesions. J Cutan Pathol. 2022;49(10):859–67.
53. Liu J, Yu W, Gao F, Qi S, Du J, Ma X, et al. CCND1 copy number increase and cyclin D1 expression in acral melanoma: a comparative study of fluorescence in situ hybridization and immunohistochemistry in a Chinese cohort. Diagn Pathol. 2021;16(1):60.
54. Torres-Cabala C, Li-Ning-Tapia E, Hwu WJ. Pathology-based biomarkers useful for clinical decisions in melanoma. Arch Med Res. 2020;51(8):827–38.
55. Ramani NS, Aung PP, Gu J, Sfamenos S, Sdringola-Maranga C, Nagarajan P, et al. TERT amplification but not activation of canonical Wnt/β-catenin pathway is involved in acral lentiginous melanoma progression to metastasis. Mod Pathol. 2020;33(10):2067–74.
56. Cho WC, Wang WL, Milton DR, Ingram DR, Nagarajan P, Curry JL, et al. Telomerase reverse transcriptase protein expression is more frequent in acral lentiginous melanoma than in other types of cutaneous melanoma. Arch Pathol Lab Med. 2021;145(7):842–50.
57. Cho WC, Li W, Gu J, Wang WL, Ning J, Sfamenos S, et al. Telomerase reverse transcriptase immunohistochemical expression is sensitive but not specific for TERT gene amplification in acral melanoma. J Cutan Pathol. 2023;50(9):845–51.
58. Ryu HJ, Kim C, Jang H, Kim SI, Shin SJ, Chung KY, et al. Nuclear localization of yes-associated protein is associated with tumor progression in cutaneous melanoma. Lab Investig. 2024;104(5):102048.
59. Ito T, Tanaka Y, Murata M, Kaku-Ito Y, Furue K, Furue M. BRAF heterogeneity in melanoma. Curr Treat Options in Oncol. 2021;22(3):20.
60. Pineda-Reyes J, Arudra SK, Aung PP, Nagarajan P, Curry JL, Tetzlaff M, et al. Dual PD-L1/SOX10 immunohistochemistry combined with digital imaging enhances stratification accuracy of patients with metastatic melanoma. Am J Surg Pathol. 2024;48(12):1551–6.
61. Ledesma DA, Marques-Piubelli ML, Li-Ning-Tapia E, Hudgens C, Gu J, Lazcano R, et al. Apoptosis pathway-associated proteins are frequently expressed in melanoma: a study of 32 cases with focus on acral lentiginous melanoma. Am J Dermatopathol. 2024;46(7):410–5.
62. Phan A, Touzet S, Dalle S, Ronger-Savlé S, Balme B, Thomas L. Acral lentiginous melanoma: a clinicoprognostic study of 126 cases. Br J Dermatol. 2006;155(3):561–9.
63. Shi K, Zhang B, Kong BY, Zhang Y, Igartua C, Mohan LS, et al. Distinct genomic features in a retrospective cohort of mucosal, acral, and vulvovaginal melanomas. J Am Acad Dermatol. 2023;88(5):1051–9.
64. Zhang X, Peng Y, Li C, Li Q, Yu Z, Pang Y, et al. Genomic heterogeneity and branched evolution of early stage primary acral melanoma shown by multiregional microdissection sequencing. J Invest Dermatol. 2019;139(7):1526–34.
65. Liu H, Gao J, Feng M, Cheng J, Tang Y, Cao Q, et al. Integrative molecular and spatial analysis reveals evolutionary dynamics and tumor-immune interplay of in situ and invasive acral melanoma. Cancer Cell. 2024;42(6):1067–85.e11.
66. Curtin JA, Fridlyand J, Kageshita T, Patel HN, Busam KJ, Kutzner H, et al. Distinct sets of genetic alterations in melanoma. N Engl J Med. 2005;353(20):2135–47.
67. Tod BM, Schneider JW, Bowcock AM, Visser WI, Kotze MJ. The tumor genetics of acral melanoma: what should a dermatologist know? JAAD Int. 2020;1(2):135–47.
68. Hayward NK, Wilmott JS, Waddell N, Johansson PA, Field MA, Nones K, et al. Whole-genome landscapes of major melanoma subtypes. Nature. 2017;545(7653):175–80.
69. Bastian BC. The molecular pathology of melanoma: an integrated taxonomy of melanocytic neoplasia. Annu Rev Pathol. 2014;9:239–71.
70. Newell F, Wilmott JS, Johansson PA, Nones K, Addala V, Mukhopadhyay P, et al. Whole-genome sequencing of acral melanoma reveals genomic complexity and diversity. Nat Commun. 2020;11(1):5259.

71. Lee M, Yoon J, Chung YJ, Lee SY, Choi JY, Shin OR, et al. Whole-exome sequencing reveals differences between nail apparatus melanoma and acral melanoma. J Am Acad Dermatol. 2018;79(3):559–61.e1.
72. Holman BN, Van Gulick RJ, Amato CM, MacBeth ML, Davies KD, Aisner DL, et al. Clinical and molecular features of subungual melanomas are site-specific and distinct from acral melanomas. Melanoma Res. 2020;30(6):562–73.
73. Kim SH, Tsao H. Acral melanoma: a review of its pathogenesis, progression, and management. Biomolecules. 2025;15(1):120.
74. Bastian BC, Kashani-Sabet M, Hamm H, Godfrey T, Moore DH 2nd, Bröcker EB, et al. Gene amplifications characterize acral melanoma and permit the detection of occult tumor cells in the surrounding skin. Cancer Res. 2000;60(7):1968–73.
75. Turner JA, Van Gulick RJ, Robinson WA, Mughal T, Tobin RP, MacBeth ML, et al. Expanding the landscape of oncogenic drivers and treatment options in acral and mucosal melanomas by targeted genomic profiling. Int J Cancer. 2024;155(10):1792–807.
76. Gottesdiener LS, O'Connor S, Busam KJ, Won H, Solit DB, Hyman DM, et al. Rates of ERBB2 alterations across melanoma subtypes and a complete response to trastuzumab emtansine in an ERBB2-amplified acral melanoma. Clin Cancer Res. 2018;24(23):5815–9.
77. LeBlanc RE, Lefferts JA, Baker ML, Linos KD. Novel LRRFIP2-RAF1 fusion identified in an acral melanoma: a review of the literature on melanocytic proliferations with RAF1 fusions and the potential therapeutic implications. J Cutan Pathol. 2020;47(12):1181–6.
78. Curtin JA, Busam K, Pinkel D, Bastian BC. Somatic activation of KIT in distinct subtypes of melanoma. J Clin Oncol. 2006;24(26):4340–6.
79. Torres-Cabala CA, Wang WL, Trent J, Yang D, Chen S, Galbincea J, et al. Correlation between KIT expression and KIT mutation in melanoma: a study of 173 cases with emphasis on the acral-lentiginous/mucosal type. Mod Pathol. 2009;22(11):1446–56.
80. Shim JH, Shin HT, Park J, Park JH, Lee JH, Yang JM, et al. Mutational profiling of acral melanomas in Korean populations. Exp Dermatol. 2017;26(10):883–8.
81. Chen YA, Teer JK, Eroglu Z, Wu JY, Koomen JM, Karreth FA, et al. Translational pathology, genomics and the development of systemic therapies for acral melanoma. Semin Cancer Biol. 2020;61:149–57.
82. Pradhan D, Jour G, Milton D, Vasudevaraja V, Tetzlaff MT, Nagarajan P, et al. Aberrant DNA methylation predicts melanoma-specific survival in patients with acral melanoma. Cancers (Basel). 2019;11(12):2031.
83. Castaneda CA, Torres-Cabala C, Castillo M, Villegas V, Casavilca S, Cano L, et al. Tumor infiltrating lymphocytes in acral lentiginous melanoma: a study of a large cohort of cases from Latin America. Clin Transl Oncol. 2017;19(12):1478–88.
84. Li J, Smalley I, Chen Z, Wu JY, Phadke MS, Teer JK, et al. Single-cell characterization of the cellular landscape of acral melanoma identifies novel targets for immunotherapy. Clin Cancer Res. 2022;28(10):2131–46.
85. Borkowska A, Szumera-Ciećkiewicz A, Spałek M, Teterycz P, Czarnecka A, Kowalik A, et al. Mutation profile of primary subungual melanomas in Caucasians. Oncotarget. 2020;11(25):2404–13.
86. Dika E, Altimari A, Patrizi A, Gruppioni E, Fiorentino M, Piraccini BM, et al. KIT, NRAS, and BRAF mutations in nail apparatus melanoma. Pigment Cell Melanoma Res. 2013;26(5):758–60.
87. Darmawan CC, Ohn J, Mun JH, Kim S, Lim Y, Jo SJ, et al. Diagnosis and treatment of nail melanoma: a review of the clinicopathologic, dermoscopic, and genetic characteristics. J Eur Acad Dermatol Venereol. 2022;36(5):651–60.
88. Millan-Esteban D, García-Casado Z, Macià A, de la Rosa I, Torrecilla-Vall-Llossera C, Penin RM, et al. Molecular profile of subungual melanoma: a MelaNostrum consortium study of 68 cases reporting BRAF, NRAS, KIT, and TERT promoter status. Dermatology. 2024;240(1):164–9.

Chapter 6
Mucosal Melanomas

Priyadharsini Nagarajan

Introduction

Primary mucosal melanomas are unusually rare tumors originating from malignant transformation of mucosal melanocytes; they comprise only 1%–3% of all melanomas [1, 2]. They can occur in any mucosal site; however, certain parts such as the sinuses, nasal cavity, anorectal canal, and vulva are most commonly affected [3]. Even though they share the cell of origin, histopathological, and immunophenotypic features with the more routine cutaneous melanoma, they are intrinsically divergent tumors, with respect to etiopathogenesis, susceptible population, molecular events, staging, and prognosis. They also frequently pose diagnostic difficulties due to their semblance to other neoplastic and/or reactive proliferations, and frequent lack of pigmentation, resulting in delayed diagnosis and, consequently, advanced stage at presentation and thus, poor patient outcome in general.

Patients with lighter skin are in general more susceptible to developing melanomas, regardless of cutaneous or mucosal origin; however, mucosal melanomas are proportionally more common in patients with pigmented skin [1, 4]. Moreover, compared to cutaneous melanomas, which show male predominance, mucosal melanomas are slightly more preponderant among women [3, 5, 6], including those that arise in the various non-genital mucosal sites [7–9]. Patients with mucosal melanomas are in general older, in the seventh decade, compared to fourth to fifth decades among cutaneous melanoma patients [1]. Activation of mitogen-activated protein kinase (MAPK) signaling pathway is a common event in melanomagenesis.

P. Nagarajan (✉)
Department of Anatomical Pathology, The University of Texas MD Anderson Cancer Center, Houston, TX, USA
e-mail: pnagarajan@mdanderson.org

V. G. Prieto, C. A. Torres-Cabala (eds.), *Precision Molecular Pathology of Melanocytic Lesions*, Molecular Pathology Library,
https://doi.org/10.1007/978-3-032-18222-7_6

Exposure to the ultraviolet component of sunlight has been attributed as the primary cause for the development of cutaneous melanoma, leading to high incidence of point mutations in MAPK-pathway genes [10], and de novo melanomas are typically characterized by high tumor mutational burden [11]. On the other hand, point mutations are relatively uncommon in mucosal melanomas [12], while there is high incidence of chromosomal amplifications, deletions, and copy number changes [13, 14].

Diagnosis

Clinical Challenges

In contrast to skin, which is amenable to easy inspection, most mucosal sites with the exception of conjunctiva are unexposed. Therefore, lesions arising in these locations are clinically occult. In addition, since majority of mucosae line organs with lumina, tumors may grow and expand unnoticed for years, until they become symptomatic due to obstruction, bleeding, or invasion into adjacent organs. Even when symptomatic, the clinical suspicion for a malignancy such as melanoma is typically low, attributed to their rarity, frequent lack of pigmentation, and relatively common occurrence of benign proliferations such as hemorrhoids or sinonasal polyps, which mucosal melanomas often resemble. In addition, complexion-associated melanosis involving oral, sinonasal, anorectal, and vulvar mucosa is also common in patients with pigmented skin, which may obscure subtly pigmented lesions [15]. Therefore, a high degree of clinical suspicion and low threshold for biopsy of a mucosal lesion is necessary for early diagnosis of mucosal melanoma, especially if the lesion is fast growing or if there is a recent change in a long-standing lesion.

Mucosal melanomas are frequently multifocal and may present as subtle changes in pigmentation; in such cases, multiple biopsies from different sites may be necessary not only for diagnosis but also for mapping out the extent of lesion, especially if the lesion is flat. Also, it is imperative that a thorough physical examination is made with accurate documentation of location, size, and number of lesions, since it may not be easy to differentiate mucosal melanomas from melanomas arising from the adjacent skin by histologic examination alone.

Histopathological Challenges

Histopathological diagnosis of mucosal melanoma is typically straightforward in majority of cases, since the features are similar to primary cutaneous melanomas. In mucosal melanomas, the in-situ component when present is typically lentiginous, i.e., characterized by proliferation of predominantly single melanocytes with variable cytologic atypia, distributed in a confluent pattern along the basal layer of epithelium. Melanomas may also arise in mucocutaneous junction or extend into the mucosa from the adjacent skin; in such cases, the intraepithelial component may display a superficial spreading pattern of growth, i.e., confluent proliferation an admixture of nested and single melanocytes with variable pagetoid distribution. The tumors are typically fairly cellular, composed of epithelioid to spindled cells characterized by variable amounts of amphophilic or eosinophilic cytoplasm, variable cytoplasmic pigmentation, ovoid or hyperchromatic nuclei, vesicular chromatin, and nucleoli.

In some cases, tumor cells may show exclusively nevoid or spindled cytomorphology and complete lack of pigmentation, raising the possibility of other malignancies such as small round blue cell tumors, neuroendocrine carcinomas, or even sarcoma. In such cases, employing a panel of immunohistochemical studies may aid in the establishment of melanocytic lineage. Also, identification of an intraepithelial/in-situ component or associated precursor lesions such as melanocytic nevus or melanosis may also support diagnosis of melanoma. In cases where the in-situ component is absent, i.e., in mucosal melanomas with a nodular pattern of growth, the possibility of metastasis from a cutaneous primary should be considered. In such cases, comparison of mutational profile and total mutational burden (TMB) between the cutaneous and mucosal tumors may help in accurate diagnosis, since primary cutaneous melanomas typically have high TMB with predominance of point mutations [10], while chromosomal alterations predominate in primary mucosal melanomas [13].

Establishment of melanocytic differentiation is the cornerstone in the immunohistochemical diagnosis of mucosal melanoma [16, 17]. However, some tumors may be de-differentiated, leading to loss of expression of conventional melanocytic markers such as GP100, Melan-A/ MART1 (Fig. 6.1) and tyrosinase, which may be accompanied by acquisition of epithelial markers such as cytokeratin [18], epithelial membrane antigen [19]; neuroendocrine markers such as synaptophysin [18]; and mesenchymal markers such as desmin [18] and CD34 [20]. S100 [21] and in particular SOX10 [22] (Fig. 6.1) remain the most sensitive immunohistochemical markers of melanocytic differentiation, compared to MITF [21]. Strong expression of PRAME [23–25], BRAFpV600E, or RASpQ61 [26] may strengthen the possibility of melanoma, in conjunction with other melanocytic markers. In addition to diagnosis, immunohistochemical studies using highly sensitive melanocytic markers such as SOX10 may aid in evaluation of margin status. Similarly, PRAME immunohistochemistry may also be employed for assessment of margin status in PRAME-positive mucosal melanomas [27]; however, the possibility of field effect should be taken into consideration in such cases.

Mucosal melanomas, with the exception of conjunctival melanomas, are located in sun-protected sites and, therefore, lack ultraviolet light-induced point mutations as well as the heavy mutational burden [28, 29]. Similar to cutaneous melanoma, genes involved in the MAPK pathway are frequently mutated in mucosal melanomas as well. However, structural chromosomal alterations, including amplifications and deletions of chromosomes, are much more common in mucosal melanomas

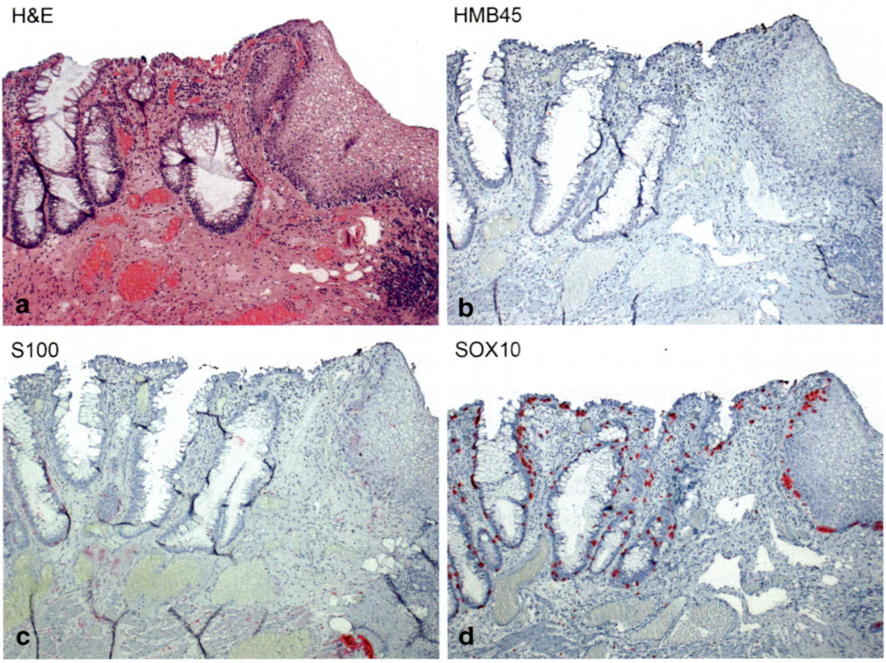

Fig. 6.1 Utility of immunohistochemical studies in determining the extent of anorectal melanoma in-situ. (**a**) Melanoma in-situ is apparent in the squamous mucosa but not in the colonic mucosa/ columnar epithelium in the H&E section (magnification 20×). (**b**–**d**) The melanoma cells are essentially negative for HMB45 (GP100, **b**) and faintly positive for S100 (**c**). But SOX10 immunohistochemical study highlights the atypical intraepithelial melanocytes involving the squamous and colonic mucosae (**d**) (magnification 20×)

[30]. In spite of these differences, DNA methylation patterns are shared to some extent between cutaneous and non-cutaneous melanomas of various sites, in association with site-specific unique features [31].

Sinonasal Melanoma

Sinonasal melanoma is a disease of older individuals, typically presenting after the age of 60 years; in a meta-analysis, the mean age at diagnosis was 67.6 years [32]. It is rare with annual incidence of 0.12 per 100,000 persons or less [33]. There is mild female predominance, and the female patients were slightly older compared to the male patients at the time of diagnosis (69.6 years vs. 64.3 years) [32]. The most commonly affected anatomic sites include nasal cavity followed by maxillary sinus and oral cavity [34]. The patients present with non-specific complaints such as nasal obstruction/ breathing difficulties, epistaxis, reduced or loss of smell, pain, and rarely visual issues [35]. The lesions may be flat, polypoid, or ulcerated, and the majority have at least focal pigmentation (Fig. 6.2).

Unlike other mucosal melanomas, in-situ component is frequently inconspicuous or absent in sinonasal melanomas (Fig. 6.2). Some studies have documented frequent expression of PRAME in sinonasal melanomas [36], which may aid in diagnosis as well as evaluation of margin status. Determination of tumor size, tumor thickness, and ulceration is challenging due to fragmentation of tissue [37] and are, therefore, not considered to be prognostically relevant [38]. However, presence of positive margins after surgery, perineural or lymphovascular invasion as well as invasion of deep soft tissue, or adjacent tissue/organs including cartilage, bone, skin, dura, and skull base correlated with worse prognosis [37]. The AJCC eighth edition sinonasal melanoma staging system utilizes only the extent of invasion as the criterion for pathological T-categorization with no further stage grouping proposed currently [39]. Patients frequently have metastatic involvement of regional lymph nodes and/or distant organs at the time of presentation [37]. Radical resective surgery remains the mainstay of treatment for local control of disease, and many patients also undergo concurrent regional lymph node dissection as well as adjuvant treatments including radiation and/or chemotherapy [9, 40].

The 5-year overall survival rate ranges from less than 20%–47% after various therapies in different cohorts [40–45]. Patients with disease localized to nasal cavity may have slightly longer overall survival [46]. Recurrence after definitive surgical resection is not infrequent and may occur in up to 32% of patients; is more common among older patients, men, patients with advanced disease as well as those with amelanotic melanomas; and is associated with shorter overall survival [9]. Distant metastasis is common, with almost 50% of patients being affected, with a mean time of 20.4 months after initial diagnosis. In multivariable analysis, older age

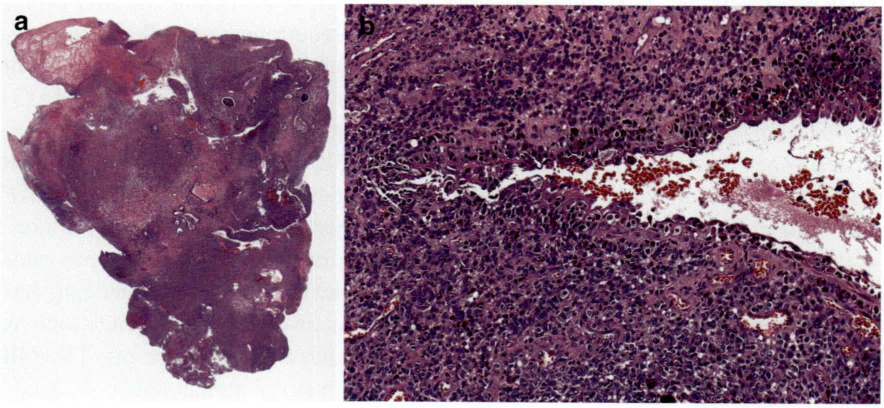

Fig. 6.2 (**a**) Sinonasal melanoma with polypoid growth pattern (**a**, magnification 0.7×). (**b**) Higher magnification (magnification 20×), showing melanoma involving the mucosal stroma (invasive component) and invaginated pseudostratified epithelium (in-situ/ intraepithelial component). Many of the intraepithelial melanocytes are pigmented, while majority of the invasive melanoma cells are amelanotic

(>67.6 years), origin of melanoma in the middle turbinate, disease stage, recurrence, distant metastasis, and treatment only with radiation correlated with shorter overall survival [9, 45].

Immunotherapy is increasingly used in the management of advanced sinonasal melanomas, in both neoadjuvant and adjuvant settings. In a multi-institutional study, nivolumab monotherapy or in combination with ipilimumab resulted in better tumor response rates compared to Pembrolizumab or other immunotherapies, such as interleukin [47]. Moreover, the tumor response was greater at primary and locoregional sites compared to metastatic sites. In another single institution study of patients with resectable sinonasal melanomas, patients with sinus and/or skull base disease were likely to be treated upfront with neoadjuvant ipilimumab and nivolumab combination therapy, while those with sinonasal melanomas localized to the nasal cavity were likely to be treated by surgical resection as the initial management strategy [48]. Studies have shown that among mucosal melanomas, sinonasal melanomas benefited the most from combination anti-PD1 and anti-CTLA4 therapy, compared to monotherapy [49]. In patients with extensive disease, immunotherapy was not associated with improved local recurrence- or progression-free survival. However, patients that showed complete pathologic and/or radiographic response after immunotherapy had longer local recurrence- and progression-free survival [48]. Recent studies have demonstrated that even though the response rates are not as promising as noted in primary cutaneous melanomas, patients treated with immune checkpoint therapy may have better overall survival [50, 51].

Chromosomal aberrations are common in sinonasal melanomas, occurring at a mean frequency of ~10 per tumor [52], with mild predominance of losses over gains. Comparative genomic hybridization analyses have revealed recurrent gain of chromosome 1q and 6p in diploid tumors; 8q, 5p13, 17q22, and 12p11 in triploid or tetraploid tumors, as well as loss of chromosome 10q (PTEN), 6q, 8p, 1p, 9p (CDKN2a), 3p, and X. Certain genomic aberrations, in particular the loss of 1p, 3/3q, and 8p may correlate with increased risk for recurrence, overall and disease-specific survival [53]. Fluorescence in-situ hybridization analyses revealed frequent gain of *RREB1* (6p25) and loss of *MYB* (6q23), followed by gain of *CCND1* (11q13) and loss of *p16/INK4A* (9q21) [53, 54]. Targeted sequencing of common melanoma-related genes revealed activation of MAPK and PI3K/Akt pathways, with frequent mutations involving *NRAS* and mutations or amplifications of *KIT* [53, 55]. *BRAF* mutations are relatively rare in sinonasal melanomas and, when present, are non-V600E variants [54, 56]. Patients with *NRAS* mutations had lower recurrence rates compared to those with *KRAS* mutations [53]. Next-generation sequencing has revealed relatively increased incidence of mutations involving other genes such as *SF3B1* [57], *NF1*, and *SPRED1* [58]. TERT promoter mutations are rare [58–60] but are more common in sinonasal rather than oral mucosal melanomas.

Conjunctival Melanoma

Conjunctival melanoma is a rare type of mucosal melanoma with an annual incidence of approximately 0.5 per million in the USA [61]. In the past decades, there has been a progressive increase in incidence worldwide [62, 63]. With a median age at diagnosis of 64 years, they are almost exclusively unilateral, and more than two-thirds are localized to the ocular apparatus at presentation [64]. Comprising 12%–22%, melanoma has the shortest disease-specific survival rate among primary conjunctival malignant neoplasms, with increased risk for local recurrence and metastasis. There is no definitive sex predilection. Ultraviolet light exposure is a major risk factor for the development of conjunctival melanoma [65]. Interpalpebral bulbar conjunctiva close to limbus is the most common site, followed by tarsus, fornix, and caruncle; multifocal involvement may be present in a third of the patients [66]. Pigmented lesion with prominent vascularity is the most common presentation, but conjunctival melanoma may be amelanotic in 10%–20% of primary cases and also when recurrent [67].

Majority of the conjunctival melanomas arise in association with pre-existing lesions, including conjunctival melanocytic intraepithelial neoplasia (C-MIN) or primary acquired melanosis (PAM) with atypia (74%–76%), nevi (7%–9%) and rarely in ethnic or complexion-associated melanosis (CAM), while only a small proportion arise de novo (15%–19%) [68–70]. Histologically, the majority of conjunctival melanomas are invasive with lentiginous (Fig. 6.3) or nodular patterns of growth, and up to 25% of the tumors may show tumor-related ulceration [7]. The tumor may extend into adjacent ocular and extraocular structures such as corneal

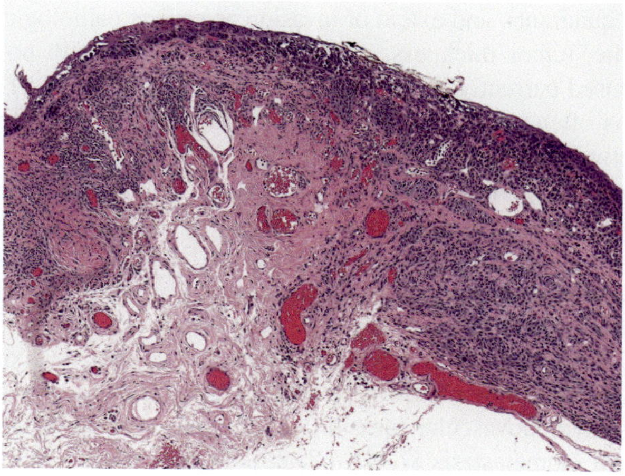

Fig. 6.3 Conjunctival melanoma showing in-situ (left) and invasive (right) components (magnification 10×). There is an asymmetric lymphohistiocytic infiltrate: moderately dense, predominantly in association with the lentiginous in-situ component. The invasive component invades the conjunctival/subepithelial stroma and displays epithelioid and nevoid cytomorphology

epithelium, leading to frequently positive limbal margin, corneal stroma, sclera, canaliculus, lacrimal sac, orbital fat, or the central nervous system [68].

Surgical excision of the mass using the "no touch" technique with "double freeze-thaw" cryotherapy of margins is the standard of care [71], although sentinel lymph node biopsies are becoming more common in thicker (greater than 2 mm) and/or larger lesions [7, 72]. The conjunctival melanocytic intraepithelial neoplasia, if present, may be treated with surgical excision and/or cryotherapy. Adjunct local therapies may include topical chemotherapy using Mitomycin-C or interferon alpha-2b and radiation using plaque brachytherapy (ruthenium-106, iodine-125, and strontium-90 are the commonly used isotopes) or proton beam [73, 74]. Studies have demonstrated that treatment of patients in institutions highly experienced in the management of ocular oncology have overall lower incidence of recurrence, metastasis, and melanoma-related death compared to those that were treated elsewhere [66, 75]. In non-metastatic locally advanced melanoma, orbital exenteration may be considered. However, there appears to be no survival benefit, likely due to the advanced nature of disease [76].

While systemic options for locally advanced or metastatic conjunctival melanoma were limited previously, the advent of immune checkpoint and targeted therapies has opened up a new avenue for management. In particular, targeting PD1/ PD-L1 axis and/or CTLA-4 has led to favorable tumor response and potential prevention of morbid surgeries such as orbital exenteration [77], irrespective of PD-L1 expression [77]. In addition, several monoclonal antibodies and small molecule inhibitors targeting signaling pathways or driver gene products, including MAPK, PI3K/AKT/ mTOR pathways, BRAF, NRAS, MEK, and KIT, can also aid in systemic control of conjunctival melanoma [78, 79].

The eighth edition AJCC staging system for conjunctival melanoma categorizes the tumor based on clinical criteria, including anatomic location, involvement of conjunctiva in quadrants, and extent of invasion as well as pathologic criteria, such as anatomic site, tumor thickness, and extent of invasion, with no further stage grouping proposed currently [80]. While the advanced categories (T3 and T4) are similar, there is often major discordance in T-categorization in early conjunctival melanomas between the clinical and pathological systems.

Local recurrence is common, likely due to the association with background conjunctival melanocytic intraepithelial neoplasia (C-MIN) and may be late, necessitating long-term patient surveillance [70]. Older age at diagnosis, presence of precursor lesion, advanced T-category, prior surgical intervention, tarsal location, forniceal involvement, and positive margins may correlate with increased risk for recurrence [66, 81, 82]. Older age, male sex, non-bulbar location, de novo development, palpebral location, nodular tumor growth pattern, greater tumor thickness, ulceration, mitotic activity, lymphovascular invasion, and orbital invasion may correlate with the development of metastasis [7, 61, 68, 82]. Greater tumor thickness, de novo development, forniceal location, nodular pattern of growth, and presence of sentinel lymph node metastasis correlated with shorter disease-specific survival [7, 68].

Similar to other mucosal melanomas, MAPK and PI3K-AKT pathways are commonly activated in conjunctival melanoma. In part due to the sun exposure, the mutational profile of conjunctival melanoma overlaps with that of cutaneous melanoma, characterized by high tumor mutational burden, particularly among those arising in bulbar conjunctiva [13, 65, 83, 84]; however, tumors of tarsal origin tend to have fewer ultraviolet light-induced C > T changes. Targeted gene sequencing has revealed frequent and mutually exclusive point mutations in *BRAF*, *NRAS*, and *NF1* genes among others such as *ACSS3*, *ATRX*, *SF3B1*, *KIT*, and *KRAS* [85]. *TERT* promoter mutations are also common and may be associated with metastasis [86, 87]. Since *ATRX* mutations have been noted in primary acquired melanosis with atypia, this may be an early event in the development of conjunctival melanoma [87]. In addition, recurrent chromosomal aberrations, such as gain of 6p and loss on 7q and 10q, have been reported in conjunctival melanomas [88]. Deletion of chr 10q11.21–26.2 region correlated with greater tumor thickness, presence of lymphovascular invasion, and *BRAF* mutations as well as metastasis.

Anorectal Melanoma

Anorectal melanoma is overall a rare malignant neoplasm with incidence of 0.3 per 1 million in the USA [89], constituting less than 2% of all anorectal malignancies [90]. Similar to some of the other types of mucosal melanomas, there is a mild female predominance [8, 89, 91, 92]. Even though anorectal melanoma may be rarely diagnosed in younger patients [8, 89], older adults, with median age of greater than 60 years, are most commonly affected, with the highest incidence in the ninth decade [89]. Most patients present with rectal bleeding, mass that is often non-pigmented, clinically resembling hemorrhoids or rarely, only pruritus. In some patients, the presenting symptoms can include fullness, pain, mucinous discharge, and changes in bowel habits. There is frequently significant delay in diagnosis [93].

Anorectal melanoma may arise in the anal canal (distal to or below the dentate line, lined by non-keratinizing stratified squamous epithelium), anorectal junction (at the dentate line, lined by squamo-columnar junctional mucosa), from the rectal canal (proximal to or above the dentate line, lined by columnar/ colonic epithelium) [8, 89, 91]. However, assigning the anatomic site can be challenging in surgical specimens, especially when the tumors are large and/or circumferential, resulting in effacement of anatomic structures. Therefore, the anatomic location of tumor is best determined during digital/ physical examination. This is particularly an issue in neoadjuvant-treated specimens with good response or minimal residual tumor, which is why mucosal tattoos are utilized more frequently nowadays to designate sites of biopsy and/or tumor [94]. Some studies have suggested that anorectal melanomas located proximal to anal canal have higher rates of systemic dissemination, compared to those arising from or below the anal canal [95], while other studies have suggested slight differences in survival based on anatomic location [91]. Rarely, anorectal melanomas may originate from the anal verge [8, 96]; establishing mucosal origin can be challenging in such cases and may necessitate molecular analyses.

Diagnosis of anorectal melanoma requires histopathological evaluation (Fig. 6.4). Therefore, a high degree of suspicion may be warranted for performing biopsies of clinically innocuous lesions. Adequate tissue without prominent crush artifact is essential for optimal histopathological evaluation. In majority of the anorectal melanomas, the diagnosis is fairly straightforward. However, in some instances, the tumor can be poorly differentiated with spindled or sarcomatoid morphology, lacking an in-situ component, melanin pigmentation of the lesional cells as well as expression of typical melanocytic markers such as MelanA/ MART1, HMB45, tyrosinase, and MITF (Fig. 6.1) [97]. In such cases, S100 and SOX10 may be positive; however, these markers are not specific for melanocytic differentiation. In addition, advanced melanomas may acquire aberrant expression of keratinocytic and/or neuroendocrine differentiation [98, 99]. Therefore, additional studies including molecular profiling may be necessary to arrive at the correct diagnosis.

Metastasis is frequent, and patients with anorectal melanomas have a shorter time to the development of metastasis and also the highest risk for developing brain metastasis, compared to other mucosal melanomas [100]. Most of the patients have advanced disease at presentation with approximately 33% and 25% of patients having regional and distant metastasis, respectively, at presentation [8]. Clinical stage at presentation, in particular the presence systemic disease is the most significant parameter affecting disease-specific survival [8, 89]. Of the primary tumor histopathological parameters, higher tumor thickness, lymphovascular invasion, and lack of regression correlated with shorter disease-specific survival [8]. Other high-risk factors include age greater than 70 years at diagnosis, level of invasion of tumor [101], especially extension beyond muscularis propria [92], and tumor size [102]. Since majority of the anorectal melanomas are ulcerated, ulceration is not a histopathologic parameter of prognostic significance in anorectal melanoma [8, 101].

The prognosis of anorectal melanoma has been dismal, with 5-year survival averaging around 20% [89, 103], with majority of patients surviving less than

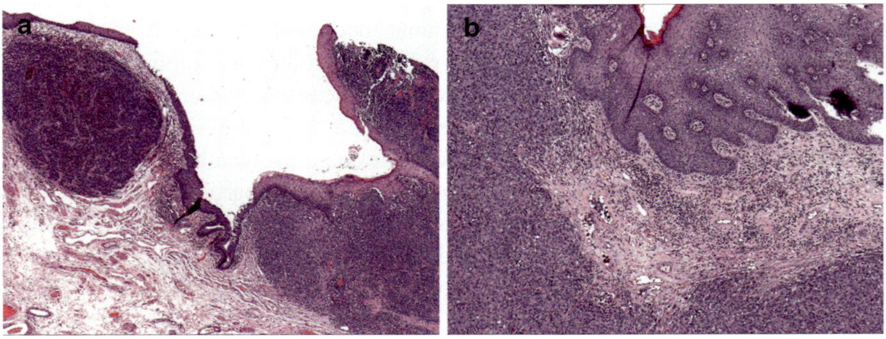

Fig. 6.4 A. Anorectal melanoma involving the squamo-columnar junctional mucosa (**a**, magnification 4×). The tumor shows focal pigmentation (nodule on the left) and abuts the overlying squamous epithelium (right). (**b**) Higher magnification of a different area of the same tumor as A shows sheets of malignant epithelioid cells in the lamina propria with focal lymphovascular invasion (magnification 8×)

2 years after diagnosis. Currently, anorectal melanomas are staged based on the extent of clinical disease as localized disease, regional, or distant metastasis [104], since there are no AJCC-approved staging systems for anorectal melanomas [105]. Minor modifications of AJCC eighth edition staging system for primary cutaneous melanomas, especially using the AJCC stage can robustly risk-stratify anorectal melanomas [8, 105]. Also, classifying melanomas based on anatomic level of invasion, regional lymph node metastatic disease burden, anatomic site of distant metastasis, and LDH levels may offer further prognostic stratification [101].

Surgical resection is the mainstay of management of early-stage anorectal melanoma [106], and complete clearance of melanoma correlates with longer overall survival [107]. Surgical management of patients with melanoma localized to the anorectum and/or regional metastasis showed longer overall and disease-specific survival compared to those that did not undergo surgery [89]. Traditionally, majority of anorectal melanomas were treated with abdominoperineal resection [108], which necessitated removal of the anal sphincter, among other morbidities, thereby significantly decreasing the quality of life. However, recent meta-analyses of retrospective studies have shown that abdominoperineal resection may provide only marginally better local control of disease, if any with lower recurrence rates [109], and there was no survival benefit compared to less extensive surgeries [110, 111]. Therefore, sphincter-sparing surgeries, such as wide local or transmucosal excision, are favored for majority of patients with anorectal melanoma.

In addition, adjuvant radiation therapy to the primary site may provide better local control [112] as well as to some extent longer survival [113]. Sentinel lymph node sampling is also increasingly employed in the management of anorectal melanomas [114]. Various combinations of adjuvant chemotherapy, biochemotherapy, *KIT*-targeted therapy, and immune-targeted therapy using interferon-1α or interleukin-2 have been used with minimal or anecdotal success [103, 115]. In patients with unresectable anorectal melanoma treated using cytotoxic chemotherapy, objective response correlated with lower mortality rates [116]. With the advent of immune checkpoint therapy, many patients with resectable mucosal melanomas undergo neoadjuvant immunotherapy [117]. Some studies have reported that a combination of anti-PD1 and anti-CTLA4 therapy might be more efficient than anti-PD1 or anti-CTLA4 monotherapy [118, 119]; however, a recent metanalysis suggested that the addition of anti-CTLA4 may not significantly improve the objective response rates (ORR) in anorectal melanomas [49]. Patients that developed objective radiological and pathological response had longer event-free and overall survival [120].

Similar to mucosal melanomas of other sites, anorectal melanomas are characterized by an overall low tumor mutational burden (median—2.6 mutations per megabase), but high incidence of chromosomal structural [10, 13, 121]. MAPK pathway is commonly affected. Common driven genes mutated include *SF3B1*, *KIT*, *NF1*, *BRAF*, *BAP1*, *NRAS*, *TP53*, *KRAS*, *CTNNB1*, *CDKN2A*, and *CDKN2B* [121–124]. Even though *KIT* mutations are fairly frequent in anorectal melanoma, there is no correlation between *KIT* mutational status and overexpression of KIT protein by immunohistochemistry [125].

Vulvovaginal Melanoma

Vulvar melanomas, accounting for less than 10% of all melanomas in women and gynecological cancers, are rare with incidence of 1.74 per 1 million person-years [126]. Primary vaginal melanomas are even more uncommon, accounting for less than 5% of vaginal malignancies [127], but they are extremely aggressive tumors with high rates of mortality. Vulvar melanomas overlap significantly with cutaneous melanomas with respect to several histologic and prognostic features and are staged according to the AJCC eighth edition primary cutaneous melanoma staging system [128, 129], while vaginal melanomas segregate with mucosal melanomas. Even though they may represent different diseases, vulvar and vaginal melanomas are often grouped and studied together due to their overall rarity and also since some of the vulvar tumors may extensively extend into other urogenital structures, including vagina, and vice versa, especially in advanced stages [130].

Vulvar and vaginal melanomas are rare, affecting predominantly older white women. Vulvar melanomas constitute less than 10% of melanomas in women and less than 10% of gynecological malignancies [131–134], while vaginal melanomas are even more infrequent, comprising less than 1% of all melanomas in women, less than 3% of vaginal cancers [135, 136]. Patients with vulvar melanoma tend to be slightly younger than those with vaginal melanomas at the time of diagnosis. The presenting symptoms include, most commonly, mass or lesion, pruritus, pain, dyspareunia, discharge, and irritation [137]. Vulvar melanomas frequently involve the following sites in the descending order of occurrence: unilateral labium majus, unilateral labium minus, both unilateral labia, clitoris, followed by bilateral labia and introitus. Vaginal melanomas may occur at any part of the vaginal canal, and urethral extension is extremely common; in some instances, it may be difficult to differentiate mucosal melanomas of vaginal from urethral origin. Multifocality and/or involvement/crossing of midline is often associated with shorter disease-specific survival in vulvar melanoma [137, 138].

Histologically, the tumors most commonly display a lentiginous pattern of growth, in which the intraepithelial component is predominated by contiguous proliferation of single melanocytes (Fig. 6.5). In primary vulvar melanomas, increasing tumor thickness, high mitotic rate, lack of regression, presence of lymphovascular invasion and satellitosis and absence of a precursor nevus correlated with shorter overall survival, while tumor thickness and mitotic rate (greater than $1/\text{mm}^2$) associated with shorter disease-specific survival [131, 137], in addition to lymph node status and distant metastasis [131, 139]. Ulceration is present in 50%–56% of primary vulvar melanomas; however, ulceration was not an independent prognostic factor [131, 137]. Compared to vulvar melanomas, vaginal melanomas have an aggressive biological behavior, including increased propensity for recurrence and death [140]. Even though some of the primary tumor features, such as involvement of the upper portion of vaginal canal, tumor size, depth of invasion, lymphovascular invasion, and margin status have been suggested to affect prognosis, only lymph node status and presence of metastasis have been significantly correlated with

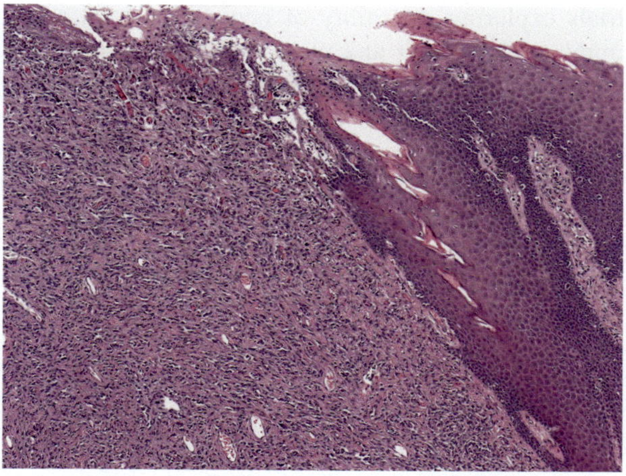

Fig. 6.5 Vulvar melanoma composed of atypical spindled cells with a subtle overlying in-situ component (magnification ×10)

patient outcome [131, 141–143]. While AJCC recommends using the primary cutaneous melanoma staging system for vulvar melanoma [128, 131], there is no standardized system for staging vaginal melanomas; the clinical stage or FIGO system is commonly employed [144].

Surgical resection is the primary modality of treatment for local control [131, 145]. Even though radical resective surgeries such as radical vulvectomy offer better local control, there are no definitive long-term survival benefits [132, 134, 146]. Similarly, sentinel lymph node biopsies are favored more currently compared to upfront inguinal lymph node dissection [147]. Similar to other mucosal melanomas, adjuvant immunotherapy is a preferred modality of treatment compared to chemotherapy with or without radiation [148]. Neoadjuvant immunotherapy is also becoming a frequent approach in patients presenting with bulky disease or advanced melanoma.

Compared to cutaneous melanomas, vulvovaginal melanomas have lower tumor mutational burden (~1.55 mutations per megabase) and show slightly increased numbers of chromosomal structural alterations [121]. *SF3B1*, *KIT*, and *NF1* mutations are more common, followed by *BRAF*, *NRAS*, *KRAS*, *ATRX*, *CDKN2A*, and *BAP1* [12, 149–152]. *TERT*-promoter mutations are extremely rare [12]. In vulvar melanomas, presence of *KIT* mutation and CD117 overexpression correlated with longer progression-free survival [153, 154].

Summary

Mucosal melanomas are unique and rare tumors compared to their cutaneous counterparts. Their aggressive clinical course has garnered more attention recently with exponentially increasing numbers of retrospective studies evaluating demographic, clinical, and histopathological features of prognostic importance as well as clinical trials exploring the utility of neoadjuvant and adjuvant treatments, particularly immune checkpoint and other molecularly-targeted therapies. In addition, next-generation sequencing has begun to unveil the similarities and differences of the molecular landscape of the various types of mucosal melanomas, in comparison with cutaneous melanomas. Thus, even though our understanding of these unusual cancers has expanded significantly in recent years, the rarity of these tumors poses a major challenge. Establishment of international mucosal melanoma consortia will aid in the collation of larger cohorts and thus refine the management of patients with mucosal melanomas.

References

1. Chang AE, Karnell LH, Menck HR. The National Cancer Data Base report on cutaneous and noncutaneous melanoma: a summary of 84,836 cases from the past decade. The American College of Surgeons Commission on Cancer and the American Cancer Society. Cancer. 1998;83(8):1664–78.
2. McLaughlin CC, et al. Incidence of noncutaneous melanomas in the U.S. Cancer. 2005;103(5):1000–7.
3. Nagarajan P, Yun SJ, Prieto VG. Mucosal melanoma: review from a pathologist point of view. Clin Dermatol. 2025;43(3):365–77.
4. Ballester Sanchez R, et al. Mucosal melanoma: an update. Actas Dermosifiliogr. 2015;106(2):96–103.
5. Carvajal RD, Spencer SA, Lydiatt W. Mucosal melanoma: a clinically and biologically unique disease entity. J Natl Compr Cancer Netw. 2012;10(3):345–56.
6. Siegel RL, Miller DR, Jemal A. Cancer statistics, 2019. CA Cancer J Clin. 2019;69:7–34.
7. Esmaeli B, et al. Greater tumor thickness, ulceration, and positive sentinel lymph node are associated with worse prognosis in patients with conjunctival melanoma: implications for future AJCC classifications. Am J Surg Pathol. 2019;43(12):1701–10.
8. Nagarajan P, et al. Prognostic model for patient survival in primary anorectal mucosal melanoma: stage at presentation determines relevance of histopathologic features. Mod Pathol. 2020;33(3):496–513.
9. Pontes FSC, et al. Sinonasal melanoma: a systematic review of the prognostic factors. Int J Oral Maxillofac Surg. 2020;49(5):549–57.
10. Hayward NK, et al. Whole-genome landscapes of major melanoma subtypes. Nature. 2017;545(7653):175–80.
11. Shain AH, et al. The genetic evolution of melanoma from precursor lesions. N Engl J Med. 2015;373(20):1926–36.
12. Wilhite AM, et al. A paradigm shift in understanding vulvovaginal melanoma as a distinct tumor type compared with cutaneous melanoma. Gynecol Oncol. 2024;188:13–21.
13. Newell F, et al. Whole-genome landscape of mucosal melanoma reveals diverse drivers and therapeutic targets. Nat Commun. 2019;10(1):3163.
14. Wang M, et al. Integrated genomic analyses of acral and mucosal melanomas nominate novel driver genes. Genome Med. 2022;14(1):65.
15. Cicek Y, Ertas U. The normal and pathological pigmentation of oral mucous membrane: a review. J Contemp Dent Pract. 2003;4(3):76–86.
16. Nagarajan P, et al. Use of new techniques in addition to IHC applied to the diagnosis of melanocytic lesions, with emphasis on CGH, FISH, and mass spectrometry. Actas Dermosifiliogr. 2017;108(1):17–30.

17. Saliba E, Bhawan J. Aberrant expression of immunohistochemical markers in malignant melanoma: a review. Dermatopathology (Basel). 2021;8(3):359–70.
18. Romano RC, Carter JM, Folpe AL. Aberrant intermediate filament and synaptophysin expression is a frequent event in malignant melanoma: an immunohistochemical study of 73 cases. Mod Pathol. 2015;28(8):1033–42.
19. Roe OD, Wahl SG. The undifferentiated carcinoma that became a melanoma: re-biopsy of a cancer of an unknown primary site: a case report. J Med Case Rep. 2017;11(1):82.
20. Breza TS, Magro CM. CD34 expression in primary cutaneous malignant melanoma: apropos of a case and review of the aberrant melanoma phenotype. J Cutan Pathol. 2005;32(10):685–9.
21. Ohsie SJ, et al. Immunohistochemical characteristics of melanoma. J Cutan Pathol. 2008;35(5):433–44.
22. Tacha D, et al. A newly developed mouse monoclonal SOX10 antibody is a highly sensitive and specific marker for malignant melanoma, including spindle cell and desmoplastic melanomas. Arch Pathol Lab Med. 2015;139(4):530–6.
23. Ronchi A, et al. PRAME immunocytochemistry for the diagnosis of melanoma metastases in cytological samples. Diagnostics (Basel). 2022;12(3):646.
24. Shah A, et al. Diagnostic utility of PRAME in rare melanoma mimics: a comparative analysis including GNET, MMNST, epithelioid MPNST, and MITF-rearranged melanocytic tumors. J Cutan Pathol. 2025;52(11):710–9.
25. Hrycaj SM, et al. PRAME expression in spindle cell melanoma, malignant peripheral nerve sheath tumour, and other cutaneous sarcomatoid neoplasms: a comparative analysis. Histopathology. 2022;81(6):818–25.
26. Kakavand H, et al. BRAF(V600E) and NRAS(Q61L/Q61R) mutation analysis in metastatic melanoma using immunohistochemistry: a study of 754 cases highlighting potential pitfalls and guidelines for interpretation and reporting. Histopathology. 2016;69(4):680–6.
27. Martin SD, et al. PRAME immunohistochemistry for distinguishing vulvar and vaginal melanoma from benign melanocytic nevi. Int J Gynecol Pathol. 2024;43(4):389–96.
28. Vergara IA, et al. Genetic drivers of non-cutaneous melanomas: challenges and opportunities in a heterogeneous landscape. Exp Dermatol. 2022;31(1):13–30.
29. Alexandrov LB, et al. The repertoire of mutational signatures in human cancer. Nature. 2020;578(7793):94–101.
30. Shteinman ER, et al. Causes, consequences and clinical significance of aneuploidy across melanoma subtypes. Front Oncol. 2022;12:988691.
31. Jurmeister P, et al. Mucosal melanomas of different anatomic sites share a common global DNA methylation profile with cutaneous melanoma but show location-dependent patterns of genetic and epigenetic alterations. J Pathol. 2022;256(1):61–70.
32. Mastoraki A, et al. Clinical evidence, diagnostic approach and challenging therapeutic modalities for malignant melanoma of the anorectum. ANZ J Surg. 2021;91(3):276–81.
33. Rojas-Lechuga MJ, et al. Survival outcomes in sinonasal mucosal melanoma: systematic review and meta-analysis. J Pers Med. 2024;14(12):1120.
34. Temmermand D, et al. Sinonasal mucosal melanoma: a population-based comparison of the EUROCARE and SEER registries. Int Arch Otorhinolaryngol. 2022;26(3):e446–52.
35. Todorovic N, et al. Primary sinonasal mucosal melanoma: a narrative review. Diagnostics (Basel). 2025;15(4):496.
36. Scheurleer WFJ, et al. PRAME staining in sinonasal mucosal melanoma: a single-center experience. Head Neck Pathol. 2023;17(2):401–8.
37. Salari B, et al. Sinonasal mucosal melanoma: an update and review of the literature. Am J Dermatopathol. 2022;44(6):424–32.
38. Williams MD, et al. Data set for the reporting of mucosal melanomas of the head and neck: explanations and recommendations of the guidelines from the international collaboration on cancer reporting. Arch Pathol Lab Med. 2019;143(5):603–9.
39. Lydiatt WM, et al. Mucosal melanoma of the head and neck. In: Amin MB, et al., editor. AJCC cancer staging manual. 8th ed. Cham: Springer Nature; 2017. p. 163–169.

40. Amit M, et al. Role of adjuvant treatment in sinonasal mucosal melanoma. J Neurol Surg B Skull Base. 2017;78(6):512–8.
41. Ganti A, et al. Treatment modalities in sinonasal mucosal melanoma: a national cancer database analysis. Laryngoscope. 2020;130(2):275–82.
42. Moreno MA, et al. Mucosal melanoma of the nose and paranasal sinuses, a contemporary experience from the MD Anderson Cancer Center. Cancer. 2010;116(9):2215–23.
43. Benlyazid A, et al. Postoperative radiotherapy in head and neck mucosal melanoma: a GETTEC study. Arch Otolaryngol Head Neck Surg. 2010;136(12):1219–25.
44. Sun S, et al. Long-term treatment outcomes and prognosis of mucosal melanoma of the head and neck: 161 cases from a single institution. Oral Oncol. 2017;74:115–22.
45. Lawaetz M, et al. Primary mucosal melanoma of the head and neck in Denmark, 1982–2012: demographic and clinical aspects. A retrospective DAHANCA study. Acta Oncol. 2016;55(8):1001–8.
46. Scheurleer WFJ, et al. Sinonasal mucosal melanoma in The Netherlands between 2001 and 2021: a clinical and epidemiological overview of 320 cases. Eur Arch Otorrinolaringol. 2024;281(10):5437–46.
47. Kshirsagar RS, et al. Outcomes of immunotherapy treatment in sinonasal mucosal melanoma. Am J Rhinol Allergy. 2025;39(2):102–8.
48. Salem AF, et al. Resectable sinonasal mucosal melanoma in the immunotherapy era: upfront surgery vs. neoadjuvant therapy. Head Neck. 2025;47(7):1848–56.
49. Dimitriou F, et al. Single-agent anti-PD-1 or combined with ipilimumab in patients with mucosal melanoma: an international, retrospective, cohort study. Ann Oncol. 2022;33(9):968–80.
50. Scherzad A, et al. Multimodal treatment and immune checkpoint inhibition in sinonasal mucosal melanoma: real-world data of a retrospective, single-center study. Eur Arch Otorrinolaringol. 2023;280(9):4215–23.
51. Lechner M, et al. International multicenter study of clinical outcomes of sinonasal melanoma shows survival benefit for patients treated with immune checkpoint inhibitors and potential improvements to the current TNM staging system. J Neurol Surg B Skull Base. 2023;84(4):307–19.
52. van Dijk M, et al. Distinct chromosomal aberrations in sinonasal mucosal melanoma as detected by comparative genomic hybridization. Genes Chromosomes Cancer. 2003;36(2):151–8.
53. Libera L, et al. KRAS/NRAS variants and copy number alterations prognostically stratify patients with sinonasal melanoma. Pathologica. 2025;117(2):121–30.
54. Turri-Zanoni M, et al. Sinonasal mucosal melanoma: molecular profile and therapeutic implications from a series of 32 cases. Head Neck. 2013;35(8):1066–77.
55. Amit M, et al. Mutation status among patients with sinonasal mucosal melanoma and its impact on survival. Br J Cancer. 2017;116(12):1564–71.
56. Zebary A, et al. KIT, NRAS and BRAF mutations in sinonasal mucosal melanoma: a study of 56 cases. Br J Cancer. 2013;109(3):559–64.
57. Wroblewska JP, et al. SF3B1, NRAS, KIT, and BRAF mutation; CD117 and cMYC expression; and tumoral pigmentation in sinonasal melanomas: an analysis with newly found molecular alterations and some population-based molecular differences. Am J Surg Pathol. 2019;43(2):168–77.
58. Chlopek M, et al. Alterations in key signaling pathways in sinonasal tract melanoma. A molecular genetics and immunohistochemical study of 90 cases and comprehensive review of the literature. Mod Pathol. 2022;35(11):1609–17.
59. Jangard M, et al. TERT promoter mutations in sinonasal malignant melanoma: a study of 49 cases. Melanoma Res. 2015;25(3):185–8.
60. Ozturk Sari S, et al. BRAF, NRAS, KIT, TERT, GNAQ/GNA11 mutation profile analysis of head and neck mucosal melanomas: a study of 42 cases. Pathology. 2017;49(1):55–61.
61. Shields CL, et al. Conjunctival melanoma: insights into classification, outcomes, and biomarkers. Clin Dermatol. 2024;42(1):46–55.

62. Yu GP, et al. Conjunctival melanoma: is it increasing in the United States? Am J Ophthalmol. 2003;135(6):800–6.
63. Triay E, et al. Time trends in the incidence of conjunctival melanoma in Sweden. Br J Ophthalmol. 2009;93(11):1524–8.
64. He LF, et al. Incidence, clinical features, and survival outcomes of primary malignant conjunctival tumor: a US population-based retrospective cohort analysis based on the SEER database (1975–2018). Transl Cancer Res. 2025;14(3):1609–25.
65. Rivolta C, et al. UV light signature in conjunctival melanoma; not only skin should be protected from solar radiation. J Hum Genet. 2016;61(4):361–2.
66. Vaidya S, et al. Conjunctival melanoma: risk factors for recurrent or new tumor in 540 patients at a single ocular oncology center. Eur J Ophthalmol. 2021;31(5):2675–85.
67. Pacheco RR, et al. Conjunctival melanoma: outcomes based on tumour origin in 629 patients at a single ocular oncology centre. Eye (Lond). 2022;36(3):603–11.
68. Shields CL, et al. Conjunctival melanoma: outcomes based on tumor origin in 382 consecutive cases. Ophthalmology. 2011;118(2):389–95. e1–2.
69. Larsen AC, et al. A retrospective review of conjunctival melanoma presentation, treatment, and outcome and an investigation of features associated with BRAF mutations. JAMA Ophthalmol. 2015;133(11):1295–303.
70. Butt K, et al. Conjunctival melanoma: a clinical review and update. Cancers (Basel). 2024;16(18):3121.
71. Shields JA, Shields CL, De Potter P. Surgical management of conjunctival tumors. The 1994 Lynn B. McMahan Lecture. Arch Ophthalmol. 1997;115(6):808–15.
72. Mor JM, et al. Sentinel lymph node biopsy in the management of conjunctival melanoma: current insights. Clin Ophthalmol. 2019;13:1297–302.
73. Kastelan S, et al. Conjunctival melanoma: comprehensive insights into clinical features, genetic alterations, and modern treatment approaches. Pathol Oncol Res. 2025;31:1612085.
74. Tzortzi P, et al. Topical chemotherapy for the treatment of melanocytic conjunctival tumors: an updated review. Eur J Ophthalmol. 2025;35(6):2336–46.
75. Damato B, Coupland SE. An audit of conjunctival melanoma treatment in Liverpool. Eye (Lond). 2009;23(4):801–9.
76. Baum SH, et al. Conjunctival and uveal melanoma: survival and risk factors following orbital exenteration. Eur J Ophthalmol. 2022;32(1):612–9.
77. Syar P, et al. Immune check point inhibitors for ocular adnexal and periocular tumors. Taiwan J Ophthalmol. 2025;15(1):14–25.
78. Grimes JM, et al. Conjunctival melanoma: current treatments and future options. Am J Clin Dermatol. 2020;21(3):371–81.
79. Li WJ, et al. Emerging techniques in the treatment of conjunctival melanoma. Curr Ophthalmol Rep. 2025;13(1):7.
80. Coupland SE, et al. Conjunctival melanoma. In: Amin MB, et al., editor. AJCC cancer staging manual. 8th ed. Cham: Springer Nature; 2017. p. 795–803.
81. Dalvin LA, et al. Conjunctival melanoma: outcomes based on age at presentation in 629 patients at a single ocular oncology center. Cornea. 2021;40(5):554–63.
82. Calis Karanfil F, et al. Factors affecting recurrence and metastasis in conjunctival melanoma. Int Ophthalmol. 2023;43(11):4203–15.
83. Swaminathan SS, et al. Molecular characteristics of conjunctival melanoma using whole-exome sequencing. JAMA Ophthalmol. 2017;135(12):1434–7.
84. Cisarova K, et al. Genomic and transcriptomic landscape of conjunctival melanoma. PLoS Genet. 2020;16(12):e1009201.
85. Scholz SL, et al. NF1 mutations in conjunctival melanoma. Br J Cancer. 2018;118(9):1243–7.
86. van Poppelen NM, et al. Molecular genetics of conjunctival melanoma and prognostic value of TERT promoter mutation analysis. Int J Mol Sci. 2021;22(11):5784.
87. van Ipenburg JA, et al. ATRX loss in the development and prognosis of conjunctival melanoma. Int J Mol Sci. 2023;24(16):12988.

88. Kenawy N, et al. Conjunctival melanoma copy number alterations and correlation with mutation status, tumor features, and clinical outcome. Pigment Cell Melanoma Res. 2019;32(4):564–75.
89. Chen H, et al. Incidence, surgical treatment, and prognosis of Anorectal melanoma from 1973 to 2011: a population-based SEER analysis. Medicine (Baltimore). 2016;95(7):e2770.
90. Metildi C, et al. Incidence and survival patterns of rare anal canal neoplasms using the surveillance epidemiology and end results registry. Am Surg. 2013;79(10):1068–74.
91. Paolino G, et al. Anorectal melanoma: systematic review of the current literature of an aggressive type of melanoma. Melanoma Res. 2024;34(6):487–96.
92. Ren M, et al. Prognostic factors in primary anorectal melanoma: a clinicopathological study of 60 cases in China. Hum Pathol. 2018;79:77–85.
93. Malaguarnera G, et al. Anorectal mucosal melanoma. Oncotarget. 2018;9(9):8785–800.
94. Acuna SA, et al. Preoperative localization of colorectal cancer: a systematic review and meta-analysis. Surg Endosc. 2017;31(6):2366–79.
95. Bello DM, et al. Anal versus rectal melanoma: does site of origin predict outcome? Dis Colon Rectum. 2013;56(2):150–7.
96. Ragnarsson-Olding BK, et al. Primary ano-rectal malignant melanomas within a population-based national patient series in Sweden during 40 years. Acta Oncol. 2009;48(1):125–31.
97. Ben-Izhak O, et al. Ki67 antigen and PCNA proliferation markers predict survival in anorectal malignant melanoma. Histopathology. 2002;41(6):519–25.
98. Mg S, et al. Amelanotic malignant melanoma with atypical divergent neuroendocrine differentiation: a report of an unusual and rare case of anorectal bleeding. Cureus. 2024;16(8):e66905.
99. Kolosov A, Leskauskaite J, Dulskas A. Primary melanoma of the anorectal region: clinical and histopathological review of 17 cases. A retrospective cohort study. Colorectal Dis. 2021;23(10):2706–13.
100. Heppt MV, et al. Prognostic factors and treatment outcomes in 444 patients with mucosal melanoma. Eur J Cancer. 2017;81:36–44.
101. Cui C, et al. An evidence-based staging system for mucosal melanoma: a proposal. Ann Surg Oncol. 2022;29(8):5221–34.
102. Wang M, et al. Tumour diameter is a predictor of mesorectal and mesenteric lymph node metastases in anorectal melanoma. Color Dis. 2013;15(9):1086–92.
103. Boer FL, et al. Trends in incidence and survival of 1496 patients with mucosal melanoma in The Netherlands (1990–2019). Cancers (Basel). 2023;15(5):1541.
104. Singer M, Mutch MG. Anal melanoma. Clin Colon Rectal Surg. 2006;19(2):78–87.
105. Nagarajan P. Mucosal melanomas of the anogenital tract: clinical and pathologic predictors of patient survival. Surg Pathol Clin. 2021;14(2):225–35.
106. Jutten E, et al. Surgical treatment of anorectal melanoma: a systematic review and meta-analysis. BJS Open. 2021;5(6):zrab107.
107. Nilsson PJ, Ragnarsson-Olding BK. Importance of clear resection margins in anorectal malignant melanoma. Br J Surg. 2010;97(1):98–103.
108. Brady MS, Kavolius JP, Quan SH. Anorectal melanoma. A 64-year experience at Memorial Sloan-Kettering Cancer Center. Dis Colon Rectum. 1995;38(2):146–51.
109. Temperley HC, et al. Optimal surgical management strategy for treatment of primary anorectal malignant melanoma-a systematic review and meta-analysis. Langenbeck's Arch Surg. 2022;407(8):3193–200.
110. Matsuda A, et al. Abdominoperineal resection provides better local control but equivalent overall survival to local excision of anorectal malignant melanoma: a systematic review. Ann Surg. 2015;261(4):670–7.
111. Smith HG, et al. Less is more: a systematic review and meta-analysis of the outcomes of radical versus conservative primary resection in anorectal melanoma. Eur J Cancer. 2020;135:113–20.
112. Kelly P, et al. Sphincter-sparing local excision and hypofractionated radiation therapy for anorectal melanoma: a 20-year experience. Cancer. 2011;117(20):4747–55.

113. Naqvi J, et al. Patterns of care and survival outcomes in the treatment of anal melanoma. J Gastrointest Cancer. 2020;51(1):211–6.
114. Mistrangelo M, et al. Feasibility and impact of sentinel lymph node biopsy in patients affected by ano-rectal melanoma. Tech Coloproctol. 2025;29(1):38.
115. Beadling C, et al. KIT gene mutations and copy number in melanoma subtypes. Clin Cancer Res. 2008;14(21):6821–8.
116. Shoushtari AN, et al. Clinical features and response to systemic therapy in a historical cohort of advanced or unresectable mucosal melanoma. Melanoma Res. 2017;27(1):57–64.
117. Ho J, et al. Neoadjuvant checkpoint inhibitor immunotherapy for resectable mucosal melanoma. Front Oncol. 2022;12:1001150.
118. Moya-Plana A, et al. Evaluation of the efficacy of immunotherapy for non-resectable mucosal melanoma. Cancer Immunol Immunother. 2019;68(7):1171–8.
119. Li J, et al. Immune checkpoint inhibitors in advanced or metastatic mucosal melanoma: a systematic review. Ther Adv Med Oncol. 2020;12:1758835920922028.
120. Sassun R, et al. Neoadjuvant immunotherapy versus adjuvant chemotherapy in anorectal melanoma. Br J Surg. 2024;111(11):znae269.
121. Rawson RV, Wilmott JS, Scolyer RA. Mucosal melanoma: a review emphasizing the molecular landscape and implications for diagnosis and management. Surg Pathol Clin. 2021;14(2):293–307.
122. Jutten E, et al. Real-world evidence of the prevalence of driver mutations in anorectal melanoma. Mol Diagn Ther. 2025;29(2):229–38.
123. Hida T, et al. Genomic landscape of cutaneous, acral, mucosal, and uveal melanoma in Japan: analysis of clinical comprehensive genomic profiling data. Int J Clin Oncol. 2024;29(12):1984–98.
124. Wroblewska JP, et al. Prognostic roles of BRAF, KIT, NRAS, IGF2R and SF3B1 mutations in mucosal melanomas. Cells. 2021;10(9):2216.
125. Santi R, et al. KIT genetic alterations in anorectal melanomas. J Clin Pathol. 2015;68(2):130–4.
126. Vyas R, et al. Epidemiology of genitourinary melanoma in the United States: 1992 through 2012. J Am Acad Dermatol. 2016;75(1):144–50.
127. Huang J, Cai M, Zhu Z. Survival and prognostic factors in primary vaginal cancer: an analysis of 2004-2014 SEER data. Transl Cancer Res. 2020;9(11):7091–102.
128. Gershenwald JE, et al. Melanoma staging: evidence-based changes in the American Joint Committee on Cancer eighth edition cancer staging manual. CA Cancer J Clin. 2017;67(6):472–92.
129. Moxley KM, et al. Malignant melanoma of the vulva: an extension of cutaneous melanoma? Gynecol Oncol. 2011;122(3):612–7.
130. Sanchez A, et al. Primary genitourinary melanoma: epidemiology and disease-specific survival in a large population-based cohort. Urol Oncol. 2016;34(4):166 e7–14.
131. Wohlmuth C, et al. Malignant melanoma of the vulva and vagina: a US population-based study of 1863 patients. Am J Clin Dermatol. 2020;21(2):285–95.
132. Trimble EL, et al. Management of vulvar melanoma. Gynecol Oncol. 1992;45(3):254–8.
133. Ragnarsson-Olding BK, et al. Malignant melanoma of the vulva in a nationwide, 25-year study of 219 Swedish females: clinical observations and histopathologic features. Cancer. 1999;86(7):1273–84.
134. Verschraegen CF, et al. Vulvar melanoma at the M. D. Anderson Cancer Center: 25 years later. Int J Gynecol Cancer. 2001;11(5):359–64.
135. Schmidt M, et al. Primary vaginal melanoma: a case report and literature review. Eur J Gynaecol Oncol. 2008;29(3):285–8.
136. Piura B, Rabinovich A, Yanai-Inbar I. Primary malignant melanoma of the vagina: case report and review of literature. Eur J Gynaecol Oncol. 2002;23(3):195–8.
137. Nagarajan P, et al. Tumor thickness and mitotic rate robustly predict melanoma-specific survival in patients with primary Vulvar melanoma: a retrospective review of 100 cases. Clin Cancer Res. 2017;23(8):2093–104.

138. Scheistroen M, et al. Malignant melanoma of the vulva. Evaluation of prognostic factors with emphasis on DNA ploidy in 75 patients. Cancer. 1995;75(1):72–80.
139. Zhou H, et al. Construction and validation of a prognostic nomogram for primary vulvar melanoma: a SEER population-based study. Jpn J Clin Oncol. 2020;50(12):1386–94.
140. Alshwayyat S, et al. Web-based predictive tool for vaginal and vulvar melanomas: a machine learning study. Future Sci OA. 2025;11(1):2540747.
141. Kalampokas E, Kalampokas T, Damaskos C. Primary vaginal melanoma, a rare and aggressive entity. A case report and review of the literature. In Vivo. 2017;31(1):133–9.
142. Joste M, et al. Vulvar and vaginal melanomas: a retrospective study spanning 19 years from a tertiary center. J Gynecol Obstet Hum Reprod. 2021;50(5):102091.
143. Ogata D, et al. Clinicopathological demographics of malignant melanomas of the vulva and vagina in Japan. Melanoma Res. 2023;33(4):300–8.
144. Hacker NF, Eifel PJ, van der Velden J. Cancer of the vagina. Int J Gynaecol Obstet. 2012;119(Suppl 2):S97–9.
145. Lu C, et al. Advances in the diagnosis and treatment of primary malignant melanoma of the vagina- a case presentation and systematic review. BMC Womens Health. 2025;25(1):444.
146. Raber G, et al. Malignant melanoma of the vulva. Report of 89 patients. Cancer. 1996;78(11):2353–8.
147. Wong SL, et al. Sentinel lymph node biopsy and Management of Regional Lymph Nodes in melanoma: American Society of Clinical Oncology and Society of Surgical Oncology clinical practice guideline update. J Clin Oncol. 2018;36(4):399–413.
148. Mitra D, et al. Gynecologic tract melanoma in the contemporary therapeutic era: high rates of local and distant disease progression. Gynecol Oncol. 2022;167(3):483–9.
149. Cai YJ, et al. Recurrent KRAS, KIT and SF3B1 mutations in melanoma of the female genital tract. BMC Cancer. 2021;21(1):677.
150. Quek C, et al. Recurrent hotspot SF3B1 mutations at codon 625 in vulvovaginal mucosal melanoma identified in a study of 27 Australian mucosal melanomas. Oncotarget. 2019;10(9):930–41.
151. Rouzbahman M, et al. Malignant melanoma of vulva and vagina: a histomorphological review and mutation analysis – a single-center study. J Low Genit Tract Dis. 2015;19(4):350–3.
152. van Engen-van Grunsven AC, et al. NRAS mutations are more prevalent than KIT mutations in melanoma of the female urogenital tract--a study of 24 cases from the Netherlands. Gynecol Oncol. 2014;134(1):10–4.
153. Dias-Santagata D, et al. KIT mutations and CD117 overexpression are markers of better progression-free survival in vulvar melanomas. Br J Dermatol. 2017;177(5):1376–84.
154. Omholt K, et al. KIT pathway alterations in mucosal melanomas of the vulva and other sites. Clin Cancer Res. 2011;17(12):3933–42.

Chapter 7
Desmoplastic Melanoma

Shira Ronen

Introduction

Desmoplastic melanoma is a rare subtype of melanoma, accounting for approximately 1%–4% of all melanoma cases. This melanoma variant may be difficult to recognize both clinically and pathologically, and it behaves differently compared to non-desmoplastic melanoma. Desmoplastic melanoma was first described by Conley et al. in 1971 as a rare morphological variant of melanoma composed of variably pleomorphic spindle melanocytes with abundant associated collagen [1]. Subsequently, in 2005, its histological definition was further expanded into two subtypes: "pure" desmoplastic melanoma, characterized by uniform desmoplasia throughout the entire tumor, and "mixed" desmoplastic melanoma, which combines desmoplasia with at least 10% of compact aggregates or nodules of melanoma cells without intervening fibrosis [2]. These subtypes are crucial in defining the behavior of desmoplastic melanoma [3].

Desmoplastic melanoma typically arises in chronically sun-exposed skin and is characterized by a very high mutation burden, with a prominent ultraviolet (UV) radiation signature. Inactivating mutations are the most common driver mutations in desmoplastic melanoma, although activating mutations in the MAPK pathway are also observed. Desmoplastic melanoma can arise de novo or within a lentigo maligna. Understanding its clinical, histological, and molecular characteristics is vital due to its rarity and the challenges associated with diagnosis and management.

S. Ronen (✉)
Pathology & Laboratory Medicine Institute, Cleveland Clinic Lerner College of Medicine of Case Western Reserve University School of Medicine, Cleveland, OH, USA
e-mail: RONENS@ccf.org

V. G. Prieto, C. A. Torres-Cabala (eds.), *Precision Molecular Pathology of Melanocytic Lesions*, Molecular Pathology Library,
https://doi.org/10.1007/978-3-032-18222-7_7

Clinical Features

Desmoplastic melanoma accounts for approximately 1%–4% of all melanomas and predominantly affects individuals with pale skin who have chronically sun-exposed skin [4]. According to previously reported statistics based on Surveillance, Epidemiology, and End Results studies in the United States, the incidence rate of desmoplastic melanoma was approximately 2.0 per million individuals, which steadily increased between 1992 and 2013 [3]. Desmoplastic melanoma has an annual increase estimated at 4.6% [5]. As the population in the United States continues to age, it is anticipated that desmoplastic melanoma will become increasingly more prevalent. The head and neck region is the most common site of involvement (51%), with the ears and bald scalp being particularly vulnerable [5]. Desmoplastic melanoma accounted for 29% of scalp melanomas in a large study. Other commonly affected sites include the extremities (30%), with the upper limbs being more frequently impacted than the lower limbs, as well as the trunk (17%) [5]. This subtype is more prevalent in males, with a male-to-female ratio of approximately 2:1 [3, 6–8]. Notably, a pooled analysis of published studies confirms that patients with desmoplastic melanoma tend to be older than those with other melanoma subtypes. The mean age for desmoplastic melanoma is approximately 63 years, with a median age ranging from 60 to 70 years, whereas the median age for non-desmoplastic melanoma is around 50 years [6–8].

Although desmoplastic melanoma typically arises in areas of chronic ultraviolet (UV) damage, it can rarely occur in sites with minimal or no evidence of sun exposure, such as acral skin, subungual locations, oral mucosa, nasal mucosa, and genital mucosa [9, 10].

Clinically, desmoplastic melanoma is often challenging to detect due to its subtle presentation. Lesions frequently appear as painless, indurated plaques or poorly demarcated areas of scar-like skin thickening. Occasionally, they may begin as a small papule or nodule [6, 7]. Due to the resemblance to scars, dermatofibromas, or nonmelanoma skin cancer, the diagnosis is often delayed, particularly as nearly half of these tumors lack pigmentation [8]. The absence of pigmentation is a major cause of clinical and histological misdiagnosis. When pigmentation is present, it is typically due to an overlying lentigo maligna. Rarely, desmoplastic melanoma can manifest in younger patients as an erythematous nodule or even as alopecia. Recurrence at the site of a prior biopsy, initially diagnosed as benign on histopathology (e.g., dermatofibroma, neurofibroma, or scar), is a relatively common presentation of desmoplastic melanoma. This can occur because the histopathological diagnosis may be challenging, especially in cases involving partial biopsies. When clinical suspicion arises, revisiting the original pathology can provide valuable insights. In rare instances, desmoplastic melanoma may also present as a metastasis from another melanoma subtype [11, 12].

Dermoscopy tends to be less effective in identifying desmoplastic melanoma unless features of an associated radial growth phase melanoma are present [13]. Features characteristic of melanocytic lesions, such as globules or a pigment network, are observed in 43%–60% of desmoplastic melanomas. However, recent studies demonstrated that at least one melanoma-specific dermoscopic feature was present in 100% of desmoplastic melanomas analyzed. These features included atypical vascular structures (observed in 81%–87% of cases), crystalline structures (shiny white lines, seen in 80%), an annular-granular pattern (present in 24%–40%), and scar-like areas (reported in 8%–67%) [7, 8, 14]. Additionally, evidence of regression, such as gray granular dots, is frequently observed in desmoplastic melanomas.

Prognosis

Because of diagnostic delays, desmoplastic melanoma is often identified at a more advanced local stage compared to other melanoma subtypes, with a mean and median Breslow thickness close to 4.0 mm in most series [5, 6]. Most desmoplastic melanomas involve at least the reticular dermis (Clark level IV), with many extending into the subcutis or deeper (Clark level V) [5]. Ulceration is observed in approximately 20% of cases, with a slightly higher incidence in "mixed" desmoplastic melanoma (24%) compared to "pure" desmoplastic melanoma (16%) [2].

The incidence of local recurrence is very high, particularly in cases with Breslow thickness >4.0 mm, where recurrence rates approach 40%, compared to 19.5% for lesions with Breslow thickness <4.0 mm [6]. Early reports indicated a local recurrence rate of 25%–60% [15–17]. More recent studies, however, have not confirmed such a concerning rate. Nonetheless, the local recurrence rate for desmoplastic melanoma in these studies remains notably higher (6–15%) compared to non-desmoplastic melanoma cases, which have a recurrence rate of less than 5% [18–21]. Neurotropism and incomplete or marginal excision (with margins <10 mm) are also associated with an increased risk of local recurrence [18–20, 22]. However, neurotropism has not been consistently identified as an independent and significant risk factor for local recurrence in the majority of studies [19, 22–25]. Prognosis is influenced by factors such as increased tumor thickness, higher mitotic rate, male sex, and older age [24].

Paradoxically, despite thick Breslow measurements, desmoplastic melanoma tends to have a better prognosis than other melanoma subtypes of similar thickness [4, 17]. Regional nodal metastasis is less frequent in desmoplastic melanoma, especially in the "pure" desmoplastic subtype, compared to other melanoma subtypes [2, 26–28]. In 2013, Hen et al. showed that sentinel lymph node positivity was observed in 13.7% of patients with desmoplastic melanoma and is significantly higher for "mixed" (24.6%) compared with "pure" (9.0%) desmoplastic melanoma [29]. The authors believe that these positive lymph node rates are sufficient to justify considering sentinel lymph node biopsy for both histologic variants, especially since the detection of sentinel lymph node disease appears to predict a higher risk of melanoma-related death. On the other hand, in 2016, Dunne et al. conducted a systematic review of 16 case series analyzing sentinel node status in 1519 patients with desmoplastic melanoma [4]. The study reported a positive sentinel node rate of 6.5% for all the patients with desmoplastic melanoma, significantly lower than the expected rate of 15–20% for non-desmoplastic melanoma. Furthermore, the rate was notably lower for "pure" desmoplastic melanoma (5.4%) compared to "mixed" desmoplastic melanoma (13.8%). Based on these findings, the authors concluded that sentinel lymph node biopsy should be considered for patients with mixed desmoplastic melanoma, similar to non-desmoplastic melanoma, but may not be necessary for "pure" desmoplastic melanoma.

When metastasis does occur, the lungs are more commonly the initial site of distant spread, followed by bone and brain [11, 17]. Given the high incidence of local recurrence with surgery alone, rare regional lymphatic involvement, and propensity for pulmonary metastases, the clinical behavior of desmoplastic melanoma appears to be similar to soft tissue sarcomas rather than other cutaneous melanomas [15].

Treatment

Desmoplastic melanoma poses challenges in recognition, both clinically and histopathologically, and exhibits distinct behavior compared to non-desmoplastic melanoma. Consequently, the standard management guidelines for non-desmoplastic melanoma may not be entirely applicable to desmoplastic melanoma, necessitating tailored approaches and specific consideration for this unique subtype. Given the very high risk of local recurrence, a wide local excision remains the cornerstone of treatment, with radiation therapy playing a role in achieving local control, particularly in cases with neurotropism [19, 22]. Although narrower excision margins are increasingly adopted for cutaneous melanoma, the optimal margins for desmoplastic melanoma remain poorly established. No clinical trials have been conducted to determine the optimal clinical or histological margin required to reduce the risk of local recurrence. Many surgeons recommend a minimum clearance margin of at least 1 cm, given the high risk of recurrence and the invasive nature of the tumor [3, 6]. Maurichi et al. reported a higher rate of local recurrence in patients with "pure" desmoplastic melanoma ≤2 mm who underwent resection with a 1 cm margin compared to those with a 2 cm margin (40% vs. 18.5%) [30]. Although it is well-established that local recurrence is closely associated with positive resection margins, current evidence does not support the need for excision margins for desmoplastic melanoma to differ from the standard recommendations for other types of cutaneous melanoma.

Several retrospective studies suggest that adjuvant radiotherapy may reduce local recurrence in specific scenarios; Guadagnolo et al. demonstrated that adjuvant radiotherapy reduced local recurrence rates in patients with desmoplastic melanoma overall but showed no benefit for those without neurotropism or with "mixed" desmoplastic melanoma [19]. Oliver et al.'s study reported 0% local recurrence in 10 patients treated with both surgery and radiotherapy compared to 12% in 78 patients treated with surgery alone [31]. Strom et al. found a significant benefit of radiotherapy for cases with involved resection margins and improved local recurrence rates for head and neck primaries with negative margins. They concluded that adjuvant radiotherapy could be safely omitted in patients with desmoplastic melanoma and clear margins who met specific criteria: non-head/neck site and ≤4 mm thickness, or no neurotropism and ≤4 mm thickness [20]. Chen et al. concluded that adjuvant radiotherapy achieves local control rates similar to those produced by adequate surgical excision in cases where sufficient margins cannot be achieved [18]. Rule et al. conducted a prospective study demonstrating that adjuvant radiotherapy following wide local excision is both efficacious and well-tolerated. Their findings suggest that adjuvant radiotherapy should be strongly considered for patients with desmoplastic melanoma who have undergone a negative wide local excision [15]. These findings highlight the potential role of radiotherapy in improving local recurrence rates for select high-risk patients, though its benefit varies depending on tumor characteristics and margin status. While no randomized controlled trials have evaluated the efficacy of adjuvant radiotherapy for desmoplastic melanoma, current recommendations suggest considering radiotherapy for patients with desmoplastic or neurotropic melanoma when adequate pathological resection margins (≥8 mm) cannot be achieved.

Since desmoplastic melanoma has a low rate of nodal metastasis, investigators have suggested that routine sentinel node biopsy may not be necessary, especially for "pure" desmoplastic melanoma [3, 24, 32, 33]. However, current recommendations still suggest considering sentinel lymph node biopsy for patients with desmoplastic melanoma, as it would be for non-desmoplastic melanoma.

The high mutation burden observed in desmoplastic melanoma correlates with favorable responses to immune checkpoint inhibitor therapy, offering promising treatment options for advanced disease [34]. Additionally, specific genetic alterations seen in desmoplastic melanoma may represent therapeutic targets, suggesting a role for therapies such as those with inhibitors of EGFR, MET, and CDK4 [35].

Histopathological Features

Desmoplastic melanoma is a dermal-based, poorly circumscribed spindle cell tumor embedded within and between fine sclerotic or mature collagen bundles, frequently exhibiting a fibromyxoid appearance (Figs. 7.1, 7.2, 7.3, 7.4 and 7.5). The cells are typically disorganized, although occasional parallel arrangements or storiform patterns may be observed (Fig. 7.3). Tumor cells often infiltrate deeply into the subcutis, extending diffusely or along fibrous septa, and may even involve the fascia [6].

Desmoplastic melanoma demonstrates significant heterogeneity in its histologic appearance, ranging from tumors with prominent stromal fibrosis throughout the lesion to melanomas in which desmoplasia is only a partial or minor component (Fig. 7.4). This heterogeneity has led to challenges in the diagnostic classification of desmoplastic melanoma. Some pathologists use the term "desmoplastic melanoma" liberally for any spindle cell melanoma with or without neurotropism, even if

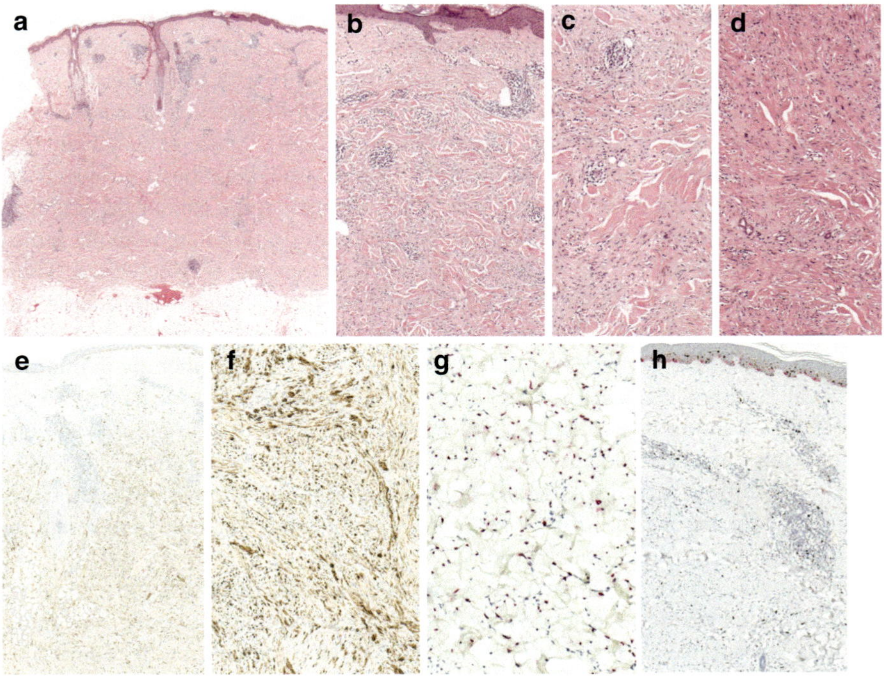

Fig. 7.1 Pure desmoplastic melanoma. (Courtesy of Dr. Phyu Aung from MD Anderson Cancer Center). Histologic features demonstrated a dermal-based, poorly circumscribed, sparse spindled cell tumor with overlying thin and atrophic epidermis (**a**). There was no evidence of in situ component (**b**). The presence of lymphoid aggregates served as a diagnostic clue in these sparsely cellular lesions. The lesional cells were embedded within and between fine sclerotic and mature collagen bundles (**c**). The spindle cells exhibited poorly defined cytoplasm and mild to moderate nuclear atypia, characterized by hyperchromatic enlarged nuclei (**d**). The lesional cells were positive for S100 (**e**, **f**) and SOX10 (**g**). Melan A/Ki67 multiple stain—Melan A was negative in desmoplastic melanoma, and the Ki-67 showed an increased proliferation index (**h**)

desmoplasia is only a focal feature. Others reserve the term for melanomas with prominent fibrosis throughout the invasive tumor component. In 2004, Busam and colleagues classified desmoplastic melanoma as either "pure" desmoplastic melanoma or "mixed" desmoplastic melanoma [2]. "Pure" desmoplastic melanoma is defined as tumors where >90% of the tumor consists of a diffuse low-density proliferation of spindle cells in a desmoplastic stroma (Figs. 7.1, 7.2, 7.3 and 7.4). In contrast, "mixed" desmoplastic melanoma is defined as tumors where <90% of the tumor is composed of a diffuse low-density spindle cell component and at least 10% of compact aggregates or nodules of melanoma cells without intervening fibrosis (Fig. 7.5). "Pure" desmoplastic melanoma accounts for close to 50% of all desmoplastic melanoma. Subclassification into "pure" and "mixed" desmoplastic melanoma is essential, as it has prognostic significance. In an analysis of 252 cases of desmoplastic melanoma, Murali et al. demonstrated that "pure" desmoplastic melanoma significantly differs from "mixed" desmoplastic melanoma in terms of

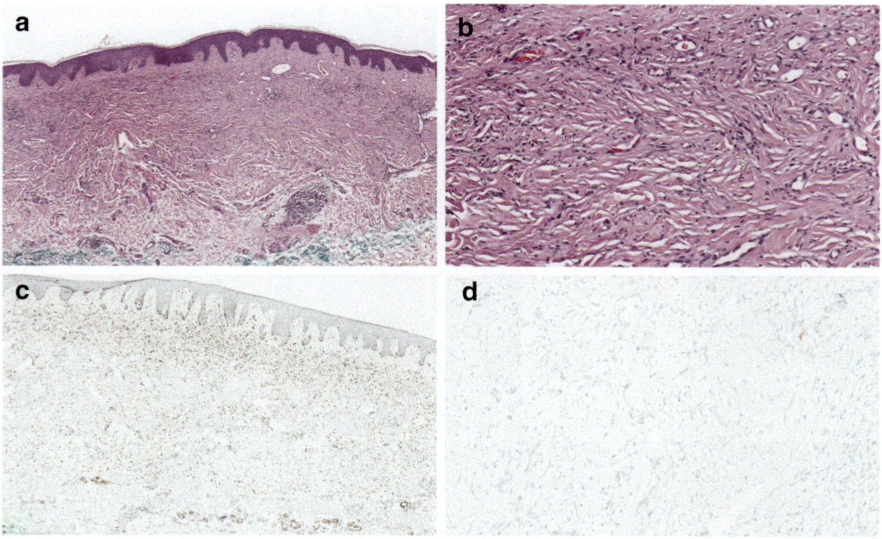

Fig. 7.2 Desmoplastic melanoma. Microscopic examination revealed a poorly defined dermal-based neoplasm with aggregates of lymphocytes at the periphery of the lesion (**a** ×100). A higher magnification showed a proliferation of spindle cells with minimal atypia and fibroblast-like appearance (**b** ×400). The presence of lymphoid aggregates prompted us to perform immunohistochemical studies and guide us to the diagnosis of desmoplastic melanoma. An immunohistochemical study for SOX10 diffusely highlights the neoplastic cells (**c** ×100), while Melan A is negative (**d** ×400)

anatomical location, Clark level, Breslow thickness, mitotic rate, perineural invasion, and locoregional recurrence rates (4% vs. 12%) [24]. Some studies have reported a lower incidence of distant metastasis and improved survival outcomes for "pure" desmoplastic melanoma compared to "mixed" desmoplastic melanoma, while others have not observed such differences [35].

The overlying epidermis is usually thin and atrophic, while the adjacent dermis demonstrates marked solar elastosis, reflecting chronic sun damage (Figs. 7.1 and 7.5). Lentigo maligna or atypical melanocytic proliferation in the epidermis may be associated with desmoplastic melanoma, but approximately half of the cases show minimal or absent junctional component (Figs. 7.4 and 7.5). In many cases, aggregates of lymphocytes and occasional plasma cells are present within or at the periphery of the tumor, serving as a diagnostic clue in sparsely cellular lesions (Figs. 7.1 and 7.3). Cytological atypia of the spindle cells can vary widely, ranging from mild to moderate and occasionally severe. Even in cases with minimal atypia, scattered hyperchromatic nuclei or elongated atypical cells are typically identifiable [8]. These cells can serve as important clues to the possible diagnosis of desmoplastic melanoma and should prompt the use of immunohistochemical stains for confirmation. The cytoplasm of the tumor cells is often poorly defined and non-pigmented, contributing to their fibroblast-like appearance, which makes the diagnosis further

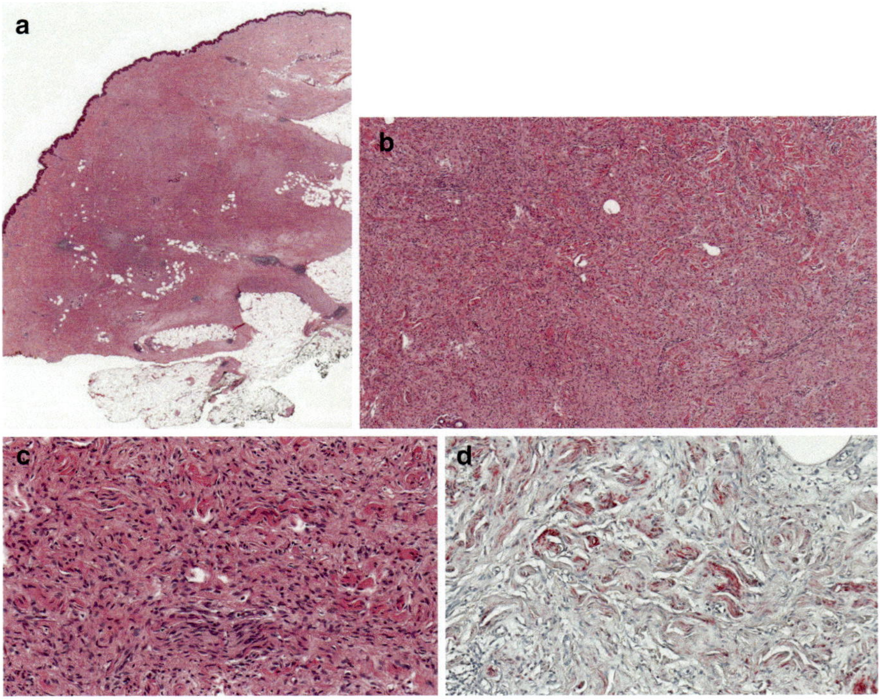

Fig. 7.3 Desmoplastic melanoma. This is another example of desmoplastic melanoma. The lesional cells infiltrated into the subcutaneous tissue, extending diffusely and along the fibrous septa (**a** ×13). The cells were mostly disorganized with occasional parallel arrangements and storiform patterns. They were embedded within sclerotic stroma with a focal fibromyxoid appearance (**b** ×100). The cells displayed mild to focal atypia with hyperchromatic nuclei (**c** ×400). The cells were diffusely positive for S100 study, further confirming the diagnosis of desmoplastic melanoma (**d** ×400)

challenging. In cases where spindle cells are sparse and widely dispersed, the presence of lymphoid aggregates may be the most striking diagnostic feature. As mentioned above, these aggregates can serve as key histological clues, guiding the pathologist toward the diagnosis of desmoplastic melanoma.

Desmoplastic melanoma rarely has an associated common acquired nevus. Lymphovascular invasion is rare. On the other hand, neurotropism, observed in about 30% of cases, is more commonly associated with the "pure" desmoplastic melanoma and is considered a hallmark feature. Neurotropism was first described by Reed and Leonard in 1979 and later expanded upon by Chen et al. and Varey et al. [18, 22, 36]. This subtype is known as desmoplastic neurotropic melanoma. It is characterized by tumor cells encircling nerves (perineural invasion) or, less commonly, invading the endoneurium (intraneural invasion). In rare instances, desmoplastic melanoma may exhibit neural transformation, where tumor cells assume nerve-like structures (variant of neurotropism). In some cases, specific named, large nerves may be affected, posing significant challenges, particularly when cranial

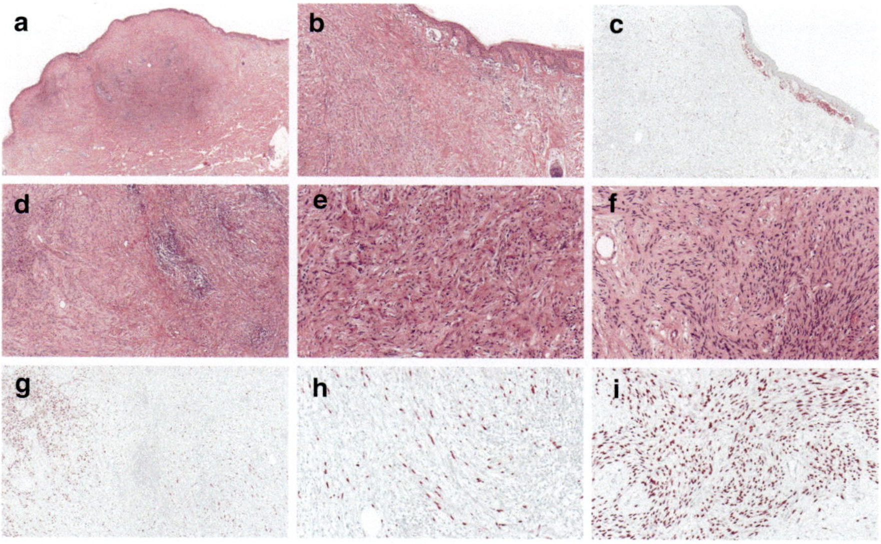

Fig. 7.4 Desmoplastic melanoma. Sections displayed spindle cells neoplasms with lymphoid aggregates within the lesion (**a** ×35). Overlying the lesion is an in-situ component, which can be observed in approximately 50% of desmoplastic melanomas (**b** ×110). An immunohistochemical study confirmed the presence of melanoma in situ (**c** ×110). This example also showed a focal area of compact aggregates of melanoma cells with minimal intervening fibrosis (**d–f**, **d** ×130, **e**, **f** ×400). This lesion was still classified as pure desmoplastic melanoma as >90% of the tumor consisted of a diffuse low-density proliferation of spindle cells, and the compact aggregates of melanoma cells consisted only of <10%. An immunohistochemical study for SOX10 highlighted both components, hypocellular (**g**) and hypercellular (**h**), within the tumor (**g** ×130, **h**, **i** ×400)

nerves and their branches are involved. This can result in tumor extension toward the skull base, complicating management and treatment strategies [19].

Metastases originating from primary cutaneous desmoplastic melanoma may consist of varying proportions of spindle and epithelioid cells, reflecting the cellular composition of the corresponding primary tumors [12].

Immunohistochemical analysis is frequently essential for confirming the diagnosis of desmoplastic melanoma, accurately assessing tumor thickness, and differentiating it from non-melanocytic mimics. The neoplastic cells in desmoplastic melanoma are positive for S100 protein and SOX10, making these markers highly sensitive for diagnosis (Figs. 7.1, 7.2, 7.3, 7.4 and 7.5) [8, 37]. In contrast, melanocytic markers such as Melan-A (Mart-1) and HMB45 antigen are typically negative, except in the non-desmoplastic areas of "mixed" desmoplastic melanomas (Figs. 7.1, 7.2 and 7.5). PRAME has been reported to be positive in approximately 35% of desmoplastic melanomas in one study, although its diagnostic utility remains under investigation [38]. Additional markers such as smooth muscle actin and CD10 may also be positive.

Diagnosis of desmoplastic melanoma can be challenging, particularly in small or superficial shave or punch biopsies, where hallmark features may be absent. The

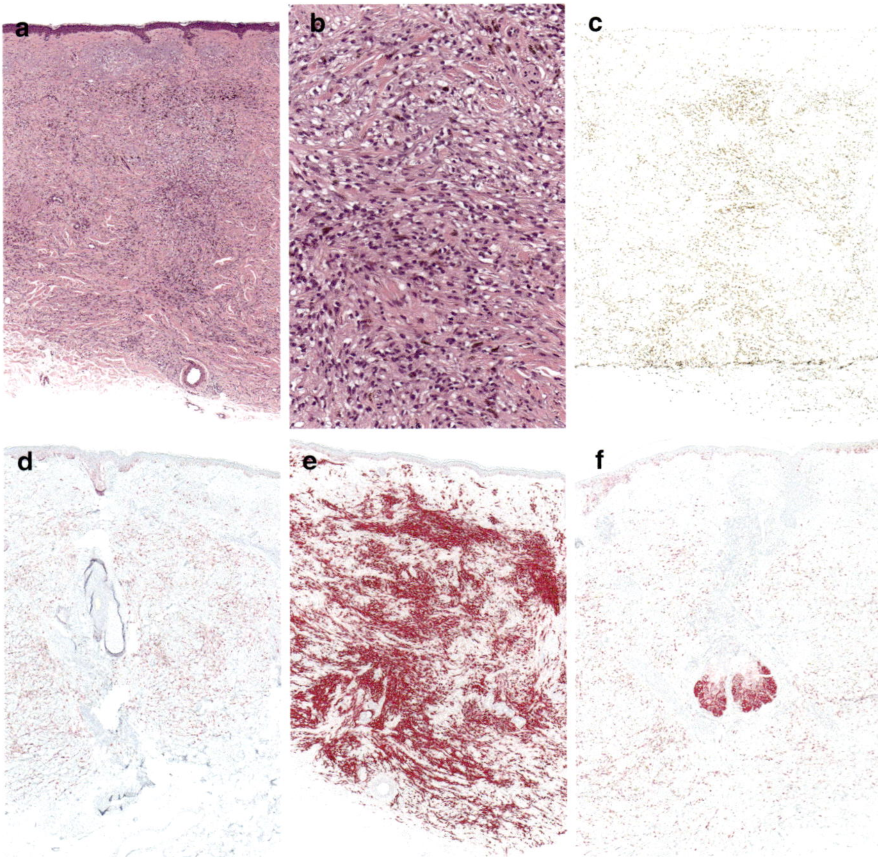

Fig. 7.5 Mixed desmoplastic melanoma. Histologic sections demonstrated a dermal-based hypercellular neoplasm on markedly sun-damaged skin (**a** ×100). The neoplastic cells were spindled with elongated to oval nuclei, prominent nucleoli, and pale eosinophilic cytoplasm. They were embedded within sclerotic stroma (**b** ×400). This is an example of a mixed desmoplastic melanoma, as >10% of the tumor was composed of compact aggregates or nodules of melanoma cells without intervening fibrosis. Immunohistochemical studies for SOX10 (**c** ×100), Melan A (**d** ×100), and HMB45 (**e** ×100) were diffusely positive within the neoplasm. Those stains also highlight an in-situ component overlying the tumor. An immunohistochemical study for PRAME was positive in more than 75% of the tumor cells, further supporting the diagnosis (**f** ×100). Melan A, HMB45, and PRAME stains can be positive in mixed desmoplastic melanomas and are typically negative in pure desmoplastic melanomas

paucicellular nature of desmoplastic melanoma may lead to misidentification as scars or benign neural lesions, whereas more cellular variants may overlap with other melanocytic or spindle cell proliferations.

Among the differential diagnoses, desmoplastic/sclerosing nevus can occasionally demonstrate perineural extension and share overlapping clinical characteristics with desmoplastic melanoma. However, it typically lacks an asymmetric infiltrative silhouette, mitotic activity, pronounced and expansive nuclear atypia, junctional component, and lymphoid infiltrates [39]. Ancillary studies, including immunohistochemistry, are recommended in diagnostically problematic cases. Desmoplastic/sclerosing nevi are consistently diffusely positive for Melan-A/MART1, a feature generally absent in desmoplastic melanoma [40]. They also typically lack significant Ki-67 expression, whereas desmoplastic melanoma often demonstrates a higher Ki-67 proliferation index [39]. Additionally, most desmoplastic melanomas show loss of p16 expression, which is retained in desmoplastic/sclerosing nevi. Exceptions do exist, as certain desmoplastic melanomas may have a very low Ki-67 proliferation index, retain p16 expression, or show Mart-1 expression. Another differential diagnosis is desmoplastic Spitz nevus, which may contain numerous spindle cells that are HMB45-negative and share age range and site distribution overlapping with desmoplastic melanoma. However, desmoplastic Spitz nevi are characteristically symmetrical; show a V-shaped silhouette, uniform cellularity and pigmentation; lack solar damage; and are often accompanied by epidermal thickening [41]. They also retain p16 expression and are usually positive for Melan A/Mart-1 [41]. Another differential consideration is sclerosing cellular blue nevi, which are also most commonly seen on the scalp. Unlike desmoplastic melanoma, these lesions lack mitotic activity and are diffusely positive for HMB45.

In cases where immunohistochemical findings are inconclusive, molecular testing can be a valuable tool and further provide definitive diagnostic support. A positive fluorescence in situ hybridization (FISH) with standard probes strongly favors melanoma, providing critical diagnostic confirmation in challenging cases [42].

Immature scars, especially in re-excision specimens, may mimic desmoplastic melanoma due to the presence of scattered spindle cells that express S100 protein and SOX10 (likely Schwann cells), along with focal lymphocytic infiltrates and occasional mitoses [8, 43]. However, their overall architecture and clinical context help differentiate them.

Desmoplastic changes can also occur in other melanoma subtypes, but these typically retain expression of melanocytic markers such as HMB45 antigen and Melan-A, at least focally. Additional differential diagnoses include dermatofibroma, atypical fibroxanthoma/pleomorphic dermal sarcoma, sarcomatoid carcinoma, and leiomyosarcoma. These entities can generally be distinguished based on their morphology and immunohistochemical profiles, using markers such as cytokeratin and smooth muscle actin to aid in diagnosis.

The fifth edition of the World Health Organization (WHO) Classification of Skin Tumors outlines essential and desirable diagnostic criteria for desmoplastic melanoma [11]. These criteria are categorized into essential features, which are critical for diagnosis, and desirable features, which support the diagnosis but are not mandatory.

Essential Diagnostic Criteria

- Malignant neoplasm in which spindled melanocytes are encased in dense collagenous stroma.
- Confirmation of melanocytic lineage by immunohistochemistry with S100 protein and SOX10 (or molecular genetic analysis in case of absence of expression of all usual melanocytic markers).
- No expression of Melan-A/Mart-1, HMB45 antigen, and tyrosinase except in non-desmoplastic areas in combined desmoplastic melanoma.
- "Pure" desmoplastic melanoma: >90% of tumor consists of a diffuse low-density proliferation of spindle cells in a desmoplastic stroma.
- "Mixed" desmoplastic melanoma: <90% of tumor is composed of a diffuse low-density spindle cell component and at least 10% of compact aggregates or nodules of melanoma cells without intervening fibrosis.

Desirable Diagnostic Criteria

- Presence of prominent solar elastosis in dermis.
- Presence of an associated atypical intraepidermal melanocytic proliferation or melanoma in situ, often of the lentigo maligna type.
- Presence of some melanin pigment in a few tumor cells.
- Cytological atypia of melanocytes.
- Evidence of mitotic activity.
- Accompanying aggregates of lymphocytes within and/or at the edge of the tumor.
- Neurotropism commonly present.
- Exclusion of other desmoplastic spindle cell neoplasms, such as desmoplastic spindle cell squamous cell carcinoma, atypical fibroxanthoma, and peripheral nerve sheath tumors (not always possible).

Molecular Findings

Since the introduction of the divergent pathways model in 2003, genomic research has consistently supported the hypothesis that melanomas associated with chronic sun damage exhibit distinct genetic characteristics compared to those originating from intermittently sun-exposed areas of the body [44, 45]. Similar to other melanomas associated with marked solar elastosis, desmoplastic melanoma carries the highest number of mutations among all cancers and has the highest mutation burden of any melanoma, with a median of 62 mutations per megabase [35, 46]. Ultraviolet radiation stimulates melanin synthesis, prompts melanocytes to enter the cell cycle, and causes oxidative stress, which leads to the formation of characteristic C > T and

CC > TT photoproducts [13]. The cellular alterations caused by ultraviolet are further amplified by its immunosuppressive effects, which weaken immune surveillance.

Although desmoplastic melanoma typically arises in sun-damaged skin with prominent solar elastosis, rare cases have been reported in acral, mucosal, and other sites without evidence of significant ultraviolet radiation damage [9, 47]. These uncommon presentations are expected to share molecular features with melanomas arising in their respective anatomic pathways.

Gene expression profiling has provided valuable insights into the molecular distinctions between desmoplastic melanoma and non-desmoplastic melanoma. Busam et al. identified decreased expression of genes involved in melanin synthesis in desmoplastic melanoma, which likely explains the amelanotic nature of many of these lesions [48]. Other genes related to neurotrophic factors and extracellular matrix production were upregulated in desmoplastic melanoma. Notably, clusterin, a glycoprotein implicated in tissue remodeling and fibrogenic processes, demonstrated high expression in desmoplastic melanoma, suggesting its role in the formation of the fibrous stroma characteristic of this melanoma subtype.

The driver mutations or the prevalence of certain genetic mutations associated with desmoplastic melanoma differ from those more commonly seen in other types of cutaneous melanoma. They lack common mutations in *BRAF V600E* and *NRAS Q61K/R*, but frequently harbor mutations that activate the MAPK and PI3K pathways [35]. Common mutations in desmoplastic melanoma include: loss-of-function mutation of *NF1*, gain-of-function mutation in *NRAS*, *PIK3CA*, *PTPN11*, and amplification in *ERBB2*, *MAP2K1*, *MAP3K1*, *BRAF*, *EGFR*, *MET*, *TERT*. For instance, *BRAF* is a serine/threonine protein kinase activated by the Ras-GTP protein, and its mutations are found in 41%–81% of primary cutaneous melanoma, but are significantly less frequent in melanomas on sun-damaged skin, where they occur in only 11%–30% of cases [13, 49–51]. Similarly, *NF1* mutations are found in 14% of all melanomas; however, a 2015 study revealed that 93% of desmoplastic melanomas analyzed carried *NF1* mutations [52].

Addo et al. were the first to describe the morphologic and genomic features of *NF1* mutant desmoplastic melanomas [53]. *NF1*-mutated desmoplastic melanomas, when compared to non-*NF*-mutated desmoplastic melanomas, exhibit distinct clinical and histologic features. They are less likely to have an associated melanoma in situ (35% vs. 47%), less likely to display an epithelioid component (35% vs. 59%), and more likely to show prominent pigmentation (35% vs. 12%). Two unique morphologic patterns, blue nevus-like pigmented desmoplastic melanomas and neurofibroma-like desmoplastic melanomas, are exclusive to the *NF*-mutated subgroup. These patterns are diagnostically significant and highlight the phenotypic diversity within *NF*-mutated melanomas.

Pigmented desmoplastic melanomas can mimic blue nevi but are distinguished by features such as nuclear atypia, mitotic activity, and asymmetry [53]. These tumors frequently harbor truncating *NF1* mutations and show a higher tumor mutation burden compared to non-*NF*-mutated desmoplastic melanomas. Neurofibroma-like desmoplastic melanomas, on the other hand, resemble benign neurofibromas but demonstrate features such as poor circumscription, nuclear atypia, and mitotic activity. These tumors also exhibit *NF1* mutations but have a lower tumor mutation burden and fewer pathogenic variants compared to other *NF*-mutated desmoplastic melanomas.

Genomic analysis reveals that *NF1* truncating mutations, *NF1* splice site variants, and *NF1* frameshift variants are exclusive to *NF*-mutated desmoplastic melanomas when compared with benign nevi [46, 53]. In contrast, missense mutations in NF1 were nonspecific and seen both in benign and malignant lesions, underscoring the importance of distinguishing between truncating and non-truncating variants. *NF2* variants were significantly more likely to be observed in benign *NF*-mutated nevi compared to *NF*-mutated melanomas [53]. *NF*-mutated desmoplastic melanomas demonstrate a higher tumor mutation burden (average 57.3 mutations per megabase) and a greater number of pathogenic variants (average 19 per case) compared to non-*NF*-mutated desmoplastic melanomas and *NF*-mutated benign nevi. Additional mutations in genes such as *p-TERT*, *TP53*, genes from the SWI/SNF, and *CDKN2A* were exclusively seen in melanomas and not in any of the benign nevi [46, 53]. CDKN2A variants were exclusively seen in the *NF*-mutated melanomas. The presence of activating mutations in BRAF or NRAS, in combination with TERT promoter hotspot mutations, strongly favored a diagnosis of desmoplastic melanoma [46]. These findings emphasize the importance of integrating genomic data with morphologic assessment to improve diagnostic accuracy.

In a study of 43 desmoplastic melanocytic neoplasms, expert pathologists evaluated H&E slides alone and then re-evaluated them with the addition of comprehensive genomic data [54]. The integration of genomic findings led to a 7% improvement in recognizing desmoplastic melanoma, with diagnostic accuracy increasing from 75% to 82%. Notably, genomic data helped identify malignant cases that were initially misclassified, including some that later resulted in metastatic disease. Key genomic alterations favoring a desmoplastic melanoma diagnosis included truncating mutations in *NF1*, *TP53*, *ARID2*, and *CDKN2A*, as well as the presence of a *BRAF* or *NRAS* mutation combined with a *TERT* promoter mutation. Truncating or frameshift mutations in *NF1* and *TP53* were strongly associated with melanoma, while missense mutations in these genes were less specific. Similarly, the raw number of pathogenic variants should not alone dictate diagnostic decisions; instead, specific combinations of mutations known to drive melanoma progression should guide interpretation.

Next-generation sequencing is a valuable tool for improving the diagnostic accuracy of desmoplastic melanomas, particularly in challenging cases. However, its utility is maximized when integrated with morphologic assessment and interpreted by pathologists with an understanding of bioinformatics and melanoma genetics.

Conclusion

Desmoplastic melanoma remains a rare and challenging subtype of melanoma, both diagnostically and therapeutically. Its histologic heterogeneity, ranging from pure desmoplasia to mixed, underscores the importance of subclassification for prognostic and therapeutic purposes. Patients with pure desmoplastic melanoma tend to have better outcomes, particularly in cases of thick, deeply infiltrating melanomas. Desmoplastic melanoma is characterized by distinct molecular features, including a high tumor mutation burden and frequent truncating mutations in tumor suppressor genes such as *NF1*, *TP53*, *CDKN2A*, and *ARID2*, which are absent in benign desmoplastic nevi. While missense mutations in *NF1* are nonspecific, truncating *NF1* mutations are strongly associated with desmoplastic melanoma, often accompanied by secondary mutations, such as TERT promoter mutations. These molecular alterations, along with genomic data, can significantly enhance diagnostic accuracy, particularly in distinguishing desmoplastic melanoma from benign or intermediate-grade desmoplastic melanocytic neoplasms, emphasizing the integration of genomic and morphologic assessment in challenging cases. Furthermore, the observed presence of a very high TMB may explain the high-response rate to neoadjuvant immunotherapy. Continued research into the molecular features and clinical behavior of desmoplastic melanoma will further refine its classification and improve patient management.

References

1. Conley J, Lattes R, Orr W. Desmoplastic malignant melanoma (a rare variant of spindle cell melanoma). Cancer. 1971;28(4):914–36.
2. Busam KJ, et al. Cutaneous desmoplastic melanoma: reappraisal of morphologic heterogeneity and prognostic factors. Am J Surg Pathol. 2004;28(11):1518–25.
3. Shi P, et al. Desmoplastic melanoma: demographic and clinicopathological features and disease-specific prognostic factors. Oncol Lett. 2019;17(6):5619–27.
4. Dunne JA, et al. Is sentinel lymph node biopsy warranted for desmoplastic melanoma? A systematic review. J Plast Reconstr Aesthet Surg. 2017;70(2):274–80.
5. Feng Z, et al. Incidence and survival of desmoplastic melanoma in the United States, 1992–2007. J Cutan Pathol. 2011;38(8):616–24.
6. Lens MB, Newton-Bishop JA, Boon AP. Desmoplastic malignant melanoma: a systematic review. Br J Dermatol. 2005;152(4):673–8.
7. Jaimes N, et al. Clinical and dermoscopic characteristics of desmoplastic melanomas. JAMA Dermatol. 2013;149(4):413–21.
8. Chen LL, et al. Desmoplastic melanoma: a review. J Am Acad Dermatol. 2013;68(5):825–33.
9. Ortega CA, et al. Nasal mucosal desmoplastic melanoma: a case report with review of the literature. Head Neck Pathol. 2022;16(3):942–6.
10. Kilpatrick SE, White WL, Browne JD. Desmoplastic malignant melanoma of the oral mucosa. An underrecognized diagnostic pitfall. Cancer. 1996;78(3):383–9.
11. Barnhill RL, Elder DE, Bastian BC, Scolyer RA, Calonje JE, Brenn T, Busam KJ, Yeh I. Desmoplastic melanoma. In: Elder DE, Barnhill RL, Bastian BC, editors. WHO

classification of tumours editorial board, skin tumours [Internet; beta version ahead of print]. Lyon: International Agency for Research on Cancer; 2023.
12. Murali R, et al. Clinical and pathological features of metastases of primary cutaneous desmoplastic melanoma. Histopathology. 2011;58(6):886–95.
13. DeWane ME, et al. Melanoma on chronically sun-damaged skin: lentigo maligna and desmoplastic melanoma. J Am Acad Dermatol. 2019;81(3):823–33.
14. Maher NG, et al. Detection of desmoplastic melanoma with dermoscopy and reflectance confocal microscopy. J Eur Acad Dermatol Venereol. 2017;31(12):2016–24.
15. Rule WG, et al. Results of NCCTG N0275 (Alliance) – a phase II trial evaluating resection followed by adjuvant radiation therapy for patients with desmoplastic melanoma. Cancer Med. 2016;5(8):1890–6.
16. Vongtama R, et al. Efficacy of radiation therapy in the local control of desmoplastic malignant melanoma. Head Neck. 2003;25(6):423–8.
17. Jaroszewski DE, et al. The clinical behavior of desmoplastic melanoma. Am J Surg. 2001;182(6):590–5.
18. Chen JY, et al. Desmoplastic neurotropic melanoma: a clinicopathologic analysis of 128 cases. Cancer. 2008;113(10):2770–8.
19. Guadagnolo BA, et al. The role of adjuvant radiotherapy in the local management of desmoplastic melanoma. Cancer. 2014;120(9):1361–8.
20. Strom T, et al. Radiotherapy influences local control in patients with desmoplastic melanoma. Cancer. 2014;120(9):1369–78.
21. Posther KE, et al. Histopathologic characteristics, recurrence patterns, and survival of 129 patients with desmoplastic melanoma. Ann Surg Oncol. 2006;13(5):728–39.
22. Varey AHR, et al. Neurotropic melanoma: an analysis of the clinicopathological features, management strategies and survival outcomes for 671 patients treated at a tertiary referral center. Mod Pathol. 2017;30(11):1538–50.
23. Foote MC, et al. Desmoplastic melanoma: the role of radiotherapy in improving local control. ANZ J Surg. 2008;78(4):273–6.
24. Murali R, et al. Prognostic factors in cutaneous desmoplastic melanoma: a study of 252 patients. Cancer. 2010;116(17):4130–8.
25. Livestro DP, et al. Biology of desmoplastic melanoma: a case-control comparison with other melanomas. J Clin Oncol. 2005;23(27):6739–46.
26. Pawlik TM, et al. Assessment of the role of sentinel lymph node biopsy for primary cutaneous desmoplastic melanoma. Cancer. 2006;106(4):900–6.
27. Hawkins WG, et al. Desmoplastic melanoma: a pathologically and clinically distinct form of cutaneous melanoma. Ann Surg Oncol. 2005;12(3):207–13.
28. George E, et al. Subclassification of desmoplastic melanoma: pure and mixed variants have significantly different capacities for lymph node metastasis. J Cutan Pathol. 2009;36(4):425–32.
29. Han D, et al. Desmoplastic melanoma: is there a role for sentinel lymph node biopsy? Ann Surg Oncol. 2013;20(7):2345–51.
30. Maurichi A, et al. Pure desmoplastic melanoma: a melanoma with distinctive clinical behavior. Ann Surg. 2010;252(6):1052–7.
31. Oliver DE, et al. Roles of adjuvant and salvage radiotherapy for desmoplastic melanoma. Melanoma Res. 2016;26(1):35–41.
32. Sims JR, et al. Head and neck desmoplastic melanoma: utility of sentinel node biopsy. Am J Otolaryngol. 2017;38(5):537–41.
33. Mohebati A, et al. The role of sentinel lymph node biopsy in the management of head and neck desmoplastic melanoma. Ann Surg Oncol. 2012;19(13):4307–13.
34. Eroglu Z, et al. High response rate to PD-1 blockade in desmoplastic melanomas. Nature. 2018;553(7688):347–50.
35. Shain AH, et al. Exome sequencing of desmoplastic melanoma identifies recurrent NFKBIE promoter mutations and diverse activating mutations in the MAPK pathway. Nat Genet. 2015;47(10):1194–9.

36. Reed RJ, Leonard DD. Neurotropic melanoma. A variant of desmoplastic melanoma. Am J Surg Pathol. 1979;3(4):301–11.
37. Busam KJ, et al. Analysis of microphthalmia transcription factor expression in normal tissues and tumors, and comparison of its expression with S-100 protein, gp100, and tyrosinase in desmoplastic malignant melanoma. Am J Surg Pathol. 2001;25(2):197–204.
38. Lezcano C, et al. PRAME expression in melanocytic tumors. Am J Surg Pathol. 2018;42(11):1456–65.
39. Harris GR, et al. Desmoplastic (sclerotic) nevus: an underrecognized entity that resembles dermatofibroma and desmoplastic melanoma. Am J Surg Pathol. 1999;23(7):786–94.
40. Kucher C, et al. Expression of Melan-A and Ki-67 in desmoplastic melanoma and desmoplastic nevi. Am J Dermatopathol. 2004;26(6):452–7.
41. Hilliard NJ, Krahl D, Sellheyer K. p16 expression differentiates between desmoplastic Spitz nevus and desmoplastic melanoma. J Cutan Pathol. 2009;36(7):753–9.
42. Gerami P, et al. Fluorescence in situ hybridization as an ancillary method for the distinction of desmoplastic melanomas from sclerosing melanocytic nevi. J Cutan Pathol. 2011;38(4):329–34.
43. Busam KJ. Desmoplastic melanoma. Clin Lab Med. 2011;31(2):321–30.
44. Whiteman DC, et al. Melanocytic nevi, solar keratoses, and divergent pathways to cutaneous melanoma. J Natl Cancer Inst. 2003;95(11):806–12.
45. Bastian BC. The molecular pathology of melanoma: an integrated taxonomy of melanocytic neoplasia. Annu Rev Pathol. 2014;9:239–71.
46. Roth A, et al. Next-generation sequencing as a potential diagnostic adjunct in distinguishing between desmoplastic melanocytic neoplasms. Am J Surg Pathol. 2023;47(3):318–25.
47. Ha JM, et al. Subungual desmoplastic malignant melanoma. J Eur Acad Dermatol Venereol. 2016;30(2):360–2.
48. Busam KJ, et al. Distinction of desmoplastic melanoma from non-desmoplastic melanoma by gene expression profiling. J Invest Dermatol. 2005;124(2):412–8.
49. Lee JH, Choi JW, Kim YS. Frequencies of BRAF and NRAS mutations are different in histological types and sites of origin of cutaneous melanoma: a meta-analysis. Br J Dermatol. 2011;164(4):776–84.
50. Kim SY, et al. Metaanalysis of BRAF mutations and clinicopathologic characteristics in primary melanoma. J Am Acad Dermatol. 2015;72(6):1036–1046.e2.
51. Curtin JA, et al. Distinct sets of genetic alterations in melanoma. N Engl J Med. 2005;353(20):2135–47.
52. Wiesner T, et al. NF1 mutations are common in desmoplastic melanoma. Am J Surg Pathol. 2015;39(10):1357–62.
53. Addo AK, et al. The morphologic spectrum of NF mutated desmoplastic melanocytic neoplasms. Am J Dermatopathol. 2025;47(9):692–8.
54. Chen A, et al. The impact of next-generation sequencing on interobserver agreement and diagnostic accuracy of desmoplastic melanocytic neoplasms. Am J Surg Pathol. 2024;48(6):708–18.

Chapter 8
Germline Mutations Associated Melanocytic Lesions

Volha Lenskaya, Richard K. Yang, and Phyu P. Aung

Introduction

Melanoma is the fifth most prevalent cancer in the United States; there were 186,680 new cases (89,070 noninvasive and 97,610 invasive) and 7990 deaths from the disease in 2023, and 200,340 new cases were expected in 2024, which would account for 5.6% of all cancer diagnoses [1, 2].

Melanoma is predominantly a sporadic malignancy; up to 90% of cutaneous cases are due to ultraviolet radiation exposure in individuals with phenotypic susceptibility, such as individuals prone to sunburn. Hereditary melanoma accounts for approximately 10% of cases, and familial aggregation is observed in approximately 7–15% of patients who have a documented family history of the disease [3, 4]. The terms *hereditary melanoma* and *familial melanoma* are often used interchangeably, and both refer to a heterogeneous group of disorders characterized by the occurrence of melanoma among relatives, who often have similar genetic alterations. Given the low incidence of hereditary melanoma and lack of a standardized definition of this disease, we have adopted broad criteria for hereditary melanoma in this chapter to ensure a thorough review of the topic.

Individuals in families predisposed to melanoma have a lifetime risk of developing the disease that is approximately 30–70 times as high as the risk in the general population [5]. Hereditary melanoma, like many cancer syndromes, has an autosomal dominant pattern of inheritance and presents as part of a hereditary melanoma syndrome or mixed cancer syndrome [6]. Leachman et al. described typical features of hereditary melanoma as unilateral lineage, multigenerational inheritance, and

V. Lenskaya · R. K. Yang · P. P. Aung (✉)
Division of Pathology and Laboratory Medicine, Department of Anatomic Pathology, The University of Texas MD Anderson Cancer Center, Houston, TX, USA
e-mail: VLenskaya@mdanderson.org; RKYang@mdanderson.org; paung@mdanderson.org

V. G. Prieto, C. A. Torres-Cabala (eds.), *Precision Molecular Pathology of Melanocytic Lesions*, Molecular Pathology Library,
https://doi.org/10.1007/978-3-032-18222-7_8

multiple primary lesions; Cakir et al. added another feature: onset of disease before age 50 years [7–9]. Familial aggregation restricted to siblings within a single generation or cutaneous melanoma present in second- or third-degree relatives indicates a multifactorial polygenic inheritance pattern [10], although large family aggregations of melanoma still suggest an autosomal dominant pattern of inheritance.

Genes that play critical roles in hereditary melanoma include *CDKN2A*, *CDK4*, *BAP1*, *POT1*, *ACD*, *TERF2IP*, *TERT*, *MC1R*, and *MITF* [11–13]. These can be divided into genes whose mutations have high penetrance for melanoma, including *CDKN2A, CDK4, BAP1*, and *POT1*, and genes whose mutations have medium or low penetrance for melanoma, including *MC1R* and *MITF*. Germline mutations in *CDKN2A* are the most common high-penetrance genetic variant in hereditary melanoma, identified in approximately 20–40% of affected families; the melanoma risk in individuals with *CDKN2A* mutations is up to 65 times the melanoma risk of individuals in the general population [14]. *CDKN2A* mutations are strongly correlated with a higher number of affected relatives, multiple primary melanomas, frequent co-occurrence of pancreatic cancer, and earlier age at melanoma diagnosis [14]. Variants in other melanoma susceptibility genes, such as *CDK4*, *BAP1*, *POT1*, *ACD*, *TERF2IP*, *TERT*, *MC1R*, and *MITF,* are infrequent but collectively explain an additional 10% of hereditary melanomas [15].

Germline mutations in genes linked to mixed cancer syndromes, including *PTEN*, *BRCA2*, *BRCA1*, *RB1*, and *TP53*, are also associated with elevated melanoma risk.

Importantly, known pathogenic germline mutations do not account for all instances of hereditary melanoma, leaving the genetic underpinnings of melanoma susceptibility unidentified in numerous affected families. The melanoma risk in individuals with predisposing mutations correlates with mutation type, environmental factors, and unknown variables, which is indicative of a polygenic inheritance pattern mediated by multiple low-risk alleles and genetic modifiers that remain to be fully elucidated [16]. One example is epistasis, the interaction between two genes in which the effect of one gene depends on the presence of another, a modifying gene. In fact, epistatic mutations have been found in hereditary melanoma [17]; certain allelic variants of *MC1R* can enhance the penetrance of *CDKN2A* mutations. These *MC1R* variants can double the melanoma risk compared to the risk in individuals carrying only the *CDKN2A* mutation [18]. Although heritable germline epimutations have been implicated in the formation of familial clusters in other neoplasms, there is currently insufficient evidence to support this hypothesis in hereditary melanoma [19].

Genetics of Hereditary Melanoma

As mentioned above, hereditary melanoma can be attributed to reported melanoma predisposition genes or to mixed cancer syndromes. The predisposition genes can be divided into three main categories according to the relative risk (RR) of developing the disease over time in individuals with mutations in the genes: high-penetrance melanoma susceptibility genes (RR > 5), which are often linked to hereditary forms of the disease; medium-penetrance melanoma susceptibility genes (RR 2–5), which are associated with moderately elevated risk of melanoma, particular when multiple susceptibility alleles interact; and low-penetrance melanoma susceptibility genes (RR < 2), which influence melanoma predisposition across the general population [4, 20]. In total, these genes explain approximately 50% of hereditary melanoma cases [21].

High-Penetrance Melanoma Susceptibility Genes

CDKN2A

CDKN2A (cyclin-dependent kinase inhibitor 2A), a tumor suppressor gene located at 9p21, was the first gene identified to confer high susceptibility to hereditary melanoma and is present in 20–40% of hereditary melanoma cases. In a study to determine the CDKN2A/CDK4/microphthalmia-associated transcription factor mutation rate among patients with multiple primary melanomas (MPM), the authors tested for *CDKN2A, CDK4*, and microphthalmia-associated transcription factor (MITF) in 587 patients with MPM and an equal number of patients with sporadic, single primary melanomas and control subjects. *CDKN2A* germline mutations were found in 19% of patients with multiple primary melanomas but only 4.4% of patients with a single primary melanoma [22]. The prevalence of germline *CDKN2A* mutations seems to increase with the number of melanoma cases within a family [23] and is 25% in people with two or more relatives affected by melanoma [24]. In *CDKN2A* germline-mutated melanomas, somatic *NRAS* mutations are more common, whereas *BRAF* mutations occur less frequently [25, 26].

CDKN2A produces two distinct proteins via alternative splicing: p16INK4a and p14ARF. p16INK4a exerts its tumor-suppressive role by inhibiting *CDK4/6*-mediated cell cycle progression, while p14ARF safeguards genomic integrity by stabilizing p53, thereby activating DNA damage responses and senescence to counteract oncogenic evasion [21].

CDKN2A is frequently somatically altered in sporadic melanomas, with biallelic inactivation of *CDKN2A* predominantly observed in invasive melanoma cases [15, 27].

Mutations in *CDKN2A* increase nevus count and density, significantly elevating melanoma risk. Families carrying *CDKN2A* mutations frequently have multiple members with numerous atypical melanocytic nevi, often more than 50. The likelihood of harboring *CDKN2A* mutations is elevated in individuals with melanocytic nevi localized to the buttocks or dorsal aspect of the feet [25]. Melanocytic nevi in *CDKN2A* mutation carriers exhibit a range of morphologies from benign-appearing lesions to atypical variants that are large with irregular borders and polychromatic pigmentation [26]. *CDKN2A* mutation carriers experience melanoma onset at a median age of 33–45 years, approximately 15 years earlier than the median age at onset of sporadic melanoma (53–61 years) [28]. Melanomas in *CDKN2A* mutation carriers tend to exhibit thinner Breslow thickness than sporadic melanomas, a finding possibly influenced by enhanced surveillance practices in genetically predisposed individuals [29]. Melanoma in *CDKN2A* mutation carriers is typically characterized by a high degree of pagetoid scatter, dense pigmentation, and non-spindle cell morphology during the vertical growth phase (Fig. 8.1) [30]. The most frequently identified type of melanoma in *CDKN2A* mutation carriers is superficial spreading melanoma [31].

The penetrance and frequency of *CDKN2A* mutations vary substantially across geographic regions and study populations. In a study of families with documented *CDKN2A* mutations and multiple cases of melanoma, the estimated *CDKN2A* mutation penetrance rates for melanoma by ages 50 years and 80 years were 32% and 91%, in Australia; 50% and 76%, in the United States; and 13% and 58%, respectively, in Europe [32]. The authors speculated that the wide variation in risk could be explained by differences in sun exposure patterns and the presence of additional genetic risk factors among families [32, 33]. In a meta-analysis by Goldstein et al. that included families in which at least three members had melanoma, 39% of families overall had germline *CDKN2A* mutations, and the proportion of families with germline *CDKN2A* mutations was 20% (32/162) in Australia, 45% (29/65) in North America, and 57% (89/157) in Europe [16]. In this study, the authors found *CDKN2A* mutation with overall rates of 72% and 81% and geographic region-specific rates of 33% and ≥75% [28].

In addition to heightened susceptibility to melanoma, *CDKN2A* mutation carriers exhibit increased susceptibility to cancers of the upper digestive system and

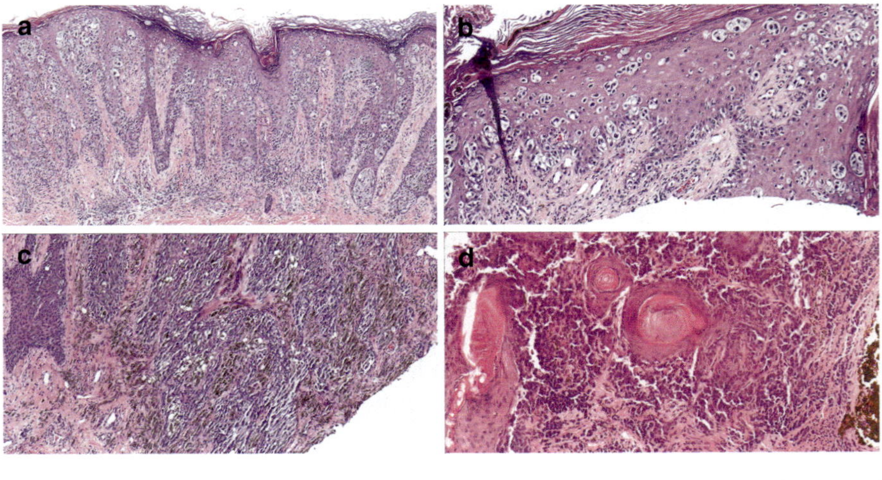

Fig. 8.1 Melanoma in a *CDKN2A* germline mutation carriers. (**a**) Superficial spreading type of melanoma, H&E (100×); (**b**) prominent pagetoid scatter of intraepithelial melanocytes, H&E (20×); (**c**) area of pigmented melanophages within melanoma, H&E (100×); (**d**) invasive melanoma component with epithelioid morphology, H&E (200×)

respiratory tract, and the susceptibility is particularly high among mutation carriers with a history of smoking. This pattern suggests that *CDKN2A* mutations may enhance sensitivity to carcinogenic compounds found in tobacco smoke [34, 35]. Therefore, *CDKN2A* mutation carriers require targeted counseling regarding smoking cessation [35].

In addition, a recent study investigated the genetic and clinical features of six individuals with cancer and *CDKN2A* mutations, including one patient with dysplastic nevus and one with melanoma, and identified c.307_308del in three patients, c.159G > C in one patient, and c.71G > C in two patients. Clinically significant variants of *CDKN2A* were associated with melanoma and pancreatic cancer in this study [36]. This highlights the need for *CDKN2A* mutation testing in patients with suspected hereditary multiple atypical nevi and melanomas.

CDK4

CDK4 (cyclin-dependent kinase 4), an oncogene located at 12q14, encodes a protein crucial for normal cell cycle regulation; when mutated, *CDK4* inhibits p16 binding, leading to *RB* phosphorylation and uncontrolled cell cycle progression [21]. Germline *CDK4* mutations, though uncommon, confer a melanoma risk comparable to that associated with *CDKN2A* mutations. *CDK4* mutations, like *CDKN2A* mutations, can disrupt G1-phase cell cycle control and mediate *RB* pathway dysregulation [21]. In a study of 17 families with *CDK4* mutations, 41.7% of affected individuals developed more than one primary melanoma. The mean age at first melanoma diagnosis in *CDK4* mutation carriers was 39 years, approximately 15 years younger than the mean age at first diagnosis in the general white population, and melanomas in *CDK4* mutation carriers usually occurred on limbs. The estimated mutation penetrance by age 50 years was 74.2%, and only 7.4% of melanomas were diagnosed in individuals aged 60 years or older. As is true for *CDKN2A*-associated melanomas, for *CDK4*-associated melanomas, superficial spreading is the most common type. A study by Tucker et al. demonstrated that precursor lesions, most commonly intradermal or dysplastic nevi, are frequently present in families with *CDK4*-associated melanoma [37].

The clinical phenotype in families with germline *CDK4* mutations is indistinguishable from that in families with *CDKN2A* mutations and is characterized by a high burden of atypical nevi, early age of melanoma onset, and a propensity for multiple primary melanomas. Therefore, in melanoma-prone families who test negative for *CDKN2A* variants, screening for *CDK4* mutations should be strongly considered.

In addition to melanoma susceptibility, germline *CDK4* mutations have been implicated in increased risk for nonmelanoma skin cancers, breast cancer, pancreatic cancer, and potentially ovarian, cervical, and gastric cancer [38], although these associations require further validation.

BAP1

BAP1 (BRCA1-associated protein 1), a tumor suppressor gene located at 3p21, encodes a deubiquitinating enzyme that is critical for regulating cell division, gene expression, signal transduction, protein trafficking, and DNA repair [11]. Dysregulation of these functions can contribute to oncogenic transformation [39, 40]. Consistent with *BAP1*'s tumor suppressor function, *BAP1*-associated tumors frequently exhibit loss of heterozygosity, reflecting the inactivation of both alleles required for tumorigenesis.

Carriers of germline *BAP1* mutations are predisposed to *BAP1* tumor predisposition syndrome (*BAP1*-TPDS), which manifests as both benign and malignant tumors. Njauw et al. found that 29% of families with both cutaneous and uveal melanomas had mutations in the *BAP1* gene, compared with only 0.52% of families with multiple cases of cutaneous melanoma alone [41]. Recent population studies confirm that the most common malignancy associated with *BAP1*-TPDS is uveal melanoma (29%), followed by mesothelioma (22%), cutaneous melanoma (18%), and renal cell carcinoma (9%); other types of cancer seen in *BAP1*-TPDS include basal cell carcinoma, hepatocellular carcinoma, and meningioma [41–44]. Approximately one quarter of patients with *BAP1* mutations and melanoma have multiple primary cutaneous melanomas [42].

BIMTs occur in up to 90% of *BAP1* mutation carriers; they tend to develop early in life (median age 31 years, range 10–56 years) and are more likely to have multiple tumors (affected family members display between 5 and 50 tumors each) [43, 44]. Morphologically, BIMTs are dome-shaped, exclusively or predominantly intradermal melanocytic tumors with epithelioid melanocytes that have round to oval vesicular nuclei and abundant amphophilic cytoplasm with a nodular or sheet-like growth pattern (Figs. 8.2 and 8.3) [45, 46]. An associated common nevus component is often present [47]. A review of 102 BIMTs found that 69% exhibited spitzoid and epithelioid cytomorphology, while 31% had smaller epithelioid cells lacking abundant eosinophilic cytoplasm [44]. Rhabdoid features were also observed. In this cohort, 12% of BIMTs were associated with a germline *BAP1* mutation [45]. Transformation of BIMT to melanoma has been reported (Fig. 8.4) [46, 48].

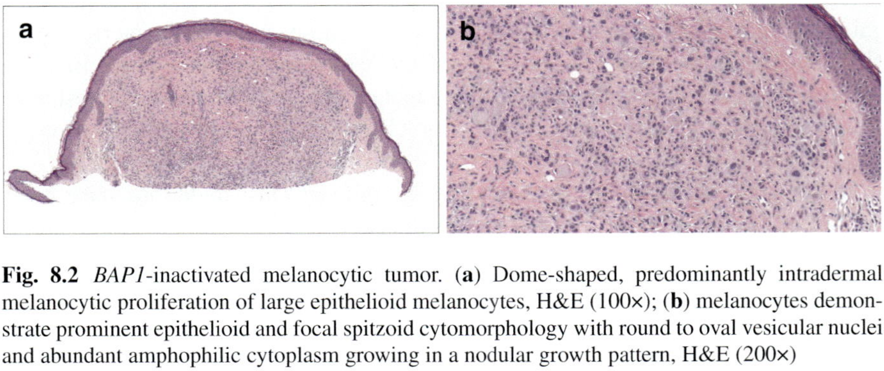

Fig. 8.2 *BAP1*-inactivated melanocytic tumor. (**a**) Dome-shaped, predominantly intradermal melanocytic proliferation of large epithelioid melanocytes, H&E (100×); (**b**) melanocytes demonstrate prominent epithelioid and focal spitzoid cytomorphology with round to oval vesicular nuclei and abundant amphophilic cytoplasm growing in a nodular growth pattern, H&E (200×)

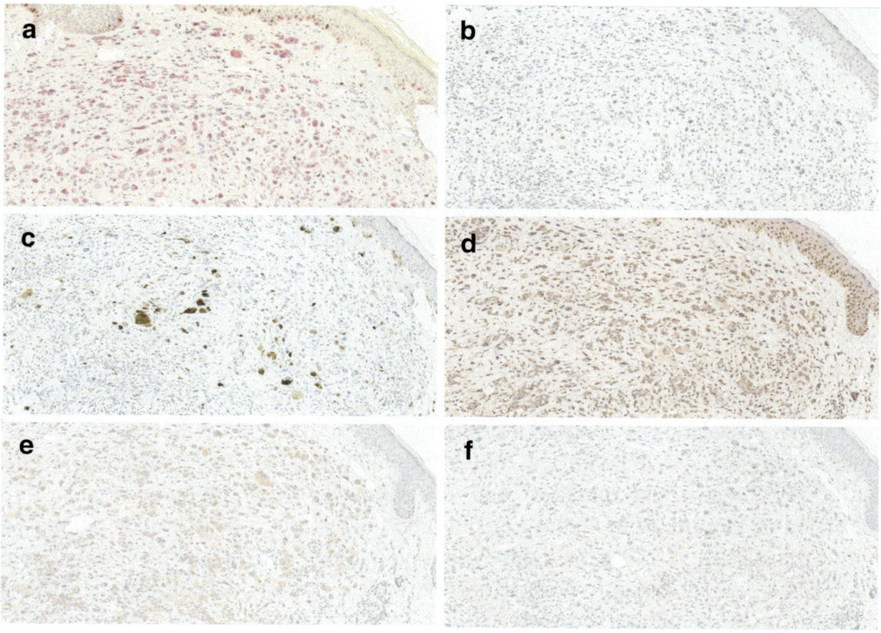

Fig. 8.3 Immunohistochemical studies for *BAP1*-inactivated melanocytic tumor. (**a**) Dual color multiplex Ki67/MART1 demonstrates low proliferative index by Ki67 and immunoreactivity for MART1 (200×); (**b**) PRAME, negative result (200×); (**c**) p16, patchy immunoreactivity (200×). (**d**) BAP1, loss of expression (200×); (**e**) BRAF V600E, patchy immunoreactivity (200×); (**f**) ALK, negative result (200X)

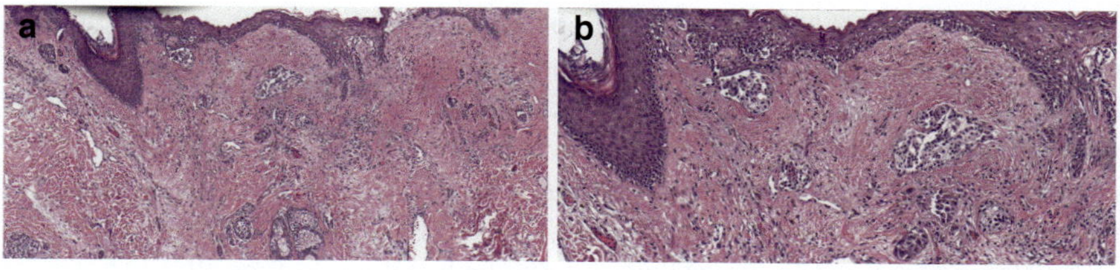

Fig. 8.4 Melanoma in a patient with *BAP1* germline mutation. (**a**) Low magnification, H&E (100×); (**b**) high magnification, H&E (200×)

Recently, Donati et al. reported a case of malignant transformation of a BIMT to a *BAP1*-inactivated melanoma with a *TERT*-p hot spot mutation in a patient with a *BAP1* germline mutation [49]. Molecular studies may facilitate discrimination between BIMTs and *BAP1*-TPDS–associated melanomas, as *BRAF V600E* mutations are present in 67–89% of BIMTs but generally absent in *BAP1*-TPDS–associated melanomas [50].

Interestingly, Lebensohn et al. found nail abnormalities consistent with onychopapillomas in 39 of 47 (83%) adults with *BAP1*-TPDS [51].

POT1

POT1 (protection of telomeres 1) encodes a protein in the shelterin complex. This complex, encoded by *POT1, TERF1, TERF2, RAP1, TIN2,* and *TPP1*, maintains chromosomal stability and telomere length by protecting against degradation and uncontrolled elongation. The loss-of-function variants in *POT1* gene result in telomere branching and elongation mediated by homology-directed repair mechanisms; homology-directed repair mechanisms may promote carcinogenesis [52–54]. Individuals carrying *POT1* missense mutations frequently have elongated telomeres, which are a recognized risk factor for melanoma [4, 53, 55]. Robles-Espinoza et al. reported that all nine *POT1* variant carriers in a familial cohort developed at least one melanoma (and one carrier developed 8 melanomas) at 25 to 80 years of age [53]. Histological analyses of melanomas in families with *POT1* mutations revealed a prevalence of spitzoid morphology (67%), indicating that telomere dysfunction might contribute to spitzoid differentiation [56]. Interestingly, the rare S270N *POT1* missense mutation was identified as a progenitor mutation in five unrelated melanoma-prone families from Italy [54]. Herrera-Mullar et al. compared tumor prevalence in 227 individuals with a pathogenic variant of *POT1* and a large number of control patients with wild-type *POT1* and found significantly higher prevalences of melanoma (odds ratio [OR] 7.03; 95% CI 4.7–10.5; $P < 0.001$) and sarcoma (OR 6.6; 95% CI 3.1–13.9; $P < 0.001$) in the individuals with *POT1* pathogenic variants [57].

POT1 mutations are associated with a multi-cancer tumor predisposition syndrome with an increased risk of several cancer types, including melanoma, chronic lymphocytic leukemia, glioma, angiosarcoma, and colorectal, thyroid, gastrointestinal stromal, and lung cancers [58]. Given the elevated risk of thyroid neoplasms in individuals with *POT1* germline mutations, Wilson et al. suggest performing thyroid ultrasound screenings in such individuals every 12 to 24 months, in addition to the standard biannual dermatological examinations and age-appropriate cancer screenings [59]. Due to the early occurrence of melanomas in *POT1* mutation carriers, Wilson et al. advise testing for *POT1* mutations in children of families with multiple *POT1* mutation carriers [60]. *POT1* pathologic variant carriers have a risk of developing sarcoma six times that of individuals with wild-type *POT1* [57].

ACD and *TERF2IP*

Germline mutations in two additional shelterin complex genes, *ACD* (adrenocortical dysplasia protein homolog) and *TERF2IP* (telomeric repeat binding factor 2–interacting protein 1), have also been identified in melanoma-prone families, implicating broader telomere dysregulation in hereditary melanoma susceptibility [21]. *ACD* enhances *POT1* binding affinity to single-stranded telomeric DNA and, in concert with *POT1*, mediates the interaction between the shelterin complex and *TERT*. Germline nonsense mutations in *ACD* and *TERF2IP* are predominantly associated with an elevated risk of multiple primary melanomas and earlier disease onset, with peak incidence occurring during adolescence [59]. Aoude et al. reported that in a cohort of 510 melanoma families, six melanomas had mutations in *ACD*, and four had mutations in *TERF2IP* [59].

Mutations in *ACD* and *TERF2IP* also predispose individuals to various other types of cancer, including hematological cancers (B cell lymphoma and leukemia) [59] and esophageal [61], breast [59], lung [61], renal [61], cervix [59], ovarian [61], colon [62], and other neoplasms [63].

TERT

TERT (telomerase reverse transcriptase) encodes a protein component of the shelterin complex, which, in conjunction with the telomerase RNA component (TERC), forms the core of the telomerase enzyme responsible for maintaining telomere length. Both somatic and germline mutations in the *TERT* promoter region have been described in neoplasms, and they seem to provoke excessive elongation of telomeres, which is linked to development of melanoma and other cancers [64]. Somatic mutations in the *TERT* promoter frequently arise as early secondary alterations following activating mutations in *BRAF* or *NRAS* and have been identified in roughly 30–70% of sporadic melanomas, with the highest prevalence observed in nodular and superficial spreading subtypes and clinically in older patients [27, 65]. Germline mutations in the *TERT* promoter are rare in hereditary melanomas and are responsible for approximately 1% of hereditary melanoma cases [66]. In a cohort study of 675 melanoma-prone families with confirmed high-penetrance melanoma susceptibility mutations in *CDKN2A, CDK4, BAP1, POT1, ACD*, and *TERF2IP*, only a single family was identified as harboring a pathogenic *TERT* promoter mutation [67].

Primary melanomas with somatic mutations in *TERT* promoter tend to be thicker, with a higher mitotic count, and appear in higher patient age at diagnosis when compared to *TERT* wild-type melanomas. Pópulo et al. analyzed a series of cases of cutaneous melanoma and found that somatic *TERT* promoter mutations were generally restricted to melanomas arising in areas with intermittent (versus chronic or no sun exposure) and melanomas of nodular or superficial spreading subtype; furthermore, somatic *TERT* promoter mutations were more common in tumors with ulceration and *BRAF V600E* mutations [66]. However, *TERT* mutation was not reported to be associated with reduced survival. Also, *TERT* mutation status does not correlate with TERT protein expression [67].

On the other hand, primary melanomas with *TERT* germline variants may be linked to early-onset melanoma and multiple primaries [68, 69]. Germline mutations in *TER*T are not associated with the same features as seen in primary melanomas with somatic *TERT* mutations [70]. *TERT* germline mutations have been reported to be associated with globular mole pattern [71].

A novel germline T > G substitution in the promoter region of *TERT* was identified in 14 affected individuals from a melanoma-prone family lacking mutations in *CDKN2A* [68]. Subsequent studies demonstrated that this T > G substitution in the

TERT promoter creates new binding sites for Ets transcription factors, including ternary complex factors ELK1 and ELK4, which leads to upregulation of expression and increased activity of *TERT*, leading to telomerase reactivation and thereby facilitating cancer initiation and progression [63, 72].

TERT promoter mutations, in addition to conferring susceptibility to early-onset melanoma, confer susceptibility to cancers of the bladder, colon, lung, prostate, testis, breast, kidney, and central nervous system (i.e., glioblastoma, glioma, and medulloblastoma) [71], raising the possibility that patients in families with confirmed TERT promoter mutation should be screened for these cancers [67].

High-Penetrance Melanoma Susceptibility Genes

While medium-penetrance variant alleles occur more frequently than high-penetrance variants do in the general population, medium-penetrance variants are unlikely to independently initiate carcinogenesis. However, the cumulative effect of multiple variant alleles or the interaction between genetic predisposition and environmental factors may increase an individual's melanoma risk beyond a critical threshold.

MC1R

MC1R (melanocortin 1 receptor) encodes a G protein–coupled receptor that regulates both hair and skin pigmentation by responding to α-melanocyte–stimulating hormone. Ultraviolet radiation activates *MC1R* via binding of α-melanocyte–stimulating hormone, triggering melanin synthesis in melanocytes. This process preferentially upregulates brown/black eumelanin production over red/yellow pheomelanin production while concurrently enhancing DNA repair mechanisms. Notably, pheomelanin has mutagenic potential due to its prooxidant properties, which promote oxidative stress and DNA damage [73, 74]. In individuals with darker skin, *MC1R* variants are linked to *BRAF* V600E–mutated melanomas occurring on non-sun-exposed areas. In contrast, *MC1R* variants show an inverse relationship with *BRAF* V600K–mutated melanomas [75–77].

MC1R variants are significant and relatively common genetic modifiers of melanoma risk and are found in up to 11% of individuals in general [78]. In sporadic melanoma cohorts, carriers of MC1R variants have a 66% increased risk of developing melanoma compared to wild-type individuals, with 28% of melanoma cases attributed to these variants [79]. There are two main *MC1R*-variant categories based on their association with the red hair color (RHC) phenotype (fair skin, red hair, freckles, and increased sensitivity to sunlight). The "R" variants are strongly associated with the red hair color phenotype and include D84E, R142H, R151C, I155T, R160W, and D294H. The "r" variants encompass essentially all other MC1R variants and generally exhibit a weaker association with the red hair color phenotype [80].

In a case-control study, 86% of patients with early-onset melanoma (diagnosed before age 40 years) carried at least one *MC1R* R or r variant, compared to 73% of unrelated controls [80]. The R alleles confer an elevated risk of melanoma that is independent of skin phototype [11]. Furthermore, a meta-analysis by Fargnoli et al. demonstrated that *CDKN2A* mutation carriers with a single *MC1R* variant have double the melanoma risk compared to those without *MC1R* variants, while carriers of multiple *MC1R* variants face over four times the risk; additionally, *MC1R* variant carriers tend to be diagnosed with melanoma at a significantly younger age [81].

The r variants (e.g., V60L) are associated with moderate melanoma risk (OR 1.69, 95% CI 1.33–2.13) while R variants (e.g., R151C, R160W, and D294H) confer the highest risk, doubling melanoma odds per allele (OR 2.23, 95% CI 1.77–2.80) [80]. Carriers of multiple *MC1R* variants had 4.6 times the melanoma risk of individuals with wild-type *MC1R* [82, 83]. Interestingly, a recent study showed that the presence of any *MC1R* variant is associated with melanoma risk independently of classic red hair color phenotype (OR 1.60, 95% CI 1.36–1.88) and suggested that studying the *MC1R* genotype might yield findings beneficial for melanoma prediction [84].

MC1R variants do not appear to correlate with high counts of acquired nevi in families with hereditary melanoma. Patients carrying *MC1R* RHC variants predominantly develop melanomas on the trunk and arms [81]. Furthermore, the carriers of RHC variants generally develop hypopigmented melanocytic lesions, called "white nevi" or "red melanomas" [85], and have larger nevi and melanomas than those seen in individuals with wild-type *MC1R*. In a cohort of 2160 melanoma patients, no significant correlation was identified between *MC1R* variant status and histopathological characteristics of the tumors [86].

Overall, even though *MC1R* variants are common in the general population, their lower penetrance for melanoma than the penetrance of *CDKN2A* underscores the role of *MC1R* variants as critical risk modifiers rather than stand-alone drivers. Clinically, *MC1R* genotyping could refine risk assessment in hereditary melanoma screening programs.

MITF

MITF (microphthalmia-associated transcription factor), a member of the *MYC* gene family, encodes a transcription factor specific to the melanocytic lineage that governs melanocyte differentiation, proliferation, and survival [87]. The most common variant of *MITF* is p.E318K, which alters its binding affinity for the ubiquitin-like protein SUMO, thus enhancing the binding of MITF protein to the hypoxia-inducible factor 1A (*HIF1A)* promoter and increasing its transcriptional activity [11]. *HIF1A* is the key pathway in renal cell carcinoma development [88, 89].

A study by Bertolotto et al. involving sequencing of the *MITF* gene in 62 patients with melanoma and renal cell carcinoma (RCC) identified the germline E318K mutation, which was associated with a more than fivefold increased risk of developing melanoma, RCC, or both. This finding helped to define the *MITF*-related melanoma and RCC predisposition syndrome [89]. Additionally, using whole-genome sequencing, Yokoyama et al. found that the *MITF* E318K variant occurs in approximately 1% of individuals of European ancestry and is linked to a two- to fivefold elevated risk of melanoma compared to non-carriers. The variant was also associated with a higher number of melanocytic nevi [90].

Reported odds ratios (ORs) for melanoma risk among carriers of the E318K variant range from approximately 1.7 (95% CI 1.1–2.7) [91] to 3.3 (95% CI 1.43–7.43) [92], depending on the study population and adjustment for confounding factors. The risk is particularly elevated in individuals with multiple primary melanomas (OR 4.5, 95% CI 1.83–11.01) and those with a high number of nevi (>200: OR 8.4, 95% CI 2.14–33.19) [90]. Individuals carrying the *MITF* E318K variant who have a personal or family history of pancreatic cancer have a 31-fold increased risk of melanoma, while those who have a personal or family history of renal cell cancer have an eightfold elevated risk [15].

Patients harboring *MITF* variants often present with darker hair, fair skin, non-blue eye color, numerous or atypical nevi, and amelanotic melanomas, reflecting the gene's role in melanocyte development and pigmentation [91]. The *MITF* E318K variant increases melanoma risk in both dark-haired and fair-haired individuals; however, its effect is significantly stronger in those with dark hair. Stratified analyses show that carriers of the E318K variant with dark hair have a higher odds ratio for melanoma than carriers with fair hair (P for interaction = 0.03) [90].

No specific histopathological markers have been identified that directly indicate the presence of *MITF* gene variants, such as E318K, in melanoma. However, some histopathological and molecular findings are worth mentioning, such as variable tumor pigmentation, heterogeneous expression of *MITF,* with high levels associated with more differentiated melanoma types and low levels associated with more invasive or undifferentiated types; and amplification of *MITF*, which is linked to poorer prognosis and increased tumor proliferation [87, 93]. A study of Italian melanoma patients reported an association of *MITF* E318K mutation with nodular-type melanoma and greater tumor thickness (Fig. 8.5) [94], although these findings were not confirmed by Australian/UK studies [89, 91]. Because transcriptional activity of *MITF* modulates target genes involved in pigmentation, including *MC1R*, a study

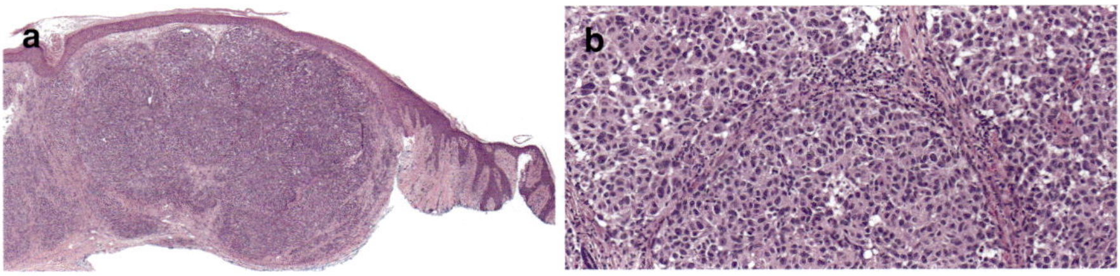

Fig. 8.5 Melanoma in a patient with *MITF* germline mutation. (**a**) Low magnification, H&E (40×); (**b**) high magnification, H&E (200×)

was conducted to investigate potential interaction between *MITF* E318K variant and *MC1R* variants in the regulation of melanoma pigmentation (amelanotic or pigmented). No significant association was observed, suggesting that the increased melanoma susceptibility associated with E318K is not dependent on the genetic determinants of red hair [90].

Low-Penetrance Melanoma Susceptibility Genes

Low-penetrance variants linked to melanoma risk have a range of functions, including the regulation of pigmentation and the formation of nevi.

Recent studies confirm that genes such as *ASIP, TYR, TYRP1, OCA2*, and *SLC45A2* play pivotal roles in human pigmentation pathways and contribute to increased melanoma susceptibility through their influence on pigmentation. Variants in these genes are associated with lighter pigmentation of skin, hair, and eye color, which reduces natural protection against ultraviolet radiation and thereby increases melanoma risk [95–98]. For example, specific *ASIP* haplotypes are linked to fair skin and heightened melanoma risk (odds ratio ~ 1.68), and variants in *TYRP1* and *SLC45A2* are associated with altered pigmentation and increased susceptibility. *OCA2* and *TYR* variants similarly influence pigmentation traits and skin cancer risk, with certain alleles correlating with fair skin and reduced tanning ability [99]. *TYR* and *TYRP1* catalyze eumelanin synthesis, while *OCA2* and *SLC45A2* regulate melanosomal pH and ion transport; variants in these genes are associated with reduced pigmentation [100].

Another group of low-penetrance genes, including *NID1, IRF4, MTAP*, and *PLA2G6*, was reported to be associated with nevus development and melanoma susceptibility [21, 96, 101]. *NID1*, involved in basement membrane remodeling, exhibits decreased expression in benign nevi and primary melanomas, with specific variants linked to reduced nevus count and melanoma risk [101]. *IRF4* encodes a transcription factor that is essential for the development of immune cells. Variants in *IRF4* are connected to nevus count and melanoma risk in children and adolescents, but not in adults. Notably, variants in the *MTAP* gene are linked to an increased risk of melanoma of the superficial spreading and nodular subtypes but not of the lentigo maligna subtype. Variants in *PLA2G6* are associated with nevus count but do not influence overall melanoma risk [102]. These findings highlight the pleiotropic effects of these genes, implicating them in pathways influencing both nevogenesis and melanoma predisposition. Although these genes were reported to be associated with a high nevus count, the exact role of these genes in nevus development and melanoma remains unclear.

Emerging Genes

ATM

ATM (ataxia telangiectasia mutated) is a cancer predisposition gene. It is established that germline pathogenic *ATM* variants are associated with increased risk of cancers of the breast, prostate, pancreas, and ovary [103]. *ATM* may also predispose to melanoma (Fig. 8.6) since genome-wide-association studies suggested that *ATM* pathogenic variants slightly increase the risk of melanoma [104] [105]. Lendinez-Sanchez et al. reported the presence of the pathogenic variant *ATM* c.3747-1G > C in two first-degree relatives affected by cutaneous melanoma, one of them diagnosed at 24 years of age [104]. Moreover, the findings of a large study by Dalmasso et al. also support the possible increase in melanoma risk for *ATM* loss-of-function variants [105].

MBD4

MBD4 (methyl-CpG binding domain 4) encodes a glycosylase involved in the DNA base excision repair pathway. *MBD4* inactivation leads to accumulation of mutations, especially in tumors with monosomy 3, a chromosomal alteration associated with high risk of metastasis in uveal melanoma [106]. Recent studies have identified *MBD4* as a novel predisposition gene for uveal melanoma [106–109]. Germline pathogenic variants in *MBD4* are associated with a distinct tumor mutational signature characterized by a high level of CpG > TpG alterations (signature SBS96) and a high tumor mutation burden resulting from failure to repair G:T mismatches caused by deamination of 5-methylcytosine [106–109].

Uveal melanomas harboring *MBD4* mutations exhibit a hypermutator phenotype with elevated tumor mutation burden, and this phenotype correlates with better responses to immune checkpoint inhibitors than are observed in uveal melanomas with low tumor mutation burden [106, 110, 111]. *MBD4* mutations, often monoallelic, are linked to a significant increase in uveal melanoma risk, with a reported RR of approximately 9 [106]. Villy et al. [112] reported that in a series of 25 families whose probands carried a monoallelic germline pathogenic variant in *MBD4*, 18

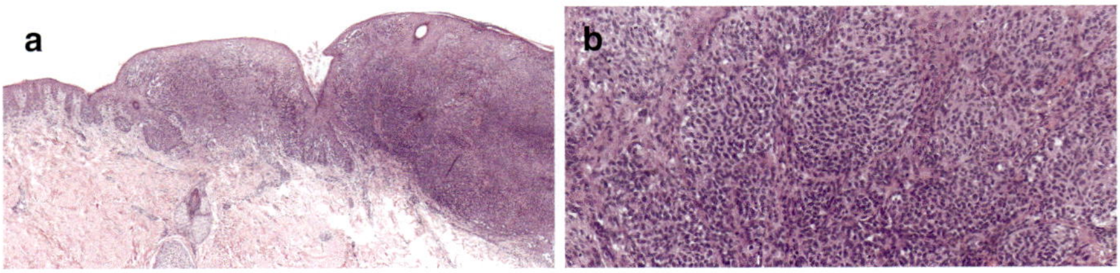

Fig. 8.6 Melanoma in a patient with *ATM* germline mutation. (**a**) Low magnification, H&E (40×); (**b**) high magnification, H&E (200×)

families presented with uveal melanoma (including a case patient with multiple uveal melanomas), and seven families presented with breast cancer. These authors suggested performing a germline genetic analysis for *MBD4* pathogenic variants in all patients with metastatic uveal melanoma [112].

MBD4 germline variants have also been implicated in increased susceptibility to other cancers, including breast, brain, and colorectal.

Genotype-Phenotype Correlations

Genes whose germline mutation is associated with increased risk of melanoma, along with the associated clinical phenotype and the anatomical sites and histopathological features of the resulting tumors, are summarized in Table 8.1. The main question that needs to be answered in future studies is whether there are phenotypic differences between hereditary and sporadic melanoma. Gillgren et al. found that hereditary melanomas are more likely to occur on the trunk than on the head and neck [113]. The pattern of metastasis does not appear to differ between hereditary and sporadic melanoma, so patients with hereditary melanoma can probably be followed up using the same program used for patients with sporadic melanoma [114].

Hereditary Syndromes

Familial Atypical Multiple Mole Melanoma Syndrome

Familial atypical multiple mole melanoma (FAMMM) syndrome is an autosomal dominant genodermatosisthat results from mutations in several genes, including the *CDKN2A* gene. The affected individuals with FAMMM have multiple melanocytic nevi, usually more than 50, and a family history of melanoma [16]. The estimated penetrance of *CDKN2A* mutations for melanoma in families with FAMMM syndrome is 30% by age 50 years and 67% by age 80 years [33]. The average age at diagnosis of melanoma is 30–40 years in patients with *CDKN2A* mutations, compared with approximately 50 years in the general population. However, while early-onset melanoma is frequently observed in *CDKN2A* mutation carriers, it is not a reliable predictor of mutation status. Studies have shown that fewer than 1% of individuals diagnosed with melanoma before age 40 years harbor *CDKN2A* mutations [115].

To be diagnosed with FAMMM syndrome, a patient must have a high total nevus count (usually >50), nevi with a lentiginous pattern or nuclear atypia, and melanomas in one or more first- or second-degree relatives [15]. Predicting *CDKN2A* mutation status solely on clinical observations remains challenging. Hereditary

Table 8.1 Summary of genes whose germline mutation is associated with melanocytic tumors

Gene	Phenotype	Histopathological features	Associated malignancies/tumors	Associated syndrome
High penetrance				
CDKN2A	Higher total nevus number and total nevus density; numerous atypical/dysplastic melanocytic nevi, often more than 50; nevi on buttocks and dorsum of feet; melanomas of head and neck area; multiple primary melanomas at age 30–40 years	Superficial spreading melanoma; high degree of pagetoid scatter, dense pigmentation, and non-spindle cell morphology during the vertical growth phase	Melanoma; pancreatic, breast, esophagus, lung, ovarian, cervical, endometrial, stomach, and colon cancers; leukemia; Hodgkin lymphoma; renal cell carcinoma; urinary bladder, prostate, and hepatic cancers; sarcomas; parotid gland, tonsillar, nasopharyngeal, and tongue cancers; and neural system tumors, including astrocytomas, neurofibromas, and schwannomas	Familial atypical multiple mole melanoma (FAMMM) syndrome; melanoma--astrocytoma syndrome
CDK4	Similar to phenotype of *CDKN2A* germline mutations: high burden of atypical nevi; predilection for multiple primary melanomas; early age of disease onset	Similar to features with *CDKN2A* germline mutations; melanomas usually harbor intradermal or dysplastic nevus	Melanoma; pancreatic, breast, ovarian, cervical, stomach, colon, lung, and prostate cancers; and lymphoma	Familial atypical multiple mole melanoma (FAMMM) syndrome
BAP1	*BAP1* tumor predisposition syndrome: uveal melanoma, cutaneous melanoma, dome--shaped skin-colored nevi, mesothelioma, and renal cell carcinoma; possibly meningioma, cholangiocarcinoma, and hepatocellular carcinoma; multiple onychopapillomas in adults	*BAP1*-inactivated nevi: predominantly intradermal, associated common nevus component often present, epithelioid nevocytes with round to oval vesicular nuclei and abundant amphophilic cytoplasm; some rhabdoid features can be present	Uveal and cutaneous melanoma, mesothelioma, basal cell carcinoma, renal cell carcinoma, hepatocellular carcinoma, cholangiocarcinoma, lung carcinoma, meningioma paraganglioma, breast cancer, neuroendocrine cancer, gastric adenocarcinoma, thyroid carcinoma, and squamous cell carcinomas	*BAP1* tumor predisposition syndrome

(continued)

Table 8.1 (continued)

Gene	Phenotype	Histopathological features	Associated malignancies/tumors	Associated syndrome
POT1	*POT1* tumor predisposition syndrome: cutaneous melanoma, chronic lymphocytic leukemia, angiosarcoma (mostly cardiac angiosarcoma), and glioma, with associations emerging for colorectal cancer, thyroid cancer, soft tissue sarcoma, osteosarcoma, breast cancer, and lung cancer; idiopathic pulmonary fibrosis	Superficial spreading type of melanoma; prevalence of spitzoid morphology	Melanoma; chronic lymphocytic leukemia; angiosarcoma; glioma; soft tissue and bone sarcomas; colorectal, thyroid, breast, lung, prostate, ovarian, renal, and brain cancers; and B cell and T cell lymphoproliferative and myeloproliferative diseases	*POT1* tumor predisposition syndrome
ACD	Multiple primary melanomas, especially in adolescence; pulmonary fibrosis; anemia, especially aplastic anemia	Superficial spreading and lentigo maligna types of melanoma	Melanoma; breast, ovarian, cervical, lung, colon, esophageal, renal, and urinary cancers; and lymphomas and leukemias	Telomeropathies
TERF2IP	Multiple primary melanomas, especially in adolescence; pulmonary fibrosis; anemia	Superficial spreading and lentigo maligna types of melanoma	Melanoma; breast, ovarian, cervical, lung, colon, esophageal, renal, and urinary cancers; and lymphomas and leukemias	Telomeropathies

(continued)

Table 8.1 (continued)

Gene	Phenotype	Histopathological features	Associated malignancies/tumors	Associated syndrome
TERT	Early-onset primary melanoma, frequently in non-UV-exposed sites	Superficial spreading and lentigo maligna types of melanoma; some associations with globular mole pattern; somatic *TERT* promoter mutations are associated with poor prognostic factors such as increased tumor thickness, ulceration, high mitotic rate, and lymph node metastasis, and occur together with *BRAF* and *CDKN2A* alterations; data on histopathologic features of melanomas associated with germline *TERT* promoter mutations are still pending	Melanoma; bladder, colon, lung, prostate, testis, breast, and kidney cancers; and central nervous system tumors (glioblastoma, glioma, and medulloblastoma)	Telomeropathies
Medium to low penetrance				
MC1R	Red hair, freckling, light skin, and UV sensitivity (losss-of--function variants); melanoma on arms and trunk; hypopigmented melanocytic lesions, called "white nevi" or "red melanomas"; larger nevi and melanomas than in individuals with wild-type *MC1R*	No distinguishing histopathological features identified to date	Melanoma	None identified

(continued)

Table 8.1 (continued)

Gene	Phenotype	Histopathological features	Associated malignancies/tumors	Associated syndrome
MITF	Darker hair, fair skin, and non-blue eyes; increased nevus count (mainly reticular pattern under dermoscopy), atypical nevi, depigmented nevi, and amelanotic melanomas; onset of melanoma before age 40 years; multiple primary melanomas; association with renal cell carcinoma in the frame of MITF--related melanoma and renal cell carcinoma predisposition syndrome	Amelanotic melanoma and depigmented nevi; increased Breslow thickness; nodular type of melanoma	Melanoma and pancreatic, breast, and kidney cancers	*MITF*-related melanoma and renal cell carcinoma predisposition syndrome
Emerging genes				
ATM	Not known	Not known	Melanoma and breast, prostate, pancreatic, gastric, colorectal, and ovarian cancers	*ATM* cancer predisposition syndrome
MBD4	Not known	Not known	Uveal melanoma	n/a

melanomas associated with *CDKN2A* mutation do not have a predilection for a certain body site. However, germline *CDKN2A* mutation carriers often present at an earlier age with melanoma diagnosis and multiple primary melanomas [116], superficial spreading melanomas without severe sunburn history [117], and acral and nodular melanomas [118]. *CDKN2A* mutation carriers have significantly more nevi than noncarriers and develop additional nevi during their lifetimes, although melanomas in patients with FAMMM often arise on normal skin [119, 120].

Germline *CDKN2A* mutations are present in at least a quarter of affected families with FAMMM and are associated with an increased risk of pancreatic cancer. The penetrance of *CDKN2A* mutations for pancreatic cancer has been estimated to be 17% by 75 years of age [121]. Few data are available on germline *CDKN2A* mutations in sporadic pancreatic cancer. Eckerle et al. reported that 66% of kindreds with *CDKN2A* mutation had at least 1 of the 10 most common *CDKN2A* mutations, and *CDKN2A* mutation frequency was greater than 60% for p.R112_L113insR and c.225_24del19; 35–50% for p.L32P, p.V126D, and p.G101W; 15–25% for p.R24P and c.-34G > T; and less than 11% for p.M53I, c.IVS2-105A > G, and c.32_33ins9–32 [122].

Rare germline *CDK4* mutations in FAMMM syndrome disrupt p16 binding, affecting cell cycle regulation and leading to overlapping cancer-related phenotypes [123].

Melanoma-Astrocytoma Syndrome

Melanoma-astrocytoma syndrome is a rare hereditary cancer syndrome characterized by the co-occurrence of cutaneous melanoma and central or peripheral nervous system tumors, most notably astrocytomas and neural tumors (neurofibromas and schwannomas), and is mechanistically linked to germline mutations in *CDKN2A* that disrupt the p14ARF transcript [123–125]. Clinical phenotypes among patients with melanoma-astrocytoma syndrome include a spectrum of neural tumors, such as glioblastoma, astrocytoma, meningioma, schwannoma, and neurofibroma, alongside cutaneous melanoma; a notable proportion of patients develop multiple neoplasms. Recent large-scale cohort studies, such as those using the UK Biobank and Geisinger MyCode databases, estimate the prevalence of melanoma-astrocytoma syndrome to be approximately 1 in 39,149 individuals in the UK Biobank and 1 in 170,503 individuals in the Geisinger MyCode cohort, with the majority of affected individuals carrying *CDKN2A* variants that specifically alter p14ARF [126]. Pathogenic variants affecting exon 1β of *CDKN2A*, which encodes p14ARF, have been identified in several families, underscoring the importance of including exon 1β in genetic testing panels for hereditary melanoma, particularly when neural system tumors are present [127, 128]. These findings highlight the necessity of comprehensive genetic evaluation in families with a history of both melanoma and neural tumors to guide surveillance and management strategies.

Melanoma-Subordinate Syndromes

Melanoma-subordinate syndromes, also known as mixed cancer syndromes, are characterized by an elevated risk of melanoma that is comparatively lower than the risk of other associated cancers within these syndromes. These syndromes result from germline mutations in genes such as *PTEN*, *TP53*, *BRCA1*, *BRCA2*, *RB1*, and genes involved in nucleotide excision repair, including those responsible for xeroderma pigmentosum (Table 8.2).

Table 8.2 Melanoma-subordinate syndromes/mixed cancer syndromes

Gene	Syndrome	Phenotype spectrum
PTEN (phosphatase and tensin homolog)	*PTEN* hamartoma tumor syndrome; Cowden syndrome; Lhermitte–Duclos disease; Bannayan–Riley–Ruvalcaba syndrome	Mucocutaneous findings: Trichilemmomas, acral keratosis, mucocutaneous neuromas, oral papillomas Thyroid findings: Thyroiditis, multinodular goiter, adenomas, thyroid cancer Breast cancer Genitourinary findings: Endometrial carcinoma, renal cell carcinoma Gastrointestinal findings: hamartomatous polyps, colorectal cancer Neurological tumors Vascular tumors (vascular malformations) Melanoma Lipomas
TP53 (tumor protein p53)	Li-Fraumeni syndrome	Soft tissue and bone sarcomas Breast carcinoma High-grade gliomas and medulloblastomas Adrenocortical carcinoma Melanoma Stomach, esophageal, colorectal, and pancreatic cancers Leukemia
BRCA1 and *BRCA2* (breast cancer gene 1 and 2)	Hereditary breast and ovarian cancer	Breast and ovarian cancer Other gynecologic cancers: fallopian tube, peritoneal, endometrial Pancreatic, prostate, colorectal, gastric, and biliary cancers Melanoma
RB1 (retinoblastoma 1)	Hereditary retinoblastoma	Retinoblastoma Pineoblastoma Osteosarcoma Soft tissue sarcomas Melanoma

(continued)

Table 8.2 (continued)

Gene	Syndrome	Phenotype spectrum
MLH1 (mutL homolog 1) *MSH2* (mutS homolog 2) *MSH6* (mutS homolog 6) *PMS2* (PMS1 homolog 2, mismatch repair system component) *EPCAM* (epithelial cell adhesion molecule)	Hereditary non-polyposis colorectal cancer (lynch syndrome)	Colorectal cancer Endometrial cancer Cancer of jejunum Genitourinary cancers: ureteral, uterine, renal pelvis Melanoma
DDB2 (damage-specific DNA--binding protein 2) *ERCC1* (ERCC excision repair 1, endonuclease non-catalytic subunit) *ERCC2* (ERCC excision repair 2, TFIIH core complex helicase subunit)	Xeroderma pigmentosum	Extreme sensitivity to light Freckling in early childhood Skin cancers in first decade of life Basal cell carcinomas Squamous cell carcinomas Melanoma Brain tumors, including medulloblastomas, glioblastomas, spinal cord astrocytomas, and schwannomas
WRN (WRN RecQ like helicase)	Werner syndrome	Thyroid cancer Meningioma Sarcoma and osteosarcoma Leukemia/myelodysplasia Melanoma
MUTYH (mutY DNA glycosylase)	*MUTYH*-associated tumor syndrome or *MUTYH*-associated polyposis	Colorectal polyposis Small intestinal, colorectal, and duodenal cancers Breast cancer Ovarian cancer Pancreatic cancer Bladder cancer Melanoma

Genetic Counseling and Management

Screening and surveillance of patients at high risk for hereditary melanoma is an evolving area. Because melanoma syndromes are uncommon, most screening and surveillance recommendations are primarily derived from limited studies or expert consensus. The patient initiating genetic counseling is referred to as the "index case" or "proband." To date, no definitive diagnostic criteria have been identified that allow for the classification of a proband as having hereditary melanoma. Furthermore, guidelines to qualify for genetic counseling vary from country to country. Predictive genetic testing, i.e., testing for a known hereditary variant, should be offered only when the variant in a melanoma predisposition gene is classified as pathogenic or likely pathogenic according to the American College of Medical Genetics and Genomics and the Association for Clinical Pathology standards [129]. While the presence of multiple atypical nevi is associated with a higher likelihood for family members to carry a genetic mutation, the presence of multiple atypical nevi is neither sufficient for diagnosing a proband with hereditary melanoma nor a definitive carrier signature, as noncarriers in families with melanoma-predisposing mutations can also exhibit this phenotype.

CDKN2A

There are no strict selection criteria to identify probands with *CDKN2A* mutations, but Leachman et al. proposed the "rule of 3's" [115], i.e., genetic testing for *CDKN2A* mutations is warranted if a family has one member with invasive cutaneous melanoma and two additional members with either cutaneous melanoma or pancreatic cancer on one side of the family or one individual with three primary cutaneous melanomas. Later, this rule was changed to the "three by 40 rule," i.e., genetic testing for *CDKN2A* mutations is warranted if an individual has three cutaneous melanomas diagnosed before age 40 years [15].

As it was mentioned above, phenotype is not an appropriate tool to establish a carrier state. Thus, three statistical predictive models have been developed to assist in identifying individuals or families with *CDKN2A* mutations: a logistic regression model, MELPREDICT, and its recent modification, GenoMELPREDICT [130, 131]; MelaPRO [132]; and CM score [133].

If genetic testing is chosen, a medical genetic counselor assesses individual medical history, ascertains a three-generation pedigree, and identifies the geographic area where the patient lives as having a high or low incidence of the mutation of interest. If the patient undergoes *CDKN2A* testing and a deleterious mutation is detected, intensive dermatologic surveillance is recommended, including a total body skin check every 3–6 months with possible additional screening tools such as dermoscopy and total body photography, along with a referral to a gastroenterologist for discussion of pancreatic cancer screening. Relatives of *CDKN2A* mutation carriers should continue intensive dermatologic surveillance and adhere to strict sun protection. Furthermore, genetic counseling and regular dermatologic assessments are recommended for all at-risk relatives, irrespective of their test outcomes, to facilitate early detection and prevention of melanoma and other associated cancers. If a patient underwent testing and received a normal *CDKN2A* result ("negative result") or a finding of a "variant of unknown significance," the follow-up depends on the individual and family history. For patients diagnosed with FAMMM, the possibility of an undetected high-risk mutation means their melanoma risk cannot be precisely calculated; thus, they should continue regular dermatologic surveillance [134, 135]. *CDKN2A* mutation carriers also require targeted counseling regarding smoking cessation.

Following appropriate candidate selection and comprehensive patient counseling, genetic testing for high-penetrance melanoma susceptibility genes is advised, especially given that cases of hereditary melanoma from inactivating *CDKN2A* mutations may benefit from *CDK4/6* inhibitor combination therapy [136].

BAP1

The likelihood of identifying a germline *BAP1* pathogenic variant in an individual is increased in individuals with a personal or family history of other *BAP1*-associated neoplasms. Thus, targeted germline *BAP1* testing is most pertinent in cases with a significant personal or family history of *BAP1*-associated neoplasms. Conversely, due to the high rate of somatic *BAP1* variants, in patients with isolated *BAP1*-related tumors without additional features indicative of a germline *BAP1* pathogenic variant (loss of BAP1 by immunohistochemistry, early age of onset, and personal/family history), in whom the detection rate is lower, testing recommendations may be country specific, or testing may be more appropriately conducted within the context of a comprehensive gene panel. Kuzbari et al. recommended that testing for *BAP1* germline variants not be conducted in a patient with a *BAP1*-mutated tumor unless there is at least a 10% chance of detecting a germline variant, calculated by germline conversion rate (GCR: defined by tumor association (pan-tumor/on-tumor) and/or by age (all ages, <30 years, <5 years) and compared this with a predefined GCR threshold of 10%) [137]. Predictive genetic testing should only be offered if the familial variant in *BAP1* is likely pathogenic or pathogenic according to American College of Medical Genetics and Genomics or Association for Clinical Pathology guidelines [138]. More recent guidelines have suggested the addition of young age of onset of a *BAP1*-associated tumor as a reason for testing for *BAP1* germline variants [139].

For individuals with a confirmed germline *BAP1* mutation, Rai et al. recommend the following surveillance tests in an appropriate clinical context: ophthalmologic surveillance annually from age 16 years to age 30 years and every 6 months after age 30 years, dermatologic surveillance every 6 months starting at age 18 years, and at 55 years, a consultation regarding the possibility of a thoraco-abdominal CT or MRI scan every 2 years with renal and chest sonography in the intervals between CT or MRI scan [42]. Individuals carrying a *BAP1* mutation should receive tailored lifestyle guidance, including advice to avoid occupations involving asbestos exposure, be aware of potential asbestos exposure during home renovations, refrain from smoking, and minimize ultraviolet exposure [140].

POT1

Heterozygous germline pathological variant in the *POT1* gene defines the *POT1* tumor predisposition syndrome, which is associated with increased lifetime risks of cutaneous melanoma, chronic lymphocytic leukemias, angiosarcoma (mostly cardiac angiosarcomas), glioma, colorectal cancer, thyroid cancer, other soft tissue sarcomas, osteosarcomas, breast cancer, and lung cancers [141]. There are no established guidelines for surveillance for individuals with *POT1* tumor predisposition syndrome. Baseline surveillance in individuals with a *POT1* germline mutation should include a dermatologic examination to check for cutaneous melanoma, a complete blood cell count, a comprehensive physical examination to check for lymphocytic leukemia, and a brain MRI scan to check for glioma. Calvete O. et al. reported that there is an association between *POT1* mutations and Li-Fraumeni-like (LFL) syndrome, particularly cardiac and breast angiosarcomas [142]. For members of families fulfilling Li-Fraumeni syndrome criteria or confirmed through genetic testing to have Li-Fraumeni-like syndrome, a whole-body MRI scan is recommended to check for angiosarcoma [57, 143]. In 2023, the recommendation was updated that screening for *POT1*-associated cancers be started at age 18 years, as most of these cancers are diagnosed in adulthood [137, 140]. For asymptomatic individuals carrying a *POT1* pathogenic variant, screening should be started at age 18 years or 2 to 5 years before the earliest diagnosis in a family member, whichever comes first. A recent study identified a specific variant, *POT1* p.(I78T), as a founder disease-causing variant associated with early-onset melanoma and additional various solid tumors with a high tumor burden among Ashkenazi Jews; the authors of the study advocated including this variant in genetic testing in appropriate populations [69].

Conclusions

Hereditary melanoma is characterized by mutations in multiple predisposition genes, including *CDKN2A*, *CDK4*, *BAP1*, *TERT*, *POT1*, *ACD*, *TERF2IP*, and *MITF*. These genetic alterations not only elevate the risk of melanoma but also predispose individuals to other types of cancer. Advances in genetic testing have enabled early identification of mutation carriers, facilitating personalized surveillance strategies aimed at early detection and prevention of melanoma and associated cancers. However, significant challenges persist in the field of hereditary melanoma. Unidentified high-penetrance genetic variants likely contribute to melanoma risk in certain families, and the roles and interactions of medium- and low-penetrance variants in melanoma susceptibility remain incompletely understood. Furthermore, genotype-phenotype correlations, including how specific genetic variants influence melanoma development, clinical features, and progression, are not fully elucidated. Ongoing research aims to address these knowledge gaps, refine testing strategies, and develop more accurate risk assessment tools and personalized management approaches for at-risk individuals and families.

References

1. American Cancer Society. Cancer facts and figures 2023. 2023: Atlanta: American Cancer Society.
2. Saginala K, et al. Epidemiology of Melanoma. Med Sci (Basel). 2021;9(4):63.

3. Debniak T. Familial malignant melanoma – overview. Hered Cancer Clin Pract. 2004;2(3):123–9.
4. Ribeiro Moura Brasil Arnaut J, et al. Molecular landscape of hereditary melanoma. Crit Rev Oncol Hematol. 2021;164:103425.
5. Hansen CB, et al. Clinical germline genetic testing for melanoma. Lancet Oncol. 2004;5(5):314–9.
6. Marzuka-Alcala A, Gabree MJ, Tsao H. Melanoma susceptibility genes and risk assessment. Methods Mol Biol. 2014;1102:381–93.
7. Anderson DE, Smith JL Jr, McBride CM. Hereditary aspects of malignant melanoma. JAMA. 1967;200(9):741–6.
8. Cakir A, et al. Phenotypic and genetic features that differ between hereditary and sporadic melanoma: results of a preliminary study from a single center from Turkey. Dermatol Pract Concept. 2023;13(3):e2023146.
9. Czene K, Lichtenstein P, Hemminki K. Environmental and heritable causes of cancer among 9.6 million individuals in the Swedish family-cancer database. Int J Cancer. 2002;99(2):260–6.
10. Tsao H. Update on familial cancer syndromes and the skin. J Am Acad Dermatol. 2000;42(6):939–69. quiz 970–2
11. Zocchi L, et al. Familial melanoma and susceptibility genes: a review of the Most common clinical and Dermoscopic phenotypic aspect, associated malignancies and practical tips for management. J Clin Med. 2021;10(16):3760.
12. Zheng C, Sarin KY. Unveiling the genetic landscape of hereditary melanoma: from susceptibility to surveillance. Cancer Treat Res Commun. 2024;40:100837.
13. Debniak T, et al. Increased risk of breast cancer in relatives of malignant melanoma patients from families with strong cancer familial aggregation. Eur J Cancer Prev. 2003;12(3):241–5.
14. Helgadottir H, et al. Germline CDKN2A mutation status and survival in familial melanoma cases. J Natl Cancer Inst. 2016;108(11):djw135.
15. Soura E, et al. Hereditary melanoma: update on syndromes and management: genetics of familial atypical multiple mole melanoma syndrome. J Am Acad Dermatol. 2016;74(3):395–407. quiz 408–10
16. Goldstein AM, et al. Features associated with germline CDKN2A mutations: a GenoMEL study of melanoma-prone families from three continents. J Med Genet. 2007;44(2):99–106.
17. Xiao F, et al. Natural and orthogonal model for estimating gene-gene interactions applied to cutaneous melanoma. Hum Genet. 2014;133(5):559–74.
18. Maccioni L, et al. Variants at the 9p21 locus and melanoma risk. BMC Cancer. 2013;13:325.
19. Salgado C, et al. Genome-wide analysis of constitutional DNA methylation in familial melanoma. Clin Epigenetics. 2020;12(1):43.
20. Domchek SM, et al. Multiplex genetic testing for cancer susceptibility: out on the high wire without a net? J Clin Oncol. 2013;31(10):1267–70.
21. Read J, Wadt KA, Hayward NK. Melanoma genetics. J Med Genet. 2016;53(1):1–14.
22. Bruno W, et al. Multiple primary melanomas (MPMs) and criteria for genetic assessment: MultiMEL, a multicenter study of the Italian Melanoma Intergroup. J Am Acad Dermatol. 2016;74(2):325–32.
23. Goldstein AM, Tucker MA. Genetic epidemiology of cutaneous melanoma: a global perspective. Arch Dermatol. 2001;137(11):1493–6.
24. Harland M, et al. Prevalence and predictors of germline CDKN2A mutations for melanoma cases from Australia, Spain and the United Kingdom. Hered Cancer Clin Pract. 2014;12(1):20.
25. Bishop JA, et al. Genotype/phenotype and penetrance studies in melanoma families with germline CDKN2A mutations. J Invest Dermatol. 2000;114(1):28–33.
26. de Snoo FA, et al. Genome-wide linkage scan for atypical nevi in p16-Leiden melanoma families. Eur J Hum Genet. 2008;16(9):1135–41.
27. Shain AH, et al. The genetic evolution of melanoma from precursor lesions. N Engl J Med. 2015;373(20):1926–36.

28. Goldstein AM, et al. High-risk melanoma susceptibility genes and pancreatic cancer, neural system tumors, and uveal melanoma across GenoMEL. Cancer Res. 2006;66(20):9818–28.
29. Aguilera P, et al. Clinical and histopathological characteristics between familial and sporadic melanoma in Barcelona, Spain. J Clin Exp Dermatol Res. 2014;5(5):231.
30. Sargen MR, et al. Histologic features of melanoma associated with CDKN2A genotype. J Am Acad Dermatol. 2015;72(3):496–507 e7.
31. Gironi LC, et al. Melanoma-prone families: new evidence of distinctive clinical and histological features of melanomas in CDKN2A mutation carriers. Arch Dermatol Res. 2018;310(10):769–84.
32. Cust AE, et al. Melanoma risk for CDKN2A mutation carriers who are relatives of population-based case carriers in Australia and the UK. J Med Genet. 2011;48(4):266–72.
33. Bishop DT, et al. Geographical variation in the penetrance of CDKN2A mutations for melanoma. J Natl Cancer Inst. 2002;94(12):894–903.
34. Helgadottir H, et al. High risk of tobacco-related cancers in CDKN2A mutation-positive melanoma families. J Med Genet. 2014;51(8):545–52.
35. McWilliams RR, et al. Prevalence of CDKN2A mutations in pancreatic cancer patients: implications for genetic counseling. Eur J Hum Genet. 2011;19(4):472–8.
36. Danishevich A, et al. CDKN2A gene mutations: implications for hereditary cancer syndromes. Biomedicine. 2023;11(12):3343.
37. Tucker MA, et al. A natural history of melanomas and dysplastic nevi: an atlas of lesions in melanoma-prone families. Cancer. 2002;94(12):3192–209.
38. Lee KC, Higgins HW 2nd, Qureshi AA. Familial risk of melanoma and links with other cancers. Melanoma Manag. 2015;2(1):83–9.
39. Marusic Z, Buljan M, Busam KJ. Histomorphologic spectrum of BAP1 negative melanocytic neoplasms in a family with BAP1-associated cancer susceptibility syndrome. J Cutan Pathol. 2015;42(6):406–12.
40. Masoomian B, Shields JA, Shields CL. Overview of BAP1 cancer predisposition syndrome and the relationship to uveal melanoma. J Curr Ophthalmol. 2018;30(2):102–9.
41. Njauw CN, et al. Germline BAP1 inactivation is preferentially associated with metastatic ocular melanoma and cutaneous-ocular melanoma families. PLoS One. 2012;7(4):e35295.
42. Rai K, et al. Comprehensive review of BAP1 tumor predisposition syndrome with report of two new cases. Clin Genet. 2016;89(3):285–94.
43. Zhang AJ, et al. BRCA1-associated protein (BAP1)-inactivated melanocytic tumors. J Cutan Pathol. 2019;46(12):965–72.
44. Haugh AM, et al. Genotypic and phenotypic features of BAP1 cancer syndrome: a report of 8 new families and review of cases in the literature. JAMA Dermatol. 2017;153(10):999–1006.
45. Garfield EM, et al. Histomorphologic spectrum of germline-related and sporadic BAP1-inactivated melanocytic tumors. J Am Acad Dermatol. 2018;79(3):525–34.
46. Wiesner T, et al. Germline mutations in BAP1 predispose to melanocytic tumors. Nat Genet. 2011;43(10):1018–21.
47. Griewank KG, et al. SF3B1 and BAP1 mutations in blue nevus-like melanoma. Mod Pathol. 2017;30(7):928–39.
48. Carbone M, et al. BAP1 and cancer. Nat Rev Cancer. 2013;13(3):153–9.
49. Donati M, Steiner P, Kazakov DV. BAP1-inactivated melanoma arising from BAP1-inactivated melanocytic tumor in a patient with BAP1 germline mutation: a case report and review of the literature. Am J Dermatopathol. 2023;45(2):117–22.
50. Grisham EA, Tadros J, Smith E. Unique Dermoscopic and histopathologic features of melanoma arising in a patient with BAP1 tumor predisposition syndrome. Cureus. 2021;13(8):e17485.
51. Lebensohn A, et al. Multiple Onychopapillomas and BAP1 tumor predisposition syndrome. JAMA Dermatol. 2024;160(8):838–45.
52. Glousker G, et al. Human shelterin protein POT1 prevents severe telomere instability induced by homology-directed DNA repair. EMBO J. 2020;39(23):e104500.

53. Robles-Espinoza CD, et al. POT1 loss-of-function variants predispose to familial melanoma. Nat Genet. 2014;46(5):478–81.
54. Shi J, et al. Rare missense variants in POT1 predispose to familial cutaneous malignant melanoma. Nat Genet. 2014;46(5):482–6.
55. Burke LS, et al. Telomere length and the risk of cutaneous malignant melanoma in melanoma-prone families with and without CDKN2A mutations. PLoS One. 2013;8(8):e71121.
56. Sargen MR, et al. Histologic features of melanoma associated with germline mutations of CDKN2A, CDK4, and POT1 in melanoma-prone families from the United States, Italy, and Spain. J Am Acad Dermatol. 2020;83(3):860–9.
57. Herrera-Mullar J, et al. Characterization of POT1 tumor predisposition syndrome: tumor prevalence in a clinically diverse hereditary cancer cohort. Genet Med. 2023;25(11):100937.
58. Shen E, et al. POT1 mutation spectrum in tumour types commonly diagnosed among POT1-associated hereditary cancer syndrome families. J Med Genet. 2020;57(10):664–70.
59. Aoude LG, et al. Nonsense mutations in the shelterin complex genes ACD and TERF2IP in familial melanoma. J Natl Cancer Inst. 2015;107(2):dju408.
60. Wilson TL, et al. A new POT1 germline mutation-expanding the spectrum of POT1-associated cancers. Fam Cancer. 2017;16(4):561–6.
61. Deregowska A, Wnuk M. RAP1/TERF2IP-A multifunctional player in cancer development. Cancers (Basel). 2021;13(23):5970.
62. Li J, et al. A rare variant P507L in TPP1 interrupts TPP1-TIN2 interaction, influences telomere length, and confers colorectal cancer risk in Chinese population. Cancer Epidemiol Biomarkers Prev. 2018;27(9):1029–35.
63. Yuan X, Dai M, Xu D. Telomere-related markers for cancer. Curr Top Med Chem. 2020;20(6):410–32.
64. Dratwa M, et al. TERT-regulation and roles in cancer formation. Front Immunol. 2020;11:589929.
65. Populo H, et al. TERT promoter mutations in skin cancer: the effects of sun exposure and X-irradiation. J Invest Dermatol. 2014;134(8):2251–7.
66. Harland M, et al. Germline TERT promoter mutations are rare in familial melanoma. Fam Cancer. 2016;15(1):139–44.
67. Hugdahl E, et al. Prognostic impact and concordance of TERT promoter mutation and protein expression in matched primary and metastatic cutaneous melanoma. Br J Cancer. 2018;118(1):98–105.
68. Horn S, et al. TERT promoter mutations in familial and sporadic melanoma. Science. 2013;339(6122):959–61.
69. Abu Shtaya A, et al. A POT1 founder variant associated with early onset recurrent melanoma and various solid malignancies. Genes (Basel). 2024;15(3):355.
70. Zaremba A, et al. Clinical and pathological characteristics of familial melanoma with germline TERT promoter variants. Pigment Cell Melanoma Res. 2022;35(6):573–86.
71. Orlow I, et al. Genetic factors associated with naevus count and dermoscopic patterns: preliminary results from the Study of Nevi in Children (SONIC). Br J Dermatol. 2015;172(4):1081–9.
72. Yuan X, Larsson C, Xu D. Mechanisms underlying the activation of TERT transcription and telomerase activity in human cancer: old actors and new players. Oncogene. 2019;38(34):6172–83.
73. Chen S, et al. Targeting MC1R depalmitoylation to prevent melanomagenesis in redheads. Nat Commun. 2019;10(1):877.
74. Tagliabue E, et al. MC1R gene variants and non-melanoma skin cancer: a pooled-analysis from the M-SKIP project. Br J Cancer. 2015;113(2):354–63.
75. Hacker E, et al. NRAS and BRAF mutations in cutaneous melanoma and the association with MC1R genotype: findings from Spanish and Austrian populations. J Invest Dermatol. 2013;133(4):1027–33.
76. Thomas NE, et al. Associations of MC1R genotype and patient phenotypes with BRAF and NRAS mutations in melanoma. J Invest Dermatol. 2017;137(12):2588–98.

77. Fargnoli MC, et al. MC1R variants increase risk of melanomas harboring BRAF mutations. J Invest Dermatol. 2008;128(10):2485–90.
78. Kanetsky PA, Hay JL. Marshaling the translational potential of MC1R for precision risk assessment of melanoma. Cancer Prev Res (Phila). 2018;11(3):121–4.
79. Pasquali E, et al. MC1R variants increased the risk of sporadic cutaneous melanoma in darker-pigmented Caucasians: a pooled-analysis from the M-SKIP project. Int J Cancer. 2015;136(3):618–31.
80. Cust AE, et al. MC1R genotypes and risk of melanoma before age 40 years: a population-based case-control-family study. Int J Cancer. 2012;131(3):E269–81.
81. Pellegrini C, et al. Characterization of melanoma susceptibility genes in high-risk patients from Central Italy. Melanoma Res. 2017;27(3):258–67.
82. Demenais F, et al. Association of MC1R variants and host phenotypes with melanoma risk in CDKN2A mutation carriers: a GenoMEL study. J Natl Cancer Inst. 2010;102(20):1568–83.
83. Manganelli M, et al. Behind the scene: exploiting MC1R in skin cancer risk and prevention. Genes. 2021;12(7):1093.
84. Tagliabue E, et al. MC1R variants as melanoma risk factors independent of at-risk phenotypic characteristics: a pooled analysis from the M-SKIP project. Cancer Manag Res. 2018;10:1143–54.
85. Bassoli S, et al. CDKN2A and MC1R variants influence dermoscopic and confocal features of benign melanocytic lesions in multiple melanoma patients. Exp Dermatol. 2013;22(6):411–6.
86. Taylor NJ, et al. Inherited variation at MC1R and histological characteristics of primary melanoma. PLoS One. 2015;10(3):e0119920.
87. Hartman ML, Czyz M. MITF in melanoma: mechanisms behind its expression and activity. Cell Mol Life Sci. 2015;72(7):1249–60.
88. Bertolotto C, et al. A SUMOylation-defective MITF germline mutation predisposes to melanoma and renal carcinoma. Nature. 2011;480(7375):94–8.
89. Yokoyama S, et al. A novel recurrent mutation in MITF predisposes to familial and sporadic melanoma. Nature. 2011;480(7375):99–103.
90. Berwick M, et al. MITF E318K's effect on melanoma risk independent of, but modified by, other risk factors. Pigment Cell Melanoma Res. 2014;27(3):485–8.
91. Sturm RA, et al. Phenotypic characterization of nevus and tumor patterns in MITF E318K mutation carrier melanoma patients. J Invest Dermatol. 2014;134(1):141–9.
92. Potrony M, et al. Prevalence of MITF p.E318K in patients with melanoma independent of the presence of CDKN2A causative mutations. JAMA Dermatol. 2016;152(4):405–12.
93. Grill C, et al. MITF mutations associated with pigment deficiency syndromes and melanoma have different effects on protein function. Hum Mol Genet. 2013;22(21):4357–67.
94. Ghiorzo P, et al. Prevalence of the E318K MITF germline mutation in Italian melanoma patients: associations with histological subtypes and family cancer history. Pigment Cell Melanoma Res. 2013;26(2):259–62.
95. Gudbjartsson DF, et al. ASIP and TYR pigmentation variants associate with cutaneous melanoma and basal cell carcinoma. Nat Genet. 2008;40(7):886–91.
96. Bishop DT, et al. Genome-wide association study identifies three loci associated with melanoma risk. Nat Genet. 2009;41(8):920–5.
97. Jannot AS, et al. Allele variations in the OCA2 gene (pink-eyed-dilution locus) are associated with genetic susceptibility to melanoma. Eur J Hum Genet. 2005;13(8):913–20.
98. Fernandez LP, et al. SLC45A2: a novel malignant melanoma-associated gene. Hum Mutat. 2008;29(9):1161–7.
99. Nan HM, et al. Genetic variants in pigmentation genes, pigmentary phenotypes, and risk of skin cancer in Caucasians. Int J Cancer. 2009;125(4):909–17.
100. Bertrand JU, et al. Melanoma risk and melanocyte biology. Acta Derm Venereol. 2020;100(11):adv00139.
101. Nan H, et al. Genome-wide association study identifies nidogen 1 (NID1) as a susceptibility locus to cutaneous nevi and melanoma risk. Hum Mol Genet. 2011;20(13):2673–9.

102. Kvaskoff M, et al. Polymorphisms in nevus-associated genes MTAP, PLA2G6, and IRF4 and the risk of invasive cutaneous melanoma. Twin Res Hum Genet. 2011;14(5):422–32.
103. Pastorino L, et al. Insights into genetic susceptibility to melanoma by gene panel testing: potential pathogenic variants in ACD, ATM, BAP1, and POT1. Cancers (Basel). 2020;12(4):1007.
104. Lendinez-Sanchez G, et al. ATM variant as a cause of hereditary cutaneous melanoma in a Spanish family: case report. Case Rep Oncol. 2024;17(1):386–91.
105. Dalmasso B, et al. Germline ATM variants predispose to melanoma: a joint analysis across the GenoMEL and MelaNostrum consortia. Genet Med. 2021;23(11):2087–95.
106. Derrien AC, et al. Germline MBD4 mutations and predisposition to uveal melanoma. J Natl Cancer Inst. 2021;113(1):80–7.
107. Rodrigues M, et al. Outlier response to anti-PD1 in uveal melanoma reveals germline MBD4 mutations in hypermutated tumors. Nat Commun. 2018;9(1):1866.
108. Degasperi A, et al. Substitution mutational signatures in whole-genome-sequenced cancers in the UK population. Science. 2022;376(6591):eabl9283.
109. Yoon JH, et al. Human thymine DNA glycosylase (TDG) and methyl-CpG-binding protein 4 (MBD4) excise thymine glycol (Tg) from a Tg:G mispair. Nucleic Acids Res. 2003;31(18):5399–404.
110. Saint-Ghislain M, et al. Deficiency is predictive of response to immune checkpoint inhibitors in metastatic uveal melanoma patients: a retrospective study. J Clin Oncol. 2022;40(16):e21601.
111. Johansson PA, et al. Prolonged stable disease in a uveal melanoma patient with germline MBD4 nonsense mutation treated with pembrolizumab and ipilimumab. Immunogenetics. 2019;71(5–6):433–6.
112. Villy MC, et al. Familial uveal melanoma and other tumors in 25 families with monoallelic germline MBD4 variants. J Natl Cancer Inst. 2024;116(4):580–7.
113. Gillgren P, et al. Body site of cutaneous malignant melanoma–a study on patients with hereditary and multiple sporadic tumours. Melanoma Res. 2003;13(3):279–86.
114. Hornbuckle J, et al. Patterns of metastases in familial and non-familial melanoma. Melanoma Res. 2003;13(1):105–9.
115. Leachman SA, et al. Selection criteria for genetic assessment of patients with familial melanoma. J Am Acad Dermatol. 2009;61(4):677.e1–14.
116. Puig S, et al. Role of the CDKN2A locus in patients with multiple primary melanomas. J Clin Oncol. 2005;23(13):3043–51.
117. Taylor NJ, et al. Phenotypic and histopathological tumor characteristics according to CDKN2A mutation status among affected members of melanoma families. J Invest Dermatol. 2016;136(5):1066–9.
118. Visconti A, et al. Body site-specific genetic effects influence naevus count distribution in women. Pigment Cell Melanoma Res. 2020;33(2):326–33.
119. Czajkowski R, et al. FAMMM syndrome: pathogenesis and management. Dermatologic Surg. 2004;30(2 Pt 2):291–6.
120. Kelly JW, et al. A high incidence of melanoma found in patients with multiple dysplastic naevi by photographic surveillance. Med J Aust. 1997;167(4):191–4.
121. Vasen HF, et al. Risk of developing pancreatic cancer in families with familial atypical multiple mole melanoma associated with a specific 19 deletion of p16 (p16-Leiden). Int J Cancer. 2000;87(6):809–11.
122. Eckerle Mize, D., et al. Familial atypical multiple mole melanoma syndrome. In Riegert-Johnson DL, et al., editors. Cancer syndromes. 2009. Bethesda.
123. Randerson-Moor JA, et al. A germline deletion of p14(ARF) but not CDKN2A in a melanoma-neural system tumour syndrome family. Hum Mol Genet. 2001;10(1):55–62.
124. Chan AK, et al. Familial melanoma-astrocytoma syndrome: synchronous diffuse astrocytoma and pleomorphic xanthoastrocytoma in a patient with germline CDKN2A/B deletion and a significant family history. Clin Neuropathol. 2017;36(5):213–21.

125. Petronzelli F, et al. CDKN2A germline splicing mutation affecting both p16(ink4) and p14(arf) RNA processing in a melanoma/neurofibroma kindred. Genes Chromosomes Cancer. 2001;31(4):398–401.
126. Sargen MR, et al. Estimated prevalence, tumor Spectrum, and Neurofibromatosis type 1-like phenotype of CDKN2A-related melanoma-astrocytoma syndrome. JAMA Dermatol. 2023;159(10):1112–8.
127. Laud K, et al. Comprehensive analysis of CDKN2A (p16INK4A/p14ARF) and CDKN2B genes in 53 melanoma index cases considered to be at heightened risk of melanoma. J Med Genet. 2006;43(1):39–47.
128. Lesueur F, et al. The contribution of large genomic deletions at the CDKN2A locus to the burden of familial melanoma. Br J Cancer. 2008;99(2):364–70.
129. American College of Medical Genetics and Genomics. Practice Guidelines. Available from: https://www.acmg.net/ACMG/Medical-Genetics-Practice-Resources/Practice-Guidelines.aspx
130. Niendorf KB, et al. MELPREDICT: a logistic regression model to estimate CDKN2A carrier probability. J Med Genet. 2006;43(6):501–6.
131. Taylor NJ, et al. Estimating CDKN2A mutation carrier probability among global familial melanoma cases using GenoMELPREDICT. J Am Acad Dermatol. 2019;81(2):386–94.
132. Wang W, et al. Estimating CDKN2A carrier probability and personalizing cancer risk assessments in hereditary melanoma using MelaPRO. Cancer Res. 2010;70(2):552–9.
133. Potjer TP, et al. CM-score: a validated scoring system to predict CDKN2A germline mutations in melanoma families from northern Europe. J Med Genet. 2018;55(10):661–8.
134. Pauley K, et al. Considerations for germline testing in melanoma: updates in behavioral change and pancreatic surveillance for carriers of CDKN2A pathogenic variants. Front Oncol. 2022;12:837057.
135. Morton RL, Francken AB, Dieng M. Surveillance and follow-up of melanoma patients. In: Balch Cutaneous Melanoma, 2020.
136. Kreuger IZM, et al. Therapeutic strategies for targeting CDKN2A loss in melanoma. J Invest Dermatol. 2023;143(1):18–25.e1.
137. Kuzbari Z, et al. Germline-focused analysis of tumour-detected variants in 49,264 cancer patients: ESMO precision medicine working group recommendations. Ann Oncol. 2023;34(3):215–27.
138. Richards S, et al. Standards and guidelines for the interpretation of sequence variants: a joint consensus recommendation of the American College of Medical Genetics and Genomics and the Association for Molecular Pathology. Genet Med. 2015;17(5):405–24.
139. Chau C, et al. Families with BAP1-tumor predisposition syndrome in The Netherlands: path to identification and a proposal for genetic screening guidelines. Cancers (Basel). 2019;11(8):1114.
140. Lalloo F, et al. Clinical practice guidelines for the diagnosis and surveillance of BAP1 tumour predisposition syndrome. Eur J Hum Genet. 2023;31(11):1261–9.
141. Andreotti V, et al. Germline POT1 variants: a critical perspective on POT1 tumor predisposition syndrome. Genes (Basel). 2024;15(1):104.
142. Calvete O, et al. A mutation in the POT1 gene is responsible for cardiac angiosarcoma in TP53-negative Li-Fraumeni-like families. Nat Commun. 2015;6:8383.
143. Henry ML, Osborne J, Else T. POT1 Tumor Predisposition. In: Adam MP, et al., editors. GeneReviews((R)). Seattle; 1993.

Chapter 9
Family of Heavily Pigmented Melanocytic Neoplasms: From Blue Nevi and *PKC*-Fused Melanocytic Neoplasms to *PRKAR1A*-Inactivated Pigmented Epithelioid Melanocytomas

Woo Cheal Cho

Blue Nevus

Clinical Features

Blue nevi (BNs) can arise at any age but most commonly occur in children and young adults, with a female predilection [1, 2]. They are broadly classified into two main subtypes: common BN (also known as dendritic BN) and cellular BN (CBN). Common BNs most frequently appear on the dorsal aspects of the distal extremities and the face, whereas CBNs are more commonly found on the buttocks, sacrococcygeal region, and scalp [1–3]. In addition to cutaneous sites, BNs may also arise in extracutaneous locations, including lymph nodes, mucosae, and soft tissues [4, 5].

Clinically, common BNs typically present as blue to gray or blue to black macules or dome-shaped papules, usually measuring less than 10 mm in diameter [1, 2]. CBNs, while similar in color and shape, generally present as larger nodules, with diameters ranging from 10 to 30 mm [2, 3]. Occasionally, BNs may lack pigmentation, referred to as amelanotic or hypomelanotic BNs. A rare variant, the plaque-type BNs, typically present at birth or in early childhood as a large plaque—often several centimeters in diameter—or as a confluence of multiple smaller macules and/or papules. These lesions most frequently occur on the scalp, although other locations have also been reported [6]. In rare cases, BNs may be clustered within a localized anatomical region, a presentation termed agminated BN.

W. C. Cho (✉)
Department of Anatomical Pathology, The University of Texas MD Anderson Cancer Center, Houston, TX, USA
e-mail: wcho@mdanderson.org

V. G. Prieto, C. A. Torres-Cabala (eds.), *Precision Molecular Pathology of Melanocytic Lesions*, Molecular Pathology Library,
https://doi.org/10.1007/978-3-032-18222-7_9

The term "atypical" CBN has been proposed to describe lesions with histopathologic features that fall between conventional CBNs and melanomas arising in blue nevi (MBNs). These lesions exhibit significant cytologic and architectural atypia that raises concern for malignancy yet falls short of the criteria required for a definitive diagnosis of melanoma (e.g., prominent cytologic atypia, increased mitotic figures, and necrosis). At present, clear diagnostic criteria for atypical CBNs are lacking, leading to occasional disagreement among experienced dermatopathologists regarding the distinction between atypical CBNs and MBNs [7]. Limited follow-up data suggest that atypical CBNs generally follow a favorable clinical course [8–10], although there have been instances of local recurrence and regional lymph node involvement [11, 12]. As such, the use of the qualifier "atypical" may be a prudent approach to convey diagnostic uncertainty and highlight the lesion's indeterminate biologic potential while avoiding the premature labeling of it as melanoma [1]. Atypical CBNs most often occur on the trunk and extremities and have been reported across a broad age range [10].

Histopathologic Features

BNs often demonstrate overlapping histopathologic features of both common BNs and CBNs, and their classification is typically based on the predominant component observed upon microscopic examination.

Common BNs are characterized by an ill-defined intradermal proliferation of spindled, dendritic melanocytes, frequently arranged in an inverted wedge-shaped configuration (Fig. 9.1a). These melanocytes often extend into the deep reticular dermis along adnexal structures and neurovascular bundles. The stroma commonly exhibits varying degrees of fibroplasia and melanin pigmentation. Pigment is present within dendritic melanocytes and, more often, in associated stromal

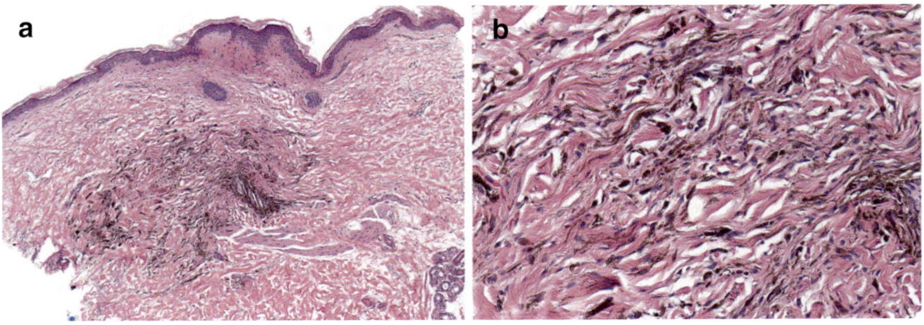

Fig. 9.1 An example of a common blue nevus showing an ill-defined intradermal proliferation of spindled, dendritic melanocytes (**a**) (hematoxylin and eosin, original magnification ×100). The lesional melanocytes exhibit slender, spindle-shaped, bluish-purple nuclei with small nucleoli, and their cytoplasm is amphophilic, with elongated, branching dendritic processes that are typically heavily pigmented (**b**) (hematoxylin and eosin, original magnification ×400)

macrophages. A junctional component is generally absent unless the lesion is part of a combined nevus. The melanocytes display slender, spindle-shaped, bluish-purple nuclei with small nucleoli, and their cytoplasm is amphophilic with elongated, branching dendritic processes that are typically heavily pigmented (Fig. 9.1b). Nuclear atypia and mitotic counts are absent or inconspicuous.

In some cases, common BNs may exhibit marked stromal fibroplasia accompanied by only a subtle proliferation of bland spindled melanocytes. This sclerosing or sclerotic variant, also known as desmoplastic BNs, can mimic desmoplastic melanomas morphologically [1, 2]. A helpful diagnostic clue is the presence of lesional dendritic melanocytes at the periphery of the lesion [2]. Another rare variant, the hypomelanotic/amelanotic BNs, contain minimal to no melanin pigment, which may lead to diagnostic confusion with non-melanocytic spindle cell neoplasms such as dermatofibromas [1, 2] (Fig. 9.2a–c). Epithelioid BNs, which may occur sporadically or in association with Carney complex (a subset of which involves mutations in the *PRKAR1A* gene), are composed predominantly of epithelioid melanocytes with heavily pigmented cytoplasm and exhibit morphologic overlap with pigmented epithelioid melanocytomas (PEMs). Additionally, an epithelioid and fusiform

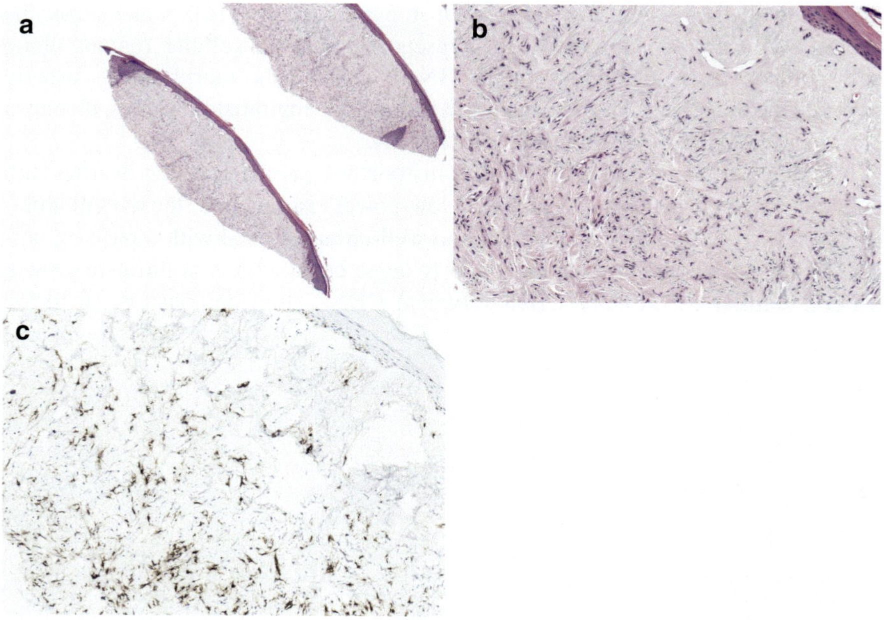

Fig. 9.2 An example of the hypopigmented/amelanotic variant of a common blue nevus showing an ill-defined intradermal proliferation of banal-appearing spindled cells (**a**) (hematoxylin and eosin, original magnification ×40); (**b**) (hematoxylin and eosin, original magnification ×200). Given the lack of significant melanin pigment in the lesional cells, this lesion may lead to diagnostic confusion with other non-melanocytic spindle cell neoplasms, such as dermatofibromas. Diffuse expression of HMB45 in the lesional cells confirms the diagnosis of blue nevus in this case (**c**) (HMB45, original magnification ×200)

variant of BNs arising in chronically sun-damaged skin—without association with Carney complex or *PRKAR1A* mutations—has also been described [13].

CBNs typically exhibit a biphasic growth pattern composed of areas resembling conventional common BNs interspersed with distinct, cellular regions of spindled to ovoid melanocytes [3] (Fig. 9.3a–b). These cellular areas frequently extend vertically into the deep reticular dermis and subcutis, often forming a bulbous or dumbbell-shaped configuration with a pushing growth pattern. Epidermal hyperplasia and a junctional melanocytic proliferation are typically absent. Occasionally, CBNs present as sharply circumscribed dermal nests or nodules composed of fusiform to ovoid melanocytes, separated by collagen bundles and admixed with numerous pigmented melanophages [10]. The stroma may show variable alterations, including myxoid, edematous, or hyalinized/fibrotic changes [1, 3].

Cytologically, the melanocytes within the cellular areas have oval to spindle-shaped, bluish to purple nuclei with finely stippled chromatin and small, visible nucleoli. Their cytoplasm is clear to amphophilic and only mildly pigmented. Mitotic counts are generally low or absent (<1–2 mitoses/mm^2), and features such as high-grade nuclear atypia, necrosis, or ulceration are typically absent [1, 2].

Rarely, CBNs may present with minimal or no melanin pigment and contain few melanophages. This hypomelanotic/amelanotic variant of CBN poses a significant diagnostic challenge both clinically and histopathologically [14]. Nonetheless, the overall architecture—particularly the presence of distinct cellular regions along with components resembling common BNs with dendritic morphology—usually supports the diagnosis. An additional rare variant, the angiomatoid CBNs, display a prominent vascular or angioma-like pattern [15].

Atypical CBNs, by definition, display histopathologic features that overlap with both conventional CBNs and MBNs. On low-power examination, the overall architecture may be relatively symmetrical and well-circumscribed with a pushing border (Fig. 9.4a), or asymmetrical and poorly demarcated with an infiltrative growth pattern. Similar to ordinary CBNs, atypical CBNs often demonstrate dendritic

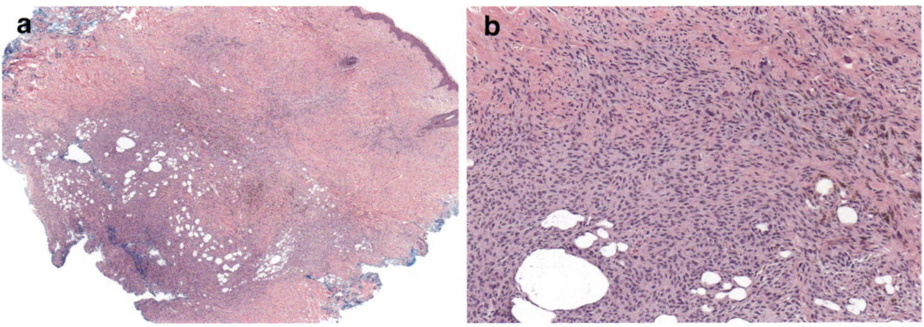

Fig. 9.3 An example of a cellular blue nevus showing conventional spindled, dendritic pigmented melanocytes admixed with distinct, cellular regions composed of spindled to ovoid melanocytes (**a**) (hematoxylin and eosin, original magnification ×40); (**b**) (hematoxylin and eosin, original magnification ×200). These cellular areas frequently extend vertically into the deep reticular dermis and subcutis (**b**)

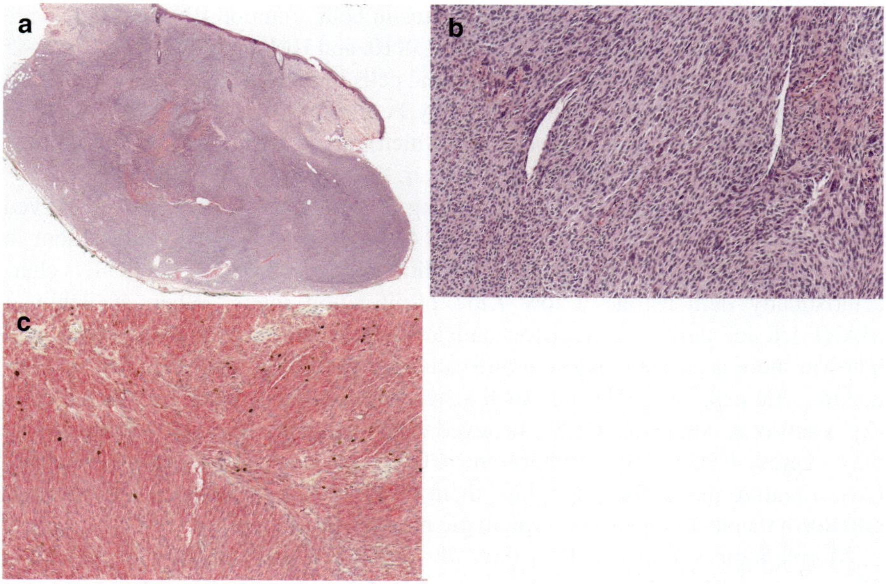

Fig. 9.4 An example of an atypical cellular blue nevus showing a dermal melanocytic proliferation with a bulbous and somewhat dumbbell-shaped configuration and a pushing growth pattern (**a**) (hematoxylin and eosin, original magnification ×20), resembling a conventional cellular blue nevus. However, the lesional melanocytes occasionally exhibit nuclear atypia and increased mitotic activity (**b**) (hematoxylin and eosin, original magnification ×200). A slightly increased Ki-67 proliferation index of approximately 2–3% is also noted in some areas (**c**) (MART-1/Ki-67, original magnification ×200)

morphology and distinct cellular areas composed of spindled to ovoid melanocytes. However, atypical CBNs also exhibit one or more worrisome features suggestive of melanoma, including large size (occasionally exceeding 50 mm in diameter), focal high-grade nuclear atypia, or increased mitotic counts—rarely up to 3–4 mitoses/mm^2, with some mitotic figures located deep within the lesion [16] (Fig. 9.4b). Atypical mitotic figures, however, are notably absent in atypical CBNs [16]. Although rare, focal ulceration or tumor necrosis may also be present [16]. Nonetheless, because distinguishing atypical CBNs from MBNs based on morphology alone is often challenging, additional immunohistochemical—and, in some cases, molecular—studies are invariably required for accurate classification.

Immunophenotypic Features

Immunohistochemical studies are generally not required for the diagnosis of common BNs. However, they can be valuable in challenging cases—such as superficial or partial biopsies—or for evaluating the aforementioned morphologic variants.

Immunophenotypically, lesional melanocytes in both common BNs and CBNs are typically positive for MART-1/Melan-A, SOX10, and HMB-45 [1, 2, 16]. HMB-45 labeling is usually diffuse across the lesional cells in both subtypes [2, 17]. In contrast, S100 expression is variable and may be completely absent, particularly in hypomelanotic/amelanotic variants [18], which may present a diagnostic pitfall if interpretation relies solely on a single marker.

Lesional melanocytes in BNs, including CBNs, consistently show preserved expression of BAP1 [19, 20] and p16. PRAME expression is typically absent in both common BNs and CBNs [21, 22]. Additionally, common BNs and CBNs characteristically demonstrate a low Ki67 proliferation index. When available, a MART-1/K-i67 dual immunohistochemical study is preferable to Ki-67 alone, as it helps to more accurately assess proliferation by excluding from the analysis non-melanocytic cells in the dermis, such as reactive lymphocytes or endothelial cells [2]. A subset of congenital CBNs, believed to be related to neurocristic hamartomas, may express CD34 [23]. Furthermore, CBNs lack nuclear β-catenin expression [24], a feature that helps distinguish them from WNT-activated deep penetrating/plexiform melanocytomas, a morphologic mimic (see below).

Morphologic variants of BNs typically retain immunoreactivity for MART-1/Melan-A and HMB-45 (Fig. 9.2c), aiding in their distinction from morphologic mimics, such as desmoplastic melanomas and dermatofibromas. Pure desmoplastic melanomas, for example, usually lack MART-1/Melan-A and HMB-45 expression but are strongly positive for S100. In contrast, dermatofibromas are negative for all melanocytic markers, including MART-1/Melan-A, HMB-45, SOX10, and S100.

Immunophenotypic data on atypical CBNs remain limited [1, 2, 10, 25]. In our experience, some atypical CBNs demonstrate diffuse MART-1/Melan-A and HMB-45 expression, while others exhibit patchy immunoreactivity for HMB-45. Ki-67 proliferation indices are typically low to intermediate, usually less than 10% (Fig. 9.4c). The diagnostic utility of p16 in atypical CBNs remains uncertain, as its expression appears to correlate variably with the degree of cytologic atypia [25]. At present, there are no robust data on the frequency or diagnostic value of PRAME expression in atypical CBNs.

Molecular Features

Common BNs and CBNs are genetically distinct from standard, epidermal-derived melanocytic nevi and cutaneous melanomas. They typically lack *BRAF* and *NRAS* mutations [26, 27]. Instead, they share genetic similarities with uveal melanomas and harbor activating mutations in *GNAQ* and *GNA11*, and less frequently in *CYSLTR2* and *PLCB4*, in a mutually exclusive pattern [28–31]. Notably, copy number aberrations are not a typical feature of common BNs or CBNs.

Although molecular testing is not required for diagnosing common BNs, CBNs, or their variants, it can be useful in cases with histopathologic or immunophenotypic features concerning for malignancy, such as in atypical CBNs. Similar to common BNs and CBNs, atypical CBNs also harbor activating mutations in *GNAQ*, *CYSLTR2*, and *PLCB4*, with these mutations occurring in a mutually exclusive manner [28–31]. However, *GNA11* mutations appear to be rare in atypical CBNs [31, 32].

Most atypical CBNs (approximately 73%) do not exhibit chromosomal aberrations on comparative genomic hybridization (CGH); when present, the number of abnormalities is typically limited to one to three—fewer than the three or more often observed in MBNs [33]. Additionally, a subset of atypical CBNs (25%) has been shown to harbor isolated copy number gains involving a single chromosome (e.g., gain of chromosome 20 or 15q), detected using whole-genome copy number microarray assays [34].

In contrast to Spitz melanocytic neoplasms, which frequently harbor gene fusions involving receptor tyrosine kinases (e.g., *ALK*, *ROS1*, *NTRK1*, *NTRK3*, *RET*, *MET*) or serine/threonine kinases (e.g., *BRAF*, *MAP3K8*) [35–40], gene fusions are rare in BNs and their malignant counterparts. However, a recent study has identified novel *GRM1* fusions in atypical CBNs and plaque-type BNs, suggesting an alternative oncogenic driver in a subset of these lesions [41]. These tumors lacked mutations in *GNAQ*, *GNA11*, *CYSLTR2*, and *PLCB4* [41]. Moreover, melanocytic neoplasms with protein kinase C (*PKC*) fusions have recently been described. These tumors often display a biphasic dermal proliferation with heavy pigmentation resembling a "combined blue and common nevus" pattern [41, 42]. Because *PKC* fusions activate the protein kinase C pathway, downstream of Gαq/11, similarly to BNs, they are now thought to be biologically aligned with the BN family rather than with *PRKAR1A*-inactivated PEMs [42–44]. A more detailed discussion of the clinical, histopathologic, and molecular features of *PKC*-fused melanocytic neoplasms is provided at the end of this chapter.

Melanoma Arising in Blue Nevus

The term MBN refers to a melanoma that develops in association with a pre-existing common BN or CBN, or at the site of a previously excised BN, also known as melanoma ex-blue nevus [1]. In contrast, the term blue nevus-like melanoma describes a melanoma that apparently arises de novo but exhibits histopathologic features closely resembling those of a common BN or CBN [1].

Clinical Features

MBNs most commonly arise on the scalp and typically affect older individuals, usually over the age of 45, with a slight male predominance [1]. Clinically, these lesions present as large—sometimes exceeding 100 mm in diameter—pigmented bluish to black nodules or plaques [1, 45].

Histopathologic Features

Histopathologically, MBNs may resemble CBNs or atypical CBNs on low-power examination. However, they typically display features characteristic of melanoma, including poor circumscription with an infiltrative border or an asymmetrical expansile growth pattern with a pushing border (Fig. 9.5a). Additional findings commonly include deep dermal and subcutaneous involvement, epidermal ulceration, a prominent host immune response with tumor-infiltrating lymphocytes, marked cytologic pleomorphism with high-grade nuclear atypia, increased dermal mitotic counts (often >3–4 mitoses/mm^2) (Fig. 9.5b), including atypical mitotic figures, and tumor necrosis, particularly in larger lesions [1]. When present, a residual pre-existing BN is often located at the tumor periphery, unless entirely overrun by melanoma.

Immunophenotypic Features

Immunophenotypically, lesional cells in MBNs often exhibit patchy immunoreactivity for HMB-45, in contrast to the diffuse expression typically observed in common BNs and CBNs. MART-1/Melan-A expression may also be patchy in tumor cells. As expected, MBNs usually demonstrate a high Ki-67 proliferation index. The diagnostic utility of BAP1 immunohistochemistry (IHC) in MBNs has been highlighted in several studies. In one study, 64% (7/11) of MBNs showed loss of BAP1 nuclear expression, whereas none (0/24) of the CBNs included in the study demonstrated BAP1 loss [46]. Similar findings were reported in a more recent study, where 75% (3/4) of MBNs lacked BAP1 nuclear expression, while 91% (10/11) of

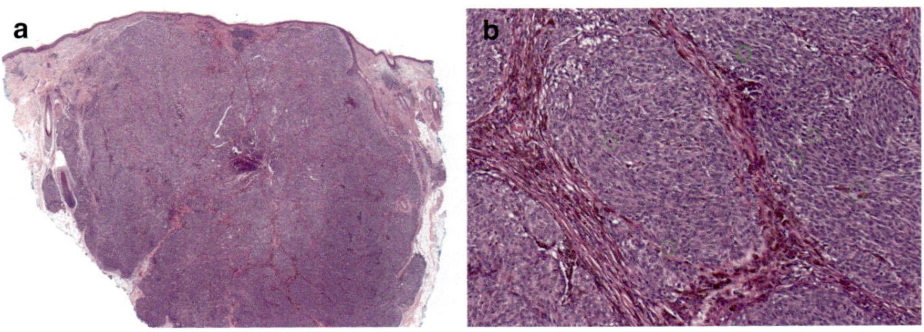

Fig. 9.5 An example of a melanoma arising in a blue nevus, showing an expansile vertical growth pattern with a pushing border (**a**) (hematoxylin and eosin, original magnification ×20). The tumor also demonstrates high cellularity, marked cytologic atypia, and increased dermal mitotic activity (**b**) (hematoxylin and eosin, original magnification ×200; green circles, mitotic figures), consistent with melanoma. This tumor harbored a *GNA11* Q209L mutation, confirmed by subsequent next-generation sequencing

common BNs/CBNs retained BAP1 expression [20]. However, these studies largely focused on unequivocal cases of CBN and MBN, and the value of BAP1 IHC in distinguishing histopathologically ambiguous lesions like atypical CBNs from MBNs remains uncertain.

MBNs also typically lack nuclear β-catenin expression [24], a helpful immunophenotypic feature that aids in differentiating MBNs from WNT-activated deep penetrating/plexiform melanocytomas. Data on the frequency of PRAME expression in MBNs remain limited. One recent study reported that approximately 63% (5/8) of MBNs expressed PRAME [47].

Molecular Features

MBNs harbor activating mutations in *GNAQ* and *GNA11*, although at a lower frequency than those seen in common BNs or CBNs. These mutations appear in a mutually exclusive pattern [28, 29]. Additional mutations in *SF3B1* or *BAP1* have been identified in MBNs already carrying *GNAQ* or *GNA11* alterations but are notably absent in their non-malignant counterparts, including atypical CBNs [31]. This observation supports the existence of a molecular signature associated with malignancy within the BN family, which could potentially serve as a diagnostic tool in cases where morphological features alone are insufficient to distinguish between atypical CBNs and MBNs or to predict clinical outcomes.

Although rare, mutations in genes commonly associated with other melanocytic neoplasms, such as *BRAF*, frequently seen in conventional melanocytic nevi and cutaneous melanomas, can also be found in MBNs [31, 32]. In one study, *BRAF* mutations were identified in 25% (3/12) of MBNs, while none of the common BNs, CBNs, or atypical CBNs in the cohort harbored these mutations [32]. These findings suggest a potential therapeutic role for *BRAF* inhibitors in select patients with MBNs exhibiting this mutation [32].

MBNs also tend to exhibit complex copy number alterations, typically showing more than three copy number aberrations. A study utilizing array-based CGH identified recurrent chromosomal deletions involving 1p, 3p, 4q, 6q, 8p, 16q, and 17q, as well as gains in 6p, 8q, and 21q [46]. Similar patterns were observed in another study, which reported recurrent gains in 1q, 4p, 6p, and 8q, and losses in 1p and 4q [34].

In recent years, fluorescence in situ hybridization (FISH) has emerged as a valuable adjunct to histopathological evaluation, particularly in diagnostically challenging melanocytic lesions. The initial four-probe FISH assay—targeting 6p25 (*RREB1*), 6q23 (*MYB*), centromere 6, and 11q13—demonstrated high diagnostic accuracy, with a sensitivity of 86.7% and specificity of 95.4% for distinguishing unequivocal melanomas from nevi [48]. When applied to histopathologically unequivocal CBNs and MBNs, the assay demonstrated 100% sensitivity and 100% specificity [49].

Although gene fusions are more commonly associated with Spitz melanocytic neoplasms, they can occasionally occur in bona fide melanomas of non-Spitz lineage [50–53]. A recent study employing next-generation sequencing on 750 non-Spitz melanomas identified gene fusions in approximately 2% of cases [50]. However, most of these investigations have focused on cutaneous melanomas outside the BN lineage or on mucosal melanomas [50–53], leaving the prevalence of gene fusions in MBNs largely undefined. Notably, a recent study has described *MYO10::GRM1* fusions co-occurring with *SF3B1* mutations in two MBNs—specifically, a melanoma arising in a nevus of Ota and another in a plaque-type BN [41], expanding the molecular landscape of MBNs.

WNT-Activated Deep Penetrating/Plexiform Melanocytoma (Nevus)

WNT-activated deep penetrating/plexiform melanocytomas (nevi) are proposed to be categorized as intermediate-grade or borderline melanocytic lesions due to their rare but documented potential to metastasize to locoregional lymph nodes [54, 55].

Clinical Features

WNT-activated deep penetrating/plexiform melanocytomas (nevi) typically present as darkly pigmented, solitary papules measuring less than 10 mm in diameter. They most commonly occur on the head and neck, extremities, or trunk, predominantly in young women [55–57]. These lesions are also relatively common in the conjunctiva, where they often appear as part of a combined nevus [58].

Histopathologic Features

As the name suggests, WNT-activated deep penetrating/plexiform melanocytomas (nevi) are characterized by two main histologic subtypes: the deep penetrating subtype and the plexiform spindled cell subtype. The deep penetrating subtype is marked by a somewhat symmetrical, ill-defined, predominantly dermal melanocytic proliferation with a wedge-shaped configuration (Fig. 9.6a–b). This lesion extends into the deep reticular dermis and subcutis (Fig. 9.6a–b). The overlying epidermis may be mildly hyperplastic, with a junctional melanocytic component often present [56, 59]. A grenz zone, an area of uninvolved papillary dermis between the epidermis and the dermal melanocytic proliferation, is commonly observed, particularly if the lesion is not part of a combined nevus [60]. The dermal proliferation consists of

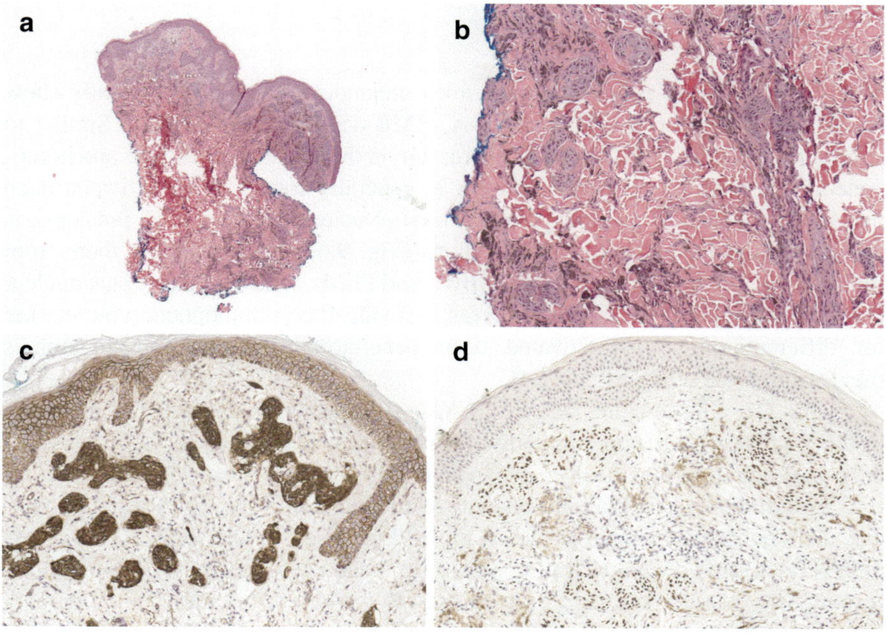

Fig. 9.6 An example of a WNT-activated deep penetrating/plexiform melanocytoma (nevus) showing a dermal proliferation composed of loose nests and, occasionally, vertically oriented fascicles of epithelioid to spindled melanocytes admixed with melanophages (**a**) (hematoxylin and eosin, original magnification ×40). The lesional melanocytes are uniformly enlarged throughout the lesion, without significant maturation with descent into the deep dermis (**b**) (hematoxylin and eosin, original magnification ×200). Immunophenotypically, lesional cells in WNT-activated deep penetrating/plexiform melanocytoma are typically diffusely positive for HMB45, with nuclear expression of β-catenin (**c**) (original magnification ×200) and LEF1 (**d**) (original magnification ×200)

loose nests and vertically oriented fascicles of epithelioid to spindled melanocytes, which often extend along skin adnexa and neurovascular bundles [56]. The plexiform spindled cell subtype is characterized by melanocytic proliferation primarily located in the superficial dermis, displaying a fascicular to plexiform architectural pattern.

Scattered melanophages with coarse pigment are found in the intervening stroma, although stromal fibroplasia is typically absent in WNT-activated deep penetrating/plexiform melanocytomas (nevi). Lesional melanocytes are uniformly enlarged throughout the lesion, with minimal maturation upon descent into the dermis. Cytologically, these melanocytes often show mild-to-moderate nuclear pleomorphism, with small to medium-sized eosinophilic nucleoli. Intranuclear pseudoinclusions and occasional mitotic figures (typically <2/mm^2) may be observed, although atypical mitoses are not present [60].

Immunophenotypic Features

WNT-activated deep penetrating/plexiform melanocytomas (nevi) typically show immunoreactivity for MART-1/Melan-A, HMB-45, S100, and SOX10. Similar to common BNs and CBNs, HMB-45 expression in these lesions is diffuse and homogeneous. The Ki-67 proliferation index is generally low in WNT-activated deep penetrating/plexiform melanocytomas (nevi). Nuclear expression of β-catenin is almost universally present in these lesions (Fig. 9.6c), distinguishing them from morphologic mimics such as CBNs, MBNs, and PEMs, which typically lack nuclear β-catenin expression. This feature serves as a valuable immunophenotypic marker for differentiating WNT-activated deep penetrating/plexiform melanocytomas (nevi) from these other lesions [24].

Cyclin D1, a protein encoded by *CCND1* and a downstream target of β-catenin in the Wnt/β-catenin signaling pathway, is often overexpressed in WNT-activated deep penetrating/plexiform melanocytomas (nevi), as evidenced by IHC. Additionally, LEF1, another downstream mediator of the Wnt/β-catenin pathway, is frequently expressed in these lesions (Fig. 9.6d). In one study, 93% (13/14) of WNT-activated deep penetrating/plexiform melanocytomas (nevi) exhibited diffuse nuclear expression of LEF1, in contrast to the absence of LEF1 immunoreactivity in all common BNs and CBNs included in the study [61]. This suggests that LEF1 IHC could serve as a potential surrogate marker for assessing the activation status of the Wnt/β-catenin signaling pathway in these melanocytomas (nevi). However, a more recent study has highlighted a potential pitfall in the use of LEF1 IHC, as some combined nevi with a BN component were found to express LEF1 [22].

Regarding PRAME, although its utility in evaluating WNT-activated deep penetrating/plexiform melanocytomas (nevi) and their morphologic mimics remains under investigation, these lesions typically lack PRAME expression. When PRAME expression is present, it is usually focal and weak [21, 22, 62].

Molecular Features

WNT-activated deep penetrating/plexiform melanocytomas (nevi) arise from the combined activation of the MAP kinase and β-catenin signaling pathways [63]. In some cases, these melanocytomas (nevi) develop from pre-existing common nevi through the sequential acquisition of mutations. Initially, mutations in the MAP kinase pathway (e.g., *BRAF* mutations) drive the formation of common nevi, followed by activation of the β-catenin pathway, typically involving *CTNNB1* mutations (with rare *APC* mutations). This second mutation triggers the phenotypic shift toward WNT-activated deep penetrating/plexiform melanocytoma (nevi) [63].

By definition, WNT-activated deep penetrating/plexiform melanocytomas do not harbor *GNAQ* or *GNA11* mutations. Therefore, if these mutations are detected in lesions with overlapping features of WNT-activated deep penetrating/plexiform melanocytomas and BNs, the lesions should be classified as BNs. Similarly, WNT-activated deep penetrating/plexiform melanocytomas (nevi) do not exhibit significant copy number alterations or other oncogenic mutations, such as *TERT* promoter mutations or *CDKN2A* inactivation. Consequently, lesions with WNT-activated deep penetrating/plexiform melanocytoma-like morphology but containing these additional oncogenic alterations may be classified as WNT-activated deep penetrating/plexiform melanocytoma (nevus)-like melanomas [63, 64]. Distinguishing WNT-activated deep penetrating/plexiform melanocytomas (nevi) from their malignant counterparts based on histopathology alone remains challenging, as diagnostic criteria for melanomas in this category are still evolving. Recent studies have proposed that features such as severe nuclear atypia, absence of a conventional nevus component, PRAME expression, complete loss of p16 expression, and the presence of *TERT* promoter mutations along with additional pathogenic mutations, support a diagnosis of WNT-activated deep penetrating/plexiform melanocytoma (nevus)-like melanoma [65]. Another recent study further suggests that these melanomas tend to be clinically larger, exhibit high-grade nuclear atypia, increased mitotic counts, a sheet-like growth pattern, subcutaneous involvement, and more frequently harbor mutations in the *TERT* promoter, *CDKN2A*, and SWI/SNF complex subunits (e.g., *ARID1A*, *ARID1B*) when compared with their melanocytoma (nevus) counterparts [66].

Pigmented Epithelioid Melanocytoma

PEMs are melanocytic tumors considered to have low to intermediate malignant potential, owing to their rare but documented capacity to metastasize to regional lymph nodes [67]. Molecularly, PEMs are defined by concurrent activation of the protein kinase A (PKA) pathway and additional alterations associated with other melanocytic lineages, including activation of the MAP kinase pathway or the presence of kinase fusions.

Clinical Features

PEMs typically present as slow-growing, pigmented nodules or papules [68]. While they can arise in various anatomic locations, including mucosal sites [69], the extremities are the most commonly affected [68]. PEMs predominantly occur in children and young adults, with reported median ages at presentation ranging from 20 to 27 years [67, 68]. There is no apparent sex predilection [67, 68].

Although PEMs have the potential to metastasize to locoregional lymph nodes—hence their designation as "melanocytomas"—they generally follow a favorable clinical course. Notably, a 5-year survival rate of 100% has been reported [67, 70].

Most PEMs occur sporadically, but a subset may arise in the context of Carney complex. In such cases, these tumors are morphologically indistinguishable from epithelioid BNs associated with Carney complex [1].

Histopathologic Features

PEMs are universally characterized by heavy pigmentation, producing a low-power impression of a densely melanized dermis (Fig. 9.7a). On low magnification, they often appear relatively symmetrical with an inverted, wedge-shaped architecture (Fig. 9.7a). These tumors predominantly consist of a dermal melanocytic proliferation with infiltrative peripheral borders that can extend into the deep dermis and subcutis. In some cases, the periphery displays a smooth, pushing border with nodular protrusions of lesional melanocytes, resembling the dumbbell configuration typically seen in CBNs. Lesional melanocytes frequently abut the overlying epidermis, which often shows hyperplasia and rarely ulcerates (Fig. 9.7a). Although uncommon, a grenz zone of uninvolved papillary dermis may be observed. A junctional component comprising singly arranged or nested dendritic melanocytes may occasionally be present. Unlike common BNs or CBNs, PEMs often exhibit epidermal hyperplasia but typically lack prominent stromal fibroplasia. Reflecting their two-step molecular evolution, a precursor component representing a common acquired nevus may also be identified [68].

Cytologically, PEMs display a mixture of three distinct melanocyte types in varying proportions: spindled dendritic cells, large epithelioid cells, and pigmented polygonal cells [1] (Fig. 9.7b). The spindled dendritic cells resemble those of common BNs but are distinguished by more abundant amphophilic cytoplasm and vesicular nuclei. The large epithelioid cells are notable for their sizable vesicular

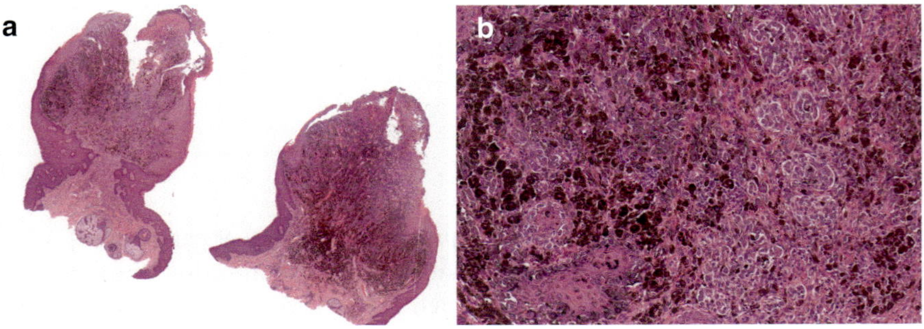

Fig. 9.7 An example of pigmented epithelioid melanocytoma showing a relatively symmetrical, wedge-shaped, heavily pigmented dermal melanocytic proliferation extending vertically into the dermis (**a**) (hematoxylin and eosin, original magnification ×20). The overlying epidermis is hyperplastic and focally ulcerated (**a**). In this case, the tumor is predominantly composed of large epithelioid cells with vesicular nuclei, prominent nucleoli, and finely pigmented cytoplasm (**b**) (hematoxylin and eosin, original magnification ×200)

nuclei, prominent nucleoli, and finely pigmented cytoplasm. In these cells, melanin tends to concentrate at the cytoplasmic periphery, sparing the perinuclear region and producing a characteristic "fried egg" appearance. These epithelioid cells may also exhibit multinucleation and variable degrees of cytologic atypia. The pigmented polygonal cells, many of which are likely tumor-associated melanophages, contain coarse melanin granules that can obscure the vesicular nuclei. Mitotic counts within the dermis are typically low, and while necrosis is rare, it may occur in larger lesions [1].

Immunophenotypic Features

PEMs demonstrate immunoreactivity for melanocytic markers, including MART-1/ Melan-A, S100, and HMB45. Expression of p16 is retained, and the Ki-67 proliferation index is typically low. In contrast to WNT-activated deep penetrating/plexiform melanocytomas (nevi), PEMs lack nuclear expression of β-catenin, a distinguishing feature [24]. Immunohistochemical loss of PRKAR1A expression—indicative of *PRKAR1A* gene inactivation—is observed in up to 82% of cases and can serve as a useful diagnostic adjunct [70]. Currently, there is limited data on the diagnostic utility of PRAME IHC in distinguishing PEMs from morphologic mimics, particularly melanomas.

Molecular Features

The molecular characterization of PEMs has evolved significantly in recent years, enabling more precise classification of these rare melanocytic neoplasms based on distinctive genetic alterations. The hallmark genetic abnormality in PEMs is the presence of inactivating mutations in the *PRKAR1A* gene, which can be identified through loss of PRKAR1A protein expression on IHC [71–73]. In many cases, *PRKAR1A* inactivation occurs alongside additional genetic alterations commonly associated with other melanocytic lineages. These include mutations seen in common acquired nevi, such as *BRAF* mutations, and kinase gene fusions characteristic of Spitz melanocytic neoplasms, including *NTRK*, *ALK*, and *RET* fusions [71–73].

Melanocytic neoplasms harboring *PKC* fusions often display histopathologic features that closely resemble PEMs. These *PKC* fusions activate the PKC pathway downstream of Gαq/11, similar to the signaling seen in BNs. Due to this biological overlap, *PKC*-fused melanocytic neoplasms are now classified within the BN family, rather than as *PRKAR1A*-inactivated PEMs, as was previously proposed [42–44].

Current data on copy number alterations in PEMs remain limited. One study involving 13 cases did not identify significant copy number aberrations [73]. However, a more recent case study described copy number gains involving chromosomes 15q and 17q [74]. *TERT* promoter mutations are typically absent in PEMs.

Nevertheless, if a lesion harbors *CDKN2A* mutations, *TERT* promoter mutations, and/or shows complex chromosomal gains and losses, it should probably be reclassified as a *PRKAR1A*-inactivated melanoma, reflecting its likely more aggressive biological behavior [75].

PKC-Fused Melanocytic Neoplasm

The detailed histopathologic and molecular characterization of *PKC*-fused melanocytic neoplasms was first described in 2023 [42]. Although these neoplasms often exhibit marked pigmentation and morphologic features that closely resemble PEMs, their underlying biology aligns more closely with the BN family. Like BNs, *PKC*-fused melanocytic neoplasms have the potential to progress to melanomas, particularly through *BAP1* inactivation, which represents a known pathway of malignant transformation within this lineage [42].

Clinical Features

In the initial series, *PKC*-fused melanocytic neoplasms were mostly observed in young adults, with a median age of 29.5 years, and demonstrated a slight male predilection [42]. These lesions typically arise on the trunk and lower extremities [42]. Reported tumor sizes range widely, from 2.5 mm to 450 mm in diameter, with a median size of 6 mm, reflecting variability in clinical presentation [42].

Histopathologic Features

In the initial series, 82% (42/51) of *PKC*-fused melanocytic neoplasms were classified as benign melanocytic nevi, 6% (3/51) as intermediate-grade melanocytic tumors, and 12% (6/51) as melanomas, based on conventional histopathologic criteria [42].

Most *PKC*-fused melanocytic neoplasms exhibit a biphasic dermal proliferation, characterized by nests of small melanocytes surrounded by fibrosis, alongside haphazardly arranged spindled and dendritic melanocytes [42]. This pattern closely resembles what has traditionally been described as "combined BNs." Most tumors are heavily pigmented, and a subset demonstrates hyperpigmented epithelioid melanocytes at the dermoepidermal junction [42]. Additional features may include hyperplastic epidermis, which is occasionally present, and, more rarely, paucicellular areas with marked sclerosis [42]. Mitotic counts are absent or very low in nevi with *PKC* fusions [42]. A recent study also identified smooth muscle hyperplasia in *PKC*-fused melanocytic neoplasms classified as BNs, suggesting a potential diagnostic histopathologic clue for this entity [76]. Rare hypopigmented variants of *PKC*-fused melanocytic neoplasms have also been recently described, expanding the known morphologic spectrum of this entity [77].

Lesions classified as intermediate grade often demonstrate confluent nests of large epithelioid melanocytes throughout the dermis, with increased mitotic counts (2–3 mitoses/mm^2) [42].

Cases categorized as melanoma show a large dermal proliferation of melanocytes arranged in nests and sheets, frequently obliterating adnexal structures and extending into the subcutis. These tumors typically exhibit significant cytologic atypia and increased mitotic counts [42].

Immunophenotypic Features

Similar to common BNs and cellular BNs, *PKC*-fused melanocytic neoplasms frequently exhibit diffuse positivity for HMB45 [42]. The Ki-67 proliferation index is typically low in lesions classified as nevi, while those designated as intermediate-grade tumors or melanomas may demonstrate an elevated Ki-67 index, reaching up to 20% [42]. A distinguishing feature of *PKC*-fused melanocytic neoplasms is the retained expression of PRKAR1A, which contrasts with the loss of PRKAR1A expression seen in *PRKAR1A*-inactivated PEMs [42]. Additionally, these tumors generally retain p16 expression, with no complete loss observed [77].

BAP1 expression is typically preserved in lesions classified as nevi or intermediate grade [42]. However, melanomas within this group may lack nuclear BAP1 expression, indicating a potential pathway of malignant progression [42].

Molecular Features

By definition, *PKC*-fused melanocytic neoplasms are characterized by gene fusions involving *PRKCA* or *PRKCB*, with a variety of identified fusion partners including *SLC11A2*, *PTPRJ*, and *ATP2B4* [42]. These tumors typically lack oncogenic mutations commonly seen in other melanocytic neoplasms, such as *BRAF*, *NRAS*, *GNAQ*, or *GNA11*, and they do not harbor other kinase gene fusions [42, 77]. Consistent with their frequent classification as BNs, significant copy number aberrations are generally absent, supporting their benign or relatively indolent biologic behavior [42]. The *TERT* promoter mutation status in these neoplasms remains largely unknown.

Summary

Our understanding of the histopathologic, immunophenotypic, and molecular features of heavily pigmented melanocytic neoplasms continues to evolve, underscoring the importance of staying current to ensure accurate classification. Certain immunohistochemical markers, such as β-catenin and PRKAR1A, serve as valuable surrogates for underlying molecular alterations and can help confirm suspected diagnoses of WNT-activated deep penetrating/plexiform melanocytomas (nevi) and PEMs, respectively. Among the entities discussed in this chapter—excluding MBNs—a common immunoprofile feature is diffuse HMB45 labeling. Additional immunophenotypic features, including diffuse PRAME expression, loss of p16, increased Ki-67 index, and/or loss of BAP1 nuclear expression, may indicate malignant potential, as in MBNs, WNT-activated deep penetrating/plexiform melanocytoma-like melanomas, and *PRKAR1A*-inactivated melanomas. In diagnostically challenging cases, molecular findings such as complex copy number aberrations, abnormal FISH results, *CDKN2A* or *BAP1* inactivation, and/or *TERT* promoter mutations can support a diagnosis of melanoma over borderline lesions or melanocytomas. Finally, certain tumors, such as *PKC*-fused melanocytic neoplasms, can only be definitively diagnosed through advanced molecular testing, including *DNA* or *RNA* sequencing—methods not always accessible in routine practice. Nonetheless, when morphologic and immunophenotypic features raise suspicion, molecular studies should be pursued to facilitate accurate classification of these rare entities.

References

1. Zembowicz A, Phadke PA. Blue nevi and variants: an update. Arch Pathol Lab Med. 2011;135(3):327–36.
2. Cho WC, Prieto VG, Aung PP. Melanocytic lesions with blue naevus-like (dendritic) morphology: an update with an emphasis on histopathological, immunophenotypic, and molecular features. Histopathology. 2021;79(3):291–305.
3. Rodriguez HA, Ackerman LV. Cellular blue nevus. Clinicopathologic study of forty-five cases. Cancer. 1968;21(3):393–405.
4. Dohse L, Ferringer T. Nodal blue nevus: a pitfall in lymph node biopsies. J Cutan Pathol. 2010;37(1):102–4.
5. Murali R, McCarthy SW, Scolyer RA. Blue nevi and related lesions: a review highlighting atypical and newly described variants, distinguishing features and diagnostic pitfalls. Adv Anat Pathol. 2009;16(6):365–82.
6. Tseng C, Wiedemeyer K, Mehta A, Rojas-Garcia P, Temple-Oberle C, Orlando A, Miller K, Gharpuray-Pandit D, Brenn T. The clinico-pathological spectrum of plaque-type blue naevi and their potential for malignant transformation. Histopathology. 2024;84(6):1047–55.
7. Barnhill RL, Argenyi Z, Berwick M, Duray PH, Erickson L, Guitart J, Horenstein MG, Lowe L, Messina J, Paine S, Piepkorn MW, Prieto V, Rabkin MS, Schmidt B, Selim A, Shea CR, Trotter MJ. Atypical cellular blue nevi (cellular blue nevi with atypical features): lack of consensus for diagnosis and distinction from cellular blue nevi and malignant melanoma ("malignant blue nevus"). Am J Surg Pathol. 2008;32(1):36–44.

8. Avidor I, Kessler E. 'Atypical' blue nevus–a benign variant of cellular blue nevus. Presentation of three cases. Dermatologica. 1977;154(1):39–44.
9. Tran TA, Carlson JA, Basaca PC, Mihm MC. Cellular blue nevus with atypia (atypical cellular blue nevus): a clinicopathologic study of nine cases. J Cutan Pathol. 1998;25(5):252–8.
10. Hung T, Argenyi Z, Erickson L, Guitart J, Horenstein MG, Lowe L, Messina J, Piepkorn MW, Prieto VG, Rabkin MS, Schmidt B, Selim MA, Shea CR, Trotter MJ, Barnhill RL. Cellular blue nevomelanocytic lesions: analysis of clinical, histological, and outcome data in 37 cases. Am J Dermatopathol. 2016;38(7):499–503.
11. Sterchi JM, Muss HB, Weidner N. Cellular blue nevus simulating metastatic melanoma: report of an unusually large lesion associated with nevus-cell aggregates in regional lymph nodes. J Surg Oncol. 1987;36(1):71–5.
12. Lamovec J. Blue nevus of the lymph node capsule. Report of a new case with review of the literature. Am J Clin Pathol. 1984;81(3):367–72.
13. Yazdan P, Haghighat Z, Guitart J, Gerami P. Epithelioid and fusiform blue nevus of chronically sun-damaged skin, an entity distinct from the epithelioid blue nevus of the Carney complex. Am J Surg Pathol. 2013;37(1):81–8.
14. Zembowicz A, Granter SR, McKee PH, Mihm MC. Amelanotic cellular blue nevus: a hypopigmented variant of the cellular blue nevus: clinicopathologic analysis of 20 cases. Am J Surg Pathol. 2002;26(11):1493–500.
15. Urso C, Tinacci G. Angiomatoid cellular blue nevus: a variant of blue nevus with an angioma-like appearance. J Cutan Pathol. 2005;32(5):385–7.
16. Zembowicz A, Mihm MC. Dermal dendritic melanocytic proliferations: an update. Histopathology. 2004;45(5):433–51.
17. Sun J, Morton TH Jr, Gown AM. Antibody HMB-45 identifies the cells of blue nevi. An immunohistochemical study on paraffin sections. Am J Surg Pathol. 1990;14(8):748–51.
18. Bhawan J, Cao SL. Amelanotic blue nevus: a variant of blue nevus. Am J Dermatopathol. 1999;21(3):225–8.
19. Zembowicz A. Blue nevi and related tumors. Clin Lab Med. 2017;37(3):401–15.
20. Chen PL, Neishaboori N, Tetzlaff MT, Chen WS, Aung PP, Curry JL, Nagarajan P, Ivan D, Hwu WJ, Prieto VG, Torres-Cabala CA. BAP-1 expression status by immunohistochemistry in cellular blue nevus and blue nevus-like melanoma. Am J Dermatopathol. 2020;42(5):313–21.
21. Lezcano C, Jungbluth AA, Nehal KS, Hollmann TJ, Busam KJ. PRAME expression in melanocytic tumors. Am J Surg Pathol. 2018;42(11):1456–65.
22. Vanderbeck K, Rothrock AT, Cho WC, Nagarajan P, Aung PP, Hudgens C, Bassett RL, Ivan D, Prieto VG, Curry JL, Torres-Cabala CA. PRAME and LEF1 in combined deep penetrating nevus and combined blue nevus: utility and pitfalls. Am J Dermatopathol. 2023;45(8):549–56.
23. Smith K, Germain M, Williams J, Skelton H. CD34-positive cellular blue nevi. J Cutan Pathol. 2001;28(3):145–50.
24. de la Fouchardière A, Caillot C, Jacquemus J, Durieux E, Houlier A, Haddad V, Pissaloux D. β-Catenin nuclear expression discriminates deep penetrating nevi from other cutaneous melanocytic tumors. Virchows Arch. 2019;474(5):539–50.
25. Chang LM, Cassarino DS. p16 expression is lost in severely atypical cellular blue nevi and melanoma compared to conventional, mildly, and moderately atypical cellular blue nevi. ISRN Dermatol. 2014;2014:348417.
26. Bastian BC. The molecular pathology of melanoma: an integrated taxonomy of melanocytic neoplasia. Annu Rev Pathol. 2014;9:239–71.
27. Shain AH, Yeh I, Kovalyshyn I, Sriharan A, Talevich E, Gagnon A, Dummer R, North J, Pincus L, Ruben B, Rickaby W, D'Arrigo C, Robson A, Bastian BC. The genetic evolution of melanoma from precursor lesions. N Engl J Med. 2015;373(20):1926–36.
28. Van Raamsdonk CD, Bezrookove V, Green G, Bauer J, Gaugler L, O'Brien JM, Simpson EM, Barsh GS, Bastian BC. Frequent somatic mutations of GNAQ in uveal melanoma and blue naevi. Nature. 2009;457(7229):599–602.
29. Van Raamsdonk CD, Griewank KG, Crosby MB, Garrido MC, Vemula S, Wiesner T, Obenauf AC, Wackernagel W, Green G, Bouvier N, Sozen MM, Baimukanova G, Roy R, Heguy A,

Dolgalev I, Khanin R, Busam K, Speicher MR, O'Brien J, Bastian BC. Mutations in GNA11 in uveal melanoma. N Engl J Med. 2010;363(23):2191–9.
30. Möller I, Murali R, Müller H, Wiesner T, Jackett LA, Scholz SL, Cosgarea I, van de Nes JA, Sucker A, Hillen U, Schilling B, Paschen A, Kutzner H, Rütten A, Böckers M, Scolyer RA, Schadendorf D, Griewank KG. Activating cysteinyl leukotriene receptor 2 (CYSLTR2) mutations in blue nevi. Mod Pathol. 2017;30(3):350–6.
31. Griewank KG, Müller H, Jackett LA, Emberger M, Möller I, van de Nes JA, Zimmer L, Livingstone E, Wiesner T, Scholz SL, Cosgarea I, Sucker A, Schimming T, Hillen U, Schilling B, Paschen A, Reis H, Mentzel T, Kutzner H, Rütten A, Murali R, Scolyer RA, Schadendorf D. SF3B1 and BAP1 mutations in blue nevus-like melanoma. Mod Pathol. 2017;30(7):928–39.
32. Yilmaz I, Gamsizkan M, Sari SO, Yaman B, Demirkesen C, Heper A, Calli AO, Narli G, Kucukodaci Z, Berber U, Demirel D, Akalin T, Demiriz M, Buyukbabani N. Molecular alterations in malignant blue nevi and related blue lesions. Virchows Arch. 2015;467(6):723–32.
33. Maize JC Jr, McCalmont TH, Carlson JA, Busam KJ, Kutzner H, Bastian BC. Genomic analysis of blue nevi and related dermal melanocytic proliferations. Am J Surg Pathol. 2005;29(9):1214–20.
34. Chan MP, Andea AA, Harms PW, Durham AB, Patel RM, Wang M, Robichaud P, Fisher GJ, Johnson TM, Fullen DR. Genomic copy number analysis of a spectrum of blue nevi identifies recurrent aberrations of entire chromosomal arms in melanoma ex blue nevus. Mod Pathol. 2016;29(3):227–39.
35. Wiesner T, He J, Yelensky R, Esteve-Puig R, Botton T, Yeh I, Lipson D, Otto G, Brennan K, Murali R, Garrido M, Miller VA, Ross JS, Berger MF, Sparatta A, Palmedo G, Cerroni L, Busam KJ, Kutzner H, Cronin MT, Stephens PJ, Bastian BC. Kinase fusions are frequent in Spitz tumours and spitzoid melanomas. Nat Commun. 2014;5:3116.
36. Yeh I, Tee MK, Botton T, Shain AH, Sparatta AJ, Gagnon A, Vemula SS, Garrido MC, Nakamaru K, Isoyama T, McCalmont TH, LeBoit PE, Bastian BC. NTRK3 kinase fusions in Spitz tumours. J Pathol. 2016;240(3):282–90.
37. Houlier A, Pissaloux D, Masse I, Tirode F, Karanian M, Pincus LB, McCalmont TH, LeBoit PE, Bastian BC, Yeh I, de la Fouchardière A. Melanocytic tumors with MAP3K8 fusions: report of 33 cases with morphological-genetic correlations. Mod Pathol. 2020;33(5):846–57.
38. Salah HT, Yang RK, Roy-Chowdhuri S, Ross MI, Aung PP, Rothrock AT, Torres-Cabala CA, Curry JL, Prieto VG, Nagarajan P, Cho WC. Spitz melanocytic neoplasms with MLPH::ALK fusions: report of two cases with previously unreported features and literature review. J Cutan Pathol. 2024;51(6):407–14.
39. Cho WC, Prieto VG, Yang RK. Spitz melanoma with SLC20A1::ALK fusion: a novel fusion previously undescribed in Spitz melanocytic neoplasm. Am J Dermatopathol. 2024;46(10):700–3.
40. Della Mura M, Sorino J, Colagrande A, Ingravallo G, Giubellino A, Fortarezza F, Yang RK, Cho WC, Cazzato G. Atypical Spitz tumor/Spitz melanocytoma revealing a VIM::NTRK3 gene fusion: clinicopathological correlation of a unique molecular finding. Am J Dermatopathol. 2025;47(11):886–90. https://doi.org/10.1097/DAD.0000000000003051.
41. Kervarrec T, Lo Bello G, Pissaloux D, Tirode F, Poulalhon N, Samimi M, Houlier A, de la Fouchardière A. GRM1 gene fusions as an alternative molecular driver in blue nevi and related melanomas. Mod Pathol. 2023;36(10):100264.
42. de la Fouchardière A, Pissaloux D, Houlier A, Paindavoine S, Tirode F, LeBoit PE, Bastian BC, Yeh I. Histologic and genetic features of 51 melanocytic neoplasms with protein kinase C fusion genes. Mod Pathol. 2023;36(11):100286.
43. Patel P, Chen A, Sharma N, Zhang Y, Quan VL, Olivares S, Gerami P. PRKC fusion melanocytic tumors, a subgroup of melanocytic tumors more closely aligned to blue nevi than to PRKAR1A-inactivated pigmented epithelioid melanocytomas. Am J Surg Pathol. 2024;48(11):1349–58.
44. Pérez-Alea M, Vivancos A, Caratú G, Matito J, Ferrer B, Hernandez-Losa J, Cortés J, Muñoz E, Garcia-Patos V, Recio JA. Genetic profile of GNAQ-mutated blue melanocytic neoplasms reveals mutations in genes linked to genomic instability and the PI3K pathway. Oncotarget. 2016;7(19):28086–95.

45. Yeh I, Fang Y, Busam KJ. Melanoma arising in a large plaque-type blue nevus with subcutaneous cellular nodules. Am J Surg Pathol. 2012;36(8):1258–63.
46. Costa S, Byrne M, Pissaloux D, Haddad V, Paindavoine S, Thomas L, Aubin F, Lesimple T, Grange F, Bonniaud B, Mortier L, Mateus C, Dreno B, Balme B, Vergier B, de la Fouchardiere A. Melanomas associated with blue nevi or mimicking cellular blue nevi: clinical, pathologic, and molecular study of 11 cases displaying a high frequency of GNA11 mutations, BAP1 expression loss, and a predilection for the scalp. Am J Surg Pathol. 2016;40(3):368–77.
47. Kline N, Menge TD, Hrycaj SM, Andea AA, Patel RM, Harms PW, Chan MP, Bresler SC. PRAME expression in challenging dermal melanocytic neoplasms and soft tissue tumors with melanocytic differentiation. Am J Dermatopathol. 2022;44(6):404–10.
48. Gerami P, Jewell SS, Morrison LE, Blondin B, Schulz J, Ruffalo T, Matushek P 4th, Legator M, Jacobson K, Dalton SR, Charzan S, Kolaitis NA, Guitart J, Lertsbarapa T, Boone S, LeBoit PE, Bastian BC. Fluorescence in situ hybridization (FISH) as an ancillary diagnostic tool in the diagnosis of melanoma. Am J Surg Pathol. 2009;33(8):1146–56.
49. Gammon B, Beilfuss B, Guitart J, Busam KJ, Gerami P. Fluorescence in situ hybridization for distinguishing cellular blue nevi from blue nevus-like melanoma. J Cutan Pathol. 2011;38(4):335–41.
50. Moran JMT, Le LP, Nardi V, Golas J, Farahani AA, Signorelli S, Onozato ML, Foreman RK, Duncan LM, Lawrence DP, Lennerz JK, Dias-Santagata D, Hoang MP. Identification of fusions with potential clinical significance in melanoma. Mod Pathol. 2022;35(12):1837–47.
51. Gao Y, Yang RK, Curry JL, Torres-Cabala CA, Cho WC. Melanoma with RNF11::BRAF fusion: a novel fusion previously undescribed in melanoma. Am J Dermatopathol. 2025;47(5):391–4.
52. Ibrahim E, Yang RK, Curry JL, Cho WC. BCR::ZNF711 and BCR::CYLC2 fusions: novel BCR fusions expanding the molecular spectrum of gene fusions in melanoma. Am J Dermatopathol. 2024;46(11):797–9.
53. Cho WC, Yang RK, Lenskaya V, Prieto VG. SBF1::BRAF-fused melanoma with prominent rhabdoid morphology and reed-sternberg-like cells: potential morphologic clues to BRAF-fused melanomas of non-Spitz lineage? Am J Dermatopathol. 2025;47(9):733–5. https://doi.org/10.1097/DAD.0000000000003048.
54. McCalmont TH, Bastian BC. An unconventional deep penetrating melanocytic nevus with microscopic involvement of regional lymph nodes. J Cutan Pathol. 2012;39(1):25–8.
55. Cosgarea I, Griewank KG, Ungureanu L, Tamayo A, Siepmann T. Deep penetrating nevus and borderline-deep penetrating nevus: a literature review. Front Oncol. 2020;10:837.
56. Seab JA Jr, Graham JH, Helwig EB. Deep penetrating nevus. Am J Surg Pathol. 1989;13(1):39–44.
57. Strazzula L, Senna MM, Yasuda M, Belazarian L. The deep penetrating nevus. J Am Acad Dermatol. 2014;71(6):1234–40.
58. Šekoranja D, Vergot K, Hawlina G, Pižem J. Combined deep penetrating nevi of the conjunctiva are relatively common lesions characterised by BRAFV600E mutation and activation of the beta catenin pathway: a clinicopathological analysis of 34 lesions. Br J Ophthalmol. 2020;104(7):1016–21.
59. Robson A, Morley-Quante M, Hempel H, McKee PH, Calonje E. Deep penetrating naevus: clinicopathological study of 31 cases with further delineation of histological features allowing distinction from other pigmented benign melanocytic lesions and melanoma. Histopathology. 2003;43(6):529–37.
60. Luzar B, Calonje E. Deep penetrating nevus: a review. Arch Pathol Lab Med. 2011;135(3):321–6.
61. Raghavan SS, Saleem A, Wang JY, Rieger KE, Brown RA, Novoa RA. Diagnostic utility of LEF1 immunohistochemistry in differentiating deep penetrating nevi from histologic mimics. Am J Surg Pathol. 2020;44(10):1413–8.
62. Lopez DR, Forcucci JA, O'Connor H, Maize JC. PReferentially expressed antigen in MElanoma (PRAME) expression in BRCA1-associated protein (BAP1)-inactivated melanocytic tumors and deep penetrating nevi: a pilot study. J Cutan Pathol. 2021;48(4):597–600.

63. Yeh I, Lang UE, Durieux E, Tee MK, Jorapur A, Shain AH, Haddad V, Pissaloux D, Chen X, Cerroni L, Judson RL, LeBoit PE, McCalmont TH, Bastian BC, de la Fouchardière A. Combined activation of MAP kinase pathway and β-catenin signaling cause deep penetrating nevi. Nat Commun. 2017;8(1):644.
64. Giubellino A, Nelson AC, He Y, Munro SA, Song KY, Glitza Oliva IC, Torres-Cabala C. Molecular characterization of biphenotypic epithelioid and plexiform melanoma with deep penetrating nevus-like features. Pigment Cell Melanoma Res. 2022;35(2):229–37.
65. Ebbelaar CF, Schrader AMR, van Dijk M, Meijers RWJ, de Leng WWJ, Bloem LT, Jansen AML, Blokx WAM. MOLecular Evaluation of Melanocytic Ambiguous Tumors (MOLEMAT) investigators. Towards diagnostic criteria for malignant deep penetrating melanocytic tumors using single nucleotide polymorphism array and next-generation sequencing. Mod Pathol. 2022;35(8):1110–20.
66. Chen L, Chen A, Sharma N, Patel P, Addo AK, Jeyakumar JE, Beydoun HM, Olivares S, Dittmann D, Vormittag-Nocito E, Dos Santos LS, Jennings L, Gerami P. Clinical, morphologic, and genomic differences in deep-penetrating nevi and deep-penetrating nevus-like melanomas. Mod Pathol. 2025;38(5):100707.
67. Mandal RV, Murali R, Lundquist KF, Ragsdale BD, Heenan P, McCarthy SW, Mihm MC Jr, Scolyer RA, Zembowicz A. Pigmented epithelioid melanocytoma: favorable outcome after 5-year follow-up. Am J Surg Pathol. 2009;33(12):1778–82.
68. Zembowicz A, Carney JA, Mihm MC. Pigmented epithelioid melanocytoma: a low-grade melanocytic tumor with metastatic potential indistinguishable from animal-type melanoma and epithelioid blue nevus. Am J Surg Pathol. 2004;28(1):31–40.
69. Bissig A, Moulin A, Spahn B, Zembowicz A, Schalenbourg A. Conjunctival pigmented epithelioid melanocytoma: a clinicopathological case report. Arch Ophthalmol. 2012;130(11):1478–9.
70. Zembowicz A, Knoepp SM, Bei T, Stergiopoulos S, Eng C, Mihm MC, Stratakis CA. Loss of expression of protein kinase a regulatory subunit 1alpha in pigmented epithelioid melanocytoma but not in melanoma or other melanocytic lesions. Am J Surg Pathol. 2007;31(11):1764–75.
71. Isales MC, Mohan LS, Quan VL, Garfield EM, Zhang B, Shi K, Arva N, Beaubier N, Yazdan P, White K, Taxter TJ, Gerami P. Distinct genomic patterns in pigmented epithelioid melanocytoma: a molecular and histologic analysis of 16 cases. Am J Surg Pathol. 2019;43(4):480–8.
72. de la Fouchardiere A, Tirode F, Castillo C, Buisson A, Boivin F, Macagno N, Pissaloux D. Attempting to solve the pigmented epithelioid melanocytoma (PEM) conundrum: PRKAR1A inactivation can occur in different genetic backgrounds (common, blue, and Spitz subgroups) with variation in their clinicopathologic characteristics. Am J Surg Pathol. 2022;46(8):1106–15.
73. Cohen JN, Joseph NM, North JP, Onodera C, Zembowicz A, LeBoit PE. Genomic analysis of pigmented epithelioid melanocytomas reveals recurrent alterations in PRKAR1A, and PRKCA genes. Am J Surg Pathol. 2017;41(10):1333–46.
74. Friedman BJ, Hernandez S, Fidai C, Jiang A, Shwayder TA, Carskadon S, Andea AA, Harms PW, Chitale D, Palanisamy N. A pediatric case of pigmented epithelioid melanocytoma with chromosomal copy number alterations in 15q and 17q and a novel NTRK3-SCAPER gene fusion. J Cutan Pathol. 2020;47(1):70–5.
75. Cohen JN, Yeh I, Mully TW, LeBoit PE, McCalmont TH. Genomic and clinicopathologic characteristics of PRKAR1A-inactivated melanomas: toward genetic distinctions of animal-type melanoma/pigment synthesizing melanoma. Am J Surg Pathol. 2020;44(6):805–16.
76. Goutas D, Hayenne P, Tirode F, Pissaloux D, Yeh I, de la Fouchardiere A. Smooth muscle hyperplasia in protein kinase C-fused blue naevi: report of 12 cases. Histopathology. 2024;85(2):347–52.
77. Li A, Umphress B, Dehner C, Jones R, Toral K, Warren S, Alomari AK. Genomic and transcriptomic characterization of protein kinase C fusion melanocytic neoplasms with distinctive hypopigmented histomorphology: a single-institution study. J Cutan Pathol. 2025;52(6):432–41. https://doi.org/10.1111/cup.14801.

Chapter 10
Family of Spitz Melanocytic Tumors: A Molecular Perspective

Jose A. Plaza and Victor G. Prieto

Introduction

Spitz neoplasms represent a diverse and complex group of melanocytic proliferations, characterized by a wide histopathologic spectrum and varying biological behaviors. Advances in molecular ancillary testing have provided clearer insights into these neoplasms, enhancing our understanding of their biology and enabling a more precise and robust classification system. In 1948, Dr. Sophie Spitz published a groundbreaking case series describing melanocytic proliferations termed "melanomas of childhood." These lesions were histopathologically characterized by unique architectural and cytological features. These lesions were typically more commonly seen in children and young adults, and they frequently appeared on extremities. Despite being cytologically atypical, most of these tumors followed an indolent clinical course, justifying their distinction from adult melanoma. Histological criteria were developed to distinguish Spitz nevi from melanoma; however, not all cases showed unequivocal histology and recognizing that there are overlapping features among these neoplasms. In 1959, Dr. Bernard Ackerman recognized that melanocytic proliferations with Spitzoid histomorphology display a broad histomorphological spectrum ranging from banal lesions (nevi) to their fully malignant counterpart (melanoma). The name Spitz nevus, now widely used, was officially established in 1967 by the Pathology Committee of the Queensland

J. A. Plaza (✉)
The Ohio State University Wexner Medical Center, Columbus, OH, USA
e-mail: JoseA.Plaza@osumc.edu

V. G. Prieto
Departments of Pathology and Dermatology, The University of Texas MD Anderson Cancer Center, Houston, TX, USA
e-mail: vprieto@mdanderson.org

V. G. Prieto, C. A. Torres-Cabala (eds.), *Precision Molecular Pathology of Melanocytic Lesions*, Molecular Pathology Library,
https://doi.org/10.1007/978-3-032-18222-7_10

Melanoma Project; this eponym honors the legacy of Dr. Spitz. A gray zone of neoplasms that histologically were difficult to predict behavior was later designated as atypical Spitz tumors. There are multiple histologic variants of Spitz nevi, and there is clear evidence in differentiating Spitz nevi from Spitz melanoma in most cases, with the understanding that there is an intermediate category, regarded as atypical Spitz tumor (AST), representing a diagnostic and prognostic gray zone. It has been shown that even among experts, the histopathologic diagnosis of AST is not fully reliable, with a relatively low interobserver agreement.

Recent molecular studies have enhanced the understanding and biological behavior of melanocytic neoplasms. While both nevi and melanomas share growth--promoting driver mutations, they differ in their genetic alterations. Nevi typically contain only a limited number of driver mutations, whereas melanomas display additional genetic changes, such as 9p21 deletions, 6p25 gains, TP53 mutations, and TERT promoter mutations. In Spitz neoplasms, driver mutations define specific histological subtypes, while other alterations influence their biological behavior. The genetic profile of Spitz melanoma differs from that of conventional (non-Spitz) melanoma. The former may exhibit activating *HRAS* mutations or various gene translocations/fusions involving *ALK, ROS1, RET, NTRK1, NTRK3, BRAF*, and *MET*, thus different from the *BRAF, NRAS*, or *NF1* mutations more commonly seen in conventional melanomas. Additionally, a subset of Spitz tumors may show BAP1 loss.

When determining the need for ancillary studies, two key factors influence the likelihood of a lesion being a true Spitz nevus or melanoma: the patient's age and the degree of spitzoid histomorphology. These factors always need to be considered in such cases, and if the patient is young and the histomorphology is typical, the probability of it being a true Spitz nevus is high, and additional molecular testing is typically unnecessary. However, for older patients, the histological features need to be more characteristic. When the histomorphology is spitzoid but somewhat equivocal, further ancillary testing, such as BRAF or NRAS IHC or molecular studies, may become essential. If the tumor carries an activating mutation in BRAF or NRAS and melanoma is part of the histologic differential diagnosis, further testing with FISH, CGH, or assessment of a TERT promoter mutation is important. In cases of benign or intermediate-grade lesions, it remains uncertain whether these have a higher risk of transformation or less stability compared to true Spitz neoplasms.

Integrating molecular data with histopathological classification enhances the accurate identification of true Spitz neoplasms within Spitzoid lesions. Moreover, establishing consistent genotype-phenotype correlations improves diagnostic precision, aiding in the classification of AST and allowing for a more refined assessment of malignancy risk. In this chapter, we will focus on the genomic and bio--morphological spectrum of Spitz tumors.

HRAS Mutations

The *RAS* proto-oncogene family consists of three members: *KRAS, NRAS*, and *HRAS*, which are located on the short arm (p) of chromosomes 12, 1, and 11, respectively. Mutations in *HRAS*, a proto-oncogene located on chromosome 11p, were the initial genetic alterations identified in Spitz neoplasms. *HRAS* is part of the *RAS* oncogene family and encodes a GTPase involved in the MAP kinase signaling pathway. Mutations in *HRAS* may lead to its continuous activation, causing abnormal expression of transcription factors that regulate cell growth and differentiation. Compared to other *RAS* proteins, *HRAS* has a stronger affinity for the PI3K-AKT pathway, which is believed to contribute to the epithelioid or spindle cell morphology observed in Spitz nevi. Activating *HRAS* mutations and copy number gains of 11p occur either exclusively or concurrently in approximately 20% of Spitz neoplasms [1–3]. The detection of *HRAS* mutations requires sequencing analysis, either classical or next-generation sequencing (NGS), while identifying 11p copy number alterations necessitates FISH or CGH analysis.

Clinically, Spitz nevi with *HRAS* mutations typically present as symmetrical, raised lesions with a plaque, or nodular-shaped silhouette, commonly on the head, neck, and extremities. Histologically, *HRAS*-mutated Spitz nevi are primarily intradermal, characterized by a desmoplastic stroma reaction ranging from low cellularity admixed with desmoplastic stroma to a bulkier cellular proliferation within the dermis (Figs. 10.1 and 10.2). A common feature of *HRAS*-mutated Spitz tumors is their infiltrative growth pattern at the base, along with minimal or absent melanin pigment. They are also distinguished by their extensive dispersion of single cells between collagen bundles. Cytologically, the cells may exhibit Spitzoid features such as vesicular nuclei and abundant eosinophilic or amphophilic cytoplasm [2, 4, 5]. Marked cytological atypia can be present in about 40% of *HRAS*-mutated cases. The proliferation rate is generally low. There may be rare deep mitotic figures in the lower half or at the base of the lesion, particularly in elderly patients. It is important to note that not all Spitz neoplasms with these genomic alterations exhibit desmoplasia. Conversely, desmoplastic features have also been observed in Spitz neoplasms with *ROS1, ALK*, and *BRAF* gene fusions.

Although Spitz nevi share many histopathologic features with melanoma, a key distinguishing factor between the two is their genomic stability. It has been proposed that RAS gene activation alone is insufficient to drive tumorigenesis and instead requires additional aberrations, such as BRAF mutations or the inactivation of p53 or p16, to promote malignant transformation; however, this hypothesis is somewhat controversial and requires further investigation. The presence of HRAS mutation appears to be associated with a favorable prognosis. To date, there are no reports of patients with HRAS-mutated Spitz tumors with distant metastases or fatal outcomes [2, 4]. Most Spitz neoplasms with activating HRAS mutations and/or copy number gains on chromosome 11p are typically histologically recognizable; however, there are cases that exhibit features within the spectrum of AST. Despite these atypical histomorphological features, the prognosis for these neoplasms is

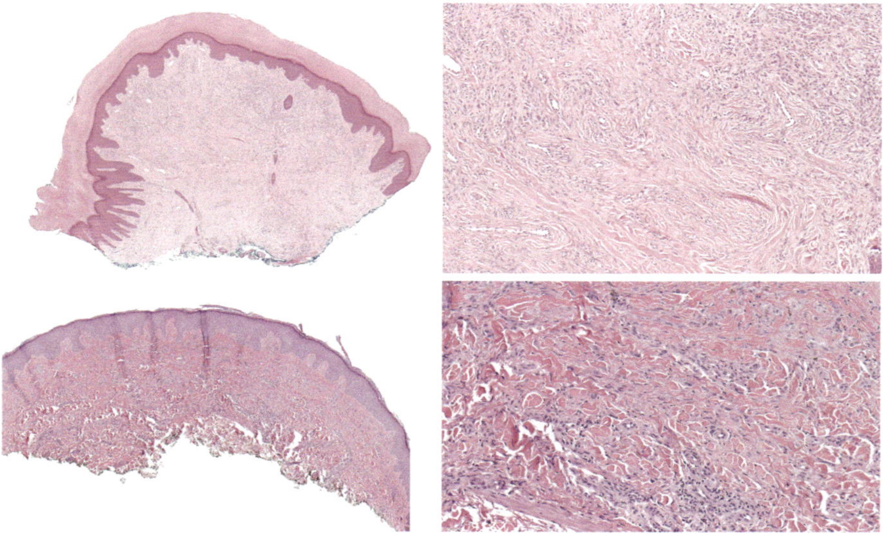

Fig. 10.1 HRAS-mutated Spitz nevi: Symmetrical, nodular lesions, predominantly intradermal, showing low cellularity with areas of desmoplastic stroma transitioning to more cellular proliferation within the dermis. Note the infiltrative growth pattern at the base without melanin pigment. A characteristic feature is the extensive dispersion of single cells between collagen bundles. The tumor cells are spindled with vesicular nuclei and eosinophilic cytoplasm (original magnification left images ×40, right images x200)

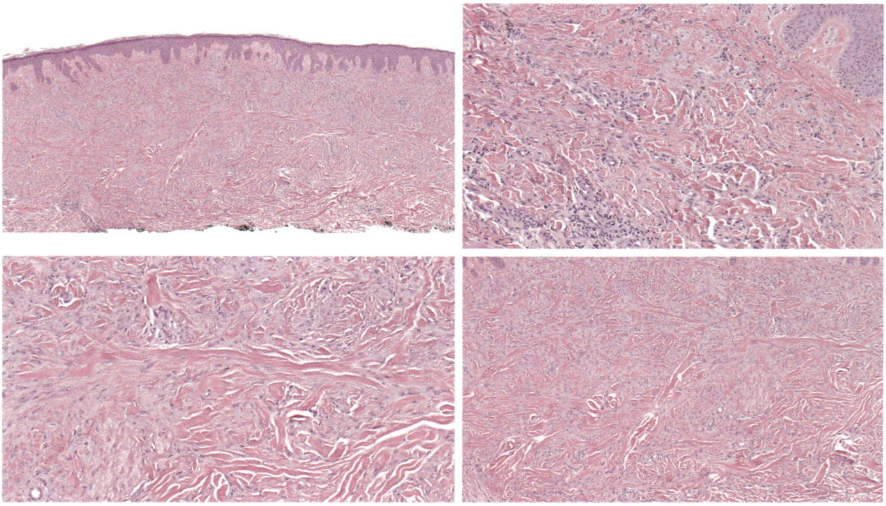

Fig. 10.2 HRAS-mutated Spitz nevi: This example shows the lesion growing as a plaque and predominantly intradermal. The tumor is low cellularity within a desmoplastic stroma and has an infiltrative growth pattern in the dermis without melanin pigment

generally favorable. In conclusion, HRAS mutation analysis appears to be a valuable tool in distinguishing Spitz nevus from Spitz melanoma. It may also serve as a foundation for a more standardized classification of Spitz tumors by integrating histological and genetic data.

ALK Fusions

The anaplastic lymphoma kinase (ALK) gene, located on chromosome 2p23, encodes a tyrosine kinase receptor that is part of the insulin receptor family. ALK fusions have also been detected in other cutaneous neoplasms, including acral melanoma, primary cutaneous anaplastic large cell lymphoma (PCALCL), and epithelioid fibrous histiocytoma. ALK fusions have been identified in approximately 10% of Spitz melanocytic neoplasms [6, 7]. Most cases with ALK fusions are classified as Spitz nevi or atypical Spitz tumors, though there are rare cases of Spitz melanoma with ALK fusion [6, 8]. Multiple ALK fusion partners have been identified, including TMP3, DCTN1, MLPH, KANK1, CLIP1, DDX3Y, EEF2, GTF3C2, MYO5A, NPM1, PPFIBP1, SPTAN1, TPR, and EHBP1 [9–12].

Clinically, ALK-fused Spitz neoplasms typically present as large, solitary papules (with a pyogenic granuloma-like appearance) on the extremities of young patients [13, 14]. Histologically, these lesions often exhibit a distinct pattern characterized by a wedge-shaped silhouette with a bulbous and/or infiltrative base. A hallmark of ALK fusions is the presence of nonpigmented (amelanotic), large spindle and epithelioid melanocytes with pericellular clefts, amphophilic cytoplasm, vesicular nuclei, and prominent nucleoli, arranged in plexiform intersecting fascicles [11, 13–15]. The tumors are usually compound but with a predominant intradermal component (Fig. 10.3). The epidermis is often hyperplastic, with rare or absent pagetoid spread. Nuclear pleomorphism can be observed in some cases. Notably, worrisome histologic features, including ulceration, deep mitotic figures (>5 mm^2), and perineural invasion, have been described in some cases, despite following indolent behavior [13, 14, 16]. Another distinct pattern associated with ALK-fused Spitz neoplasms is their angiomatoid pattern. However, while these histomorphologic features are highly sensitive for predicting ALK fusions, they are not entirely specific, as other molecular subtypes of Spitz neoplasms, such as NTRK1-fused cases, may share overlapping characteristics. ALK-fusion Spitz tumors serve as a prime example of why conventional criteria for classifying melanocytic tumors as malignant may not be applicable to Spitz neoplasms.

ALK immunostudies using the monoclonal antibodies D5F3 and 5A4 serve as excellent surrogate markers for ALK fusions and are cost-effective and reliable ancillary diagnostic tools. Most cases show diffuse, strong, and granular staining in the cytoplasm of melanocytes, with variable presence in the membrane or nucleus (including a rare nucleolar pattern) [6, 13, 14]. Next-generation sequencing (NGS) and fluorescence in situ hybridization (FISH) using a break-apart probe targeting ALK are additional ancillary diagnostic techniques for detecting ALK fusions [17].

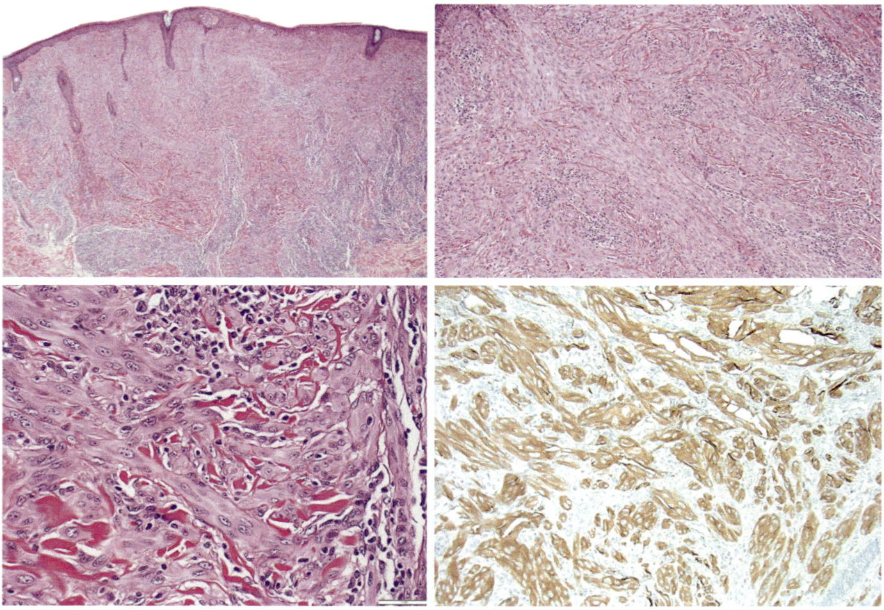

Fig. 10.3 ALK-fused Spitz neoplasm: The lesion shows a distinct pattern characterized by a wedge-shaped silhouette with an infiltrative base. Note the amelanotic large spindle and epithelioid melanocytes with pericellular clefts, amphophilic cytoplasm, vesicular nuclei, and prominent nucleoli, arranged in plexiform intersecting fascicles. The epidermis is hyperplastic. The high power shows nuclear pleomorphism with a vesicular nucleus. Immunohistochemistry detects ALK expression (original magnification X20, x40, and x400)

To the best of our knowledge, no cases of ALK-fused Spitz melanocytic neoplasms have been reported with associated systemic metastases or death from the disease.

ROS1 Fusions

ROS1 is a proto-oncogene located on chromosome 6q22.1 that encodes a tyrosine kinase receptor participating in several signaling pathways (Ras-Raf-MEK1/2-ERK1/2, JAK3-STAT3, and PI3K-AKT-mTOR). ROS1 fusions are among the most common alterations observed in Spitz melanocytic neoplasms (7%–17%) [6, 18–20]. Although clinical outcomes data for Spitz tumors with ROS1 fusions are limited, published follow-up reports show no recurrences or metastases after complete excision of the primary tumors. Thus, these tumors are likely indolent or belong to a considerably lower risk category compared to Spitz neoplasms with BRAF or MAP 3K8 fusions, which tend to be more aggressive (see below) [21–24].

Clinically, Spitz tumors with ROS1 fusions generally present as dome-shaped, well-circumscribed, pink to red papules found across various body regions, most frequently on the lower extremities. These lesions are more common in females and typically occur in individuals under 40 years of age [19, 20, 25]. They may present as a plaque-like or nodule, without significant deep infiltration, and a mixture of epithelioid and spindle cells. Key observations included the consistent absence of severe cytologic atypia, the lack of larger cell types, the presence of maturation, frequent Kamino bodies, and reduced or absent mitotic activity. Additionally, transepidermal elimination is reported not only in the central part of the lesion but also involving the follicular infundibulum and acrosyringium. In these areas, the melanocytes are almost invariably pyknotic and appear as large, ascending cells, exhibiting a full-thickness breach toward the epidermal surface [20]. An intriguing and novel observation is the presence of a ROS1 fusion in some desmoplastic Spitz neoplasms [19]. This finding not only underscores the diverse range of microscopic features associated with ROS1 fusions but also further confirms that the desmoplastic phenotype in Spitz neoplasms is not exclusively linked to HRAS aberrations. There are also reports of ROS1 fusions in pigmented spindle cell nevi of Reed [6, 26]. PWWP2A was also the most frequent rearrangement in ROS1 Spitz neoplasms. These tumors usually lack homozygous 9p21 deletion or TERT-p mutations.

ROS1 fusions can be detected by FISH studies utilizing a break-apart probe targeting ROS1. Immunohistochemistry with the monoclonal antibody D4D6 against ROS1 has demonstrated positivity in 97.4% of ROS1-fused Spitz nevi, with 100% specificity compared to FISH. Various IHC staining patterns have been observed, including diffuse granular cytoplasmic staining, dot-like staining, and nuclear staining [25]. RNA NGS cannot detect all ROS1 alterations.

NTRK Fusions

The Neurotrophic Tropomyosin Receptor Kinase (NTRK) proto-oncogene family consists of three members: NTRK1, NTRK2, and NTRK3, located on chromosomes 1q, 9q, and 15q, respectively. These are oncogenic alterations that can be therapeutically targeted and are found in a wide variety of neoplasms in different organs (including colorectal carcinomas, lung cancer, thyroid cancer, sarcomas, melanomas, gliomas, etc.) [27–29]. These genes encode the receptor tyrosine kinase proteins TRKA, TRKB, and TRKC. Normally expressed in the nervous system, these receptors are activated upon binding with ligands such as NGF, BDNF, and NT-3/4. TRK activation triggers autophosphorylation of intracellular tyrosine residues, leading to signal transmission through various pathways that regulate gene transcription involved in neuronal survival and differentiation. NTRK gene fusions result in the formation of TRK chimeric proteins with oncogenic properties, as they combine constitutive expression with ligand-independent activation due to the preservation of the kinase domain. In Spitz neoplasms, fusions involving NTRK1, NTRK2, and NTRK3 have been identified, although alterations in NTRK1 are by far the most common.

NTRK1 fusions have been observed in up to 16% of Spitz tumors, with most cases occurring in Spitz nevi and atypical Spitz tumors. Histopathologically, these tumors exhibit classic Spitzoid characteristics, including a compound or dermal exophytic, symmetric lesions characterized by thin, elongated (filigree-like) rete ridges and a flat-base or wedge-shaped silhouette (Figs. 10.4 and 10.5) [30, 31]. They often display lentiginous proliferation, nests, and rosette-like structures, cytologic atypia, along with marked maturation of epithelioid and/or spindle melanocytes [6, 14]. Kamino bodies are commonly present, while mitotic figures are rare [6]. Like ALK-fused Spitz neoplasms, some cases exhibit a plexiform pattern marked by intersecting fascicles of spindle melanocytes [15, 30].

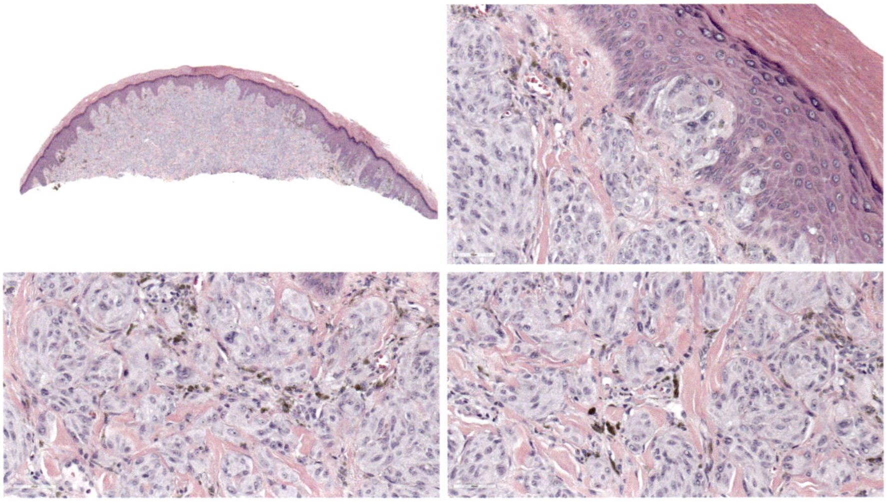

Fig. 10.4 NTRK Spitz tumor: This is a compound neoplasm showing epidermal hyperplasia and a dome-shaped silhouette. This lesion is composed of epithelioid melanocytes with defined borders, pale cytoplasm, and pleomorphic nuclei, arranged in large, lobulated, coalescing nests (original magnifications x20 and x400)

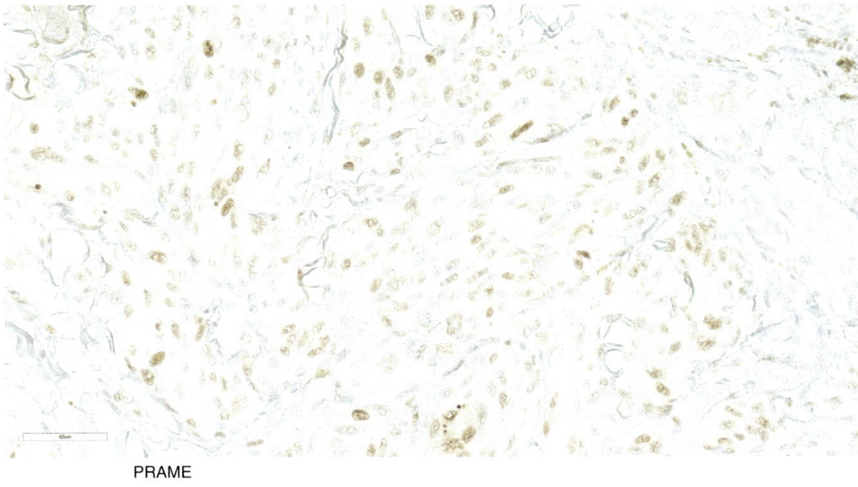

Fig. 10.5 NTRK Spitz tumor: PRAME expression as weak and strong nuclear labeling (PRAME, original magnification x400)

Only a few Spitz tumors with NTRK2 rearrangements have been documented since the first reported case featuring an NTRK2::TGF fusion in a pigmented spindle cell nevus of Reed [32–35]. There are also cases with an NTRK2 fusion involving the SQSTM1 gene (5q) [34]. These lesions are usually junctional and symmetrical (horizontal confluence), with a hyperplastic epidermis and large melanocytic nests exhibiting peripheral clefts, composed of pigmented spindle and epithelioid melanocytes with ample eosinophilic cytoplasm and elongated nuclei [34, 35]. Visible dendritic processes and Kamino bodies are usually noted. Rare cases can show a dermal component.

NTRK3-fused Spitz neoplasms are rare, with the most common fusions being ETV6::NTRK3, MYO5A::NTRK3, and MYH9::NTRK3 [34]. Histopathologically, they are primarily compound or intradermal, exhibiting epidermal hyperplasia and a dome-shaped silhouette. Their histomorphology varies depending on the specific fusion [36]. Lesions with ETV6-NTRK3 fusions predominantly consist of epithelioid melanocytes with well-defined borders, pale to eosinophilic cytoplasm, and pleomorphic nuclei, arranged in large, lobulated, coalescing nests. Some of these tumors had features reminiscent of those seen in BAP1-inactivated neoplasms. ETV6-rearranged Spitz tumors are more commonly observed in younger patients and typically occur on the head and neck area [26]. In contrast, MYO5A-NTRK3-fused lesions are more commonly seen in patients between 20 and 50 years of age and are more commonly located on the trunk and extremities. Histopathologically, they are composed of uniformly spindled melanocytes arranged in a fascicular to plexiform growth pattern, occasionally displaying neuroid features and Verocay body-like appearance and rosette-like formations [26]. Lesions with MYH9-NTRK3 fusions are characterized by large epithelioid melanocytes arranged in a syncytial pattern, with desmoplastic stroma and peripheral collagen trapping [31, 36].

Immunohistochemical analysis commonly uses the monoclonal antibody EPR17341, which targets a C-terminal epitope common to both wild-type and chimeric TRK proteins. Cases that are positive for immunohistochemistry may undergo NGS or RT PCR analysis to confirm the presence of an NTRK fusion. This approach has been validated in a large AST series, demonstrating the reliability of pan-TRK immunohistochemistry as a screening method [37]. NGS has shown some limitations in confirming gene fusions, leading to the recommendation of FISH testing for pan-TRK-IHC positive cases that are not confirmed by NGS. Additionally, the pan-TRK immunostaining pattern can provide insights into the specific NTRK fusion involved. Cases with NTRK1 or NTRK2 fusions typically exhibit strong and diffuse cytoplasmic expression [38]. Strong, diffuse nuclear staining is highly indicative of an ETV6-NTRK3 fusion, while linear staining in dendritic melanocyte processes suggests a MYO5A-NTRK3 fusion [36].

The prognosis for Spitz neoplasms with NTRK1 or NTRK3 fusions remains consistently favorable [39]. While rare cases of neoplastic cellular deposits in regional lymph nodes have been observed, there are no reported instances of distant metastases or other adverse outcomes. Spitz melanomas with pan-NTRK fusions generally exhibit indolent behavior, with lymph node metastasis being rare [12].

MAP 2K1 Mutations

MAP 2K1 is a proto-oncogene located on chromosome 15p that encodes a protein kinase with serine-threonine and tyrosine activity, playing a key role in the RAF-MEK-ERK signaling pathway. Activating mutations in MAP 2K1 have been identified in melanocytic neoplasms, including Spitz neoplasms, deep penetrating nevi, pigmented epithelioid melanocytomas, and melanomas, and in other non-melanocytic tumors such as colorectal cancer, lung adenocarcinoma, serous ovarian cancer, thyroid cancer, histiocytic sarcoma, Langerhans cell histiocytosis, Erdheim-Chester disease, and hairy cell leukemia [40–48].

Spitz neoplasms harboring MAP 2K1 mutations generally manifest as small, flat, or slightly papular pigmented lesions, predominantly found on the lower extremities of young patients, with a marked female bias. Certain histopathologic characteristics appear to be recurrent, such as a compound or intradermal wedge-shaped morphology, showing a plexiform growth and a concentric organization of tumoral nests around adnexal structures and neurovascular bundles. These tumoral nests consist of large epithelioid and spindled cells with vesicular nuclei and display moderate nuclear pleomorphism (Fig. 10.6). Other histological findings may include notable pigmentation, with stromal melanin deposition and numerous melanophages, slight epidermal hyperplasia, low mitotic activity, and inadequate maturation in dermis. In some instances, cytologic features typical of a Spitz neoplasm alongside those of a dysplastic nevus have been observed, a combination sometimes referred to as a SPARK nevus [49]. The diverse histomorphologic presentations seen in MAP 2K1-mutated Spitz neoplasms are thought to be influenced by secondary genetic alterations, as many cases also present with additional mutations in well-known oncogenes and tumor suppressor genes such as BRAF, IDH1, BAP1, and NF1 [50].

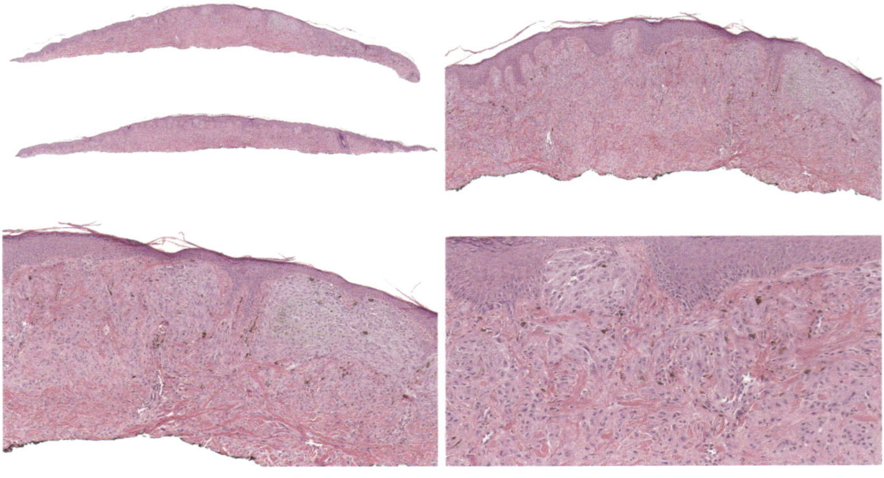

Fig. 10.6 MAP 2K1 Spitz tumor: This is an intradermal neoplasm, showing a plexiform growth with accentuation around adnexal structures. The tumor nests are composed of large epithelioid and spindled cells with vesicular nuclei and display moderate nuclear pleomorphism (original magnifications x20, x40, x100, x200)

RET Fusions

The Rearranged during Transfection (RET) proto-oncogene, located on chromosome 10q, encodes a tyrosine kinase receptor involved in several signaling pathways, including PI3K-AKT, RAF-MEK1/2-ERK1/2, and PLCγ1. RET fusions are identified in approximately 3–4% of Spitz neoplasms, [6, 18, 51] with fusion partners such as CCDC6, KIF5B, LMNA, GOLGA5, and MYO5A [6, 26, 52]. Its detection requires NGS or FISH.

The limited number of RET-rearranged Spitz neoplasms reported to date typically present as compound, symmetric lesions featuring epidermal hyperplasia, a plaque-like silhouette, and large expansile nests of dishesive, intermediate-sized, and monotonous epithelioid melanocytes showing mild to moderate nuclear atypia. In addition, cases show transepidermal elimination of nests, lobulated nests, rosette-like structures, and Kamino bodies. Given the heterogeneous histopathology of these RET Spitz neoplasms, one study subdivided the Spitz tumors into six groups according to the 5′ fusion partners [51]. Lesions with KIF5B fusion partners were predominantly composed of small, nevoid melanocytes resembling conventional type B melanocytes. The presence of junctional nests of spindled melanocytes indicated a Spitzoid component. MYO5A fusion partners were associated with spindled melanocytes arranged in broad, intersecting fascicles, producing a multinodular or plexiform architecture that extended deep into the dermis and involved subcutaneous fat. These tumors sometimes exhibited pseudo-Verocay bodies and rosette-like structures, contributing to a neuroid appearance. Lesions with OPTN 5′ fusions demonstrated transepidermal elimination and floating intraepidermal nests, features reminiscent of ROS1-fused Spitz tumors. Tumors harboring CCDC6 and LMNA fusions showed similar histologic patterns, with epithelioid melanocytes arranged in confluent nests, often with areas of cellular dishesion. Melanocytes frequently exhibited eccentric nuclei, resembling rhabdoid melanocytes seen in BAP1-inactivated melanocytic tumors. The final group comprised lesions with less commonly encountered 5′ fusion partners—NCOA4, ERC1, MYH9, and AGAP3. These tumors were generally composed of large epithelioid melanocytes and demonstrated multiple atypical features, including pagetoid spread, marked nuclear pleomorphism, giant multinucleated melanocytes, increased mitotic activity with atypical mitoses, and a sheet-like growth pattern, supporting a diagnosis of AST.

Although RET fusions have been observed in Spitz nevi, atypical Spitz tumors, and malignant Spitz tumors (MST), the prognosis appears favorable, with no adverse outcomes reported in available follow-up data.

MAP 3K8 Mutations

MAP 3K8 is a proto-oncogene located at 10p11 that encodes the serine/threonine kinase Tpl2/COT, which is involved in several signaling pathways, including MEK-1, MKK6, SAPK, NFAT, and NF-κB. MAP 3K8 truncation may lead to an increased activity of the MEK1/2 and ERK1/2 pathways, influencing cell proliferation and differentiation. Fusions or truncations involving MAP 3K8 have been identified in various neoplasms, including lung cancer, thymoma, nasopharyngeal carcinoma, and breast cancer. Rearrangements in MAP 3K8 are now recognized as the most common driver of Spitzoid melanoma [23, 53].

Clinically, MAP 3K8-fused Spitz neoplasms typically present as pigmented, exophytic lesions on the lower extremities and can occur in patients of all ages, with a slight female predominance [9, 24]. Histologically, these tumors are generally nodular or dome-shaped, asymmetric, and characterized by overlying epidermal hyperplasia. The junctional component often has a predominantly nested pattern, with epithelioid melanocytes, featuring large, uniform nuclei, prominent nucleoli, and abundant eosinophilic cytoplasm [9, 23, 24, 53]. Common histologic features include severe cytologic atypia, deep mitotic figures, lack of maturation, scattered multinucleated giant melanocytes, epidermal ulceration, and pagetoid spread. These tumors frequently exhibit inactivation of p16, which might contribute to the highly atypical histomorphologic features of these neoplasms. However, inactivation of p16 does not definitively diagnose malignancy. There are rare cases of MAP 3K8-fused Spitz neoplasms that metastasize to lymph nodes [53, 54]. Some may exhibit additional genomic alterations with prognostic relevance, particularly biallelic inactivation or homozygous deletion of CDKN2A/B and complex structural rearrangement of TERT, which can be associated with a more aggressive clinical course [18, 23]. Detection of MAP 3K8 fusions can be achieved through RNA or DNA-based NGS and/or FISH analysis.

BRAF Fusions

BRAF fusions arise from genomic rearrangements that position the 3′ end of the BRAF gene—which encodes the kinase domain—adjacent to the 5′ end of various fusion partner genes. This rearrangement eliminates the BRAF's auto-inhibitory domain, resulting in a fusion kinase that is constitutively active. Additionally, BRAF expression becomes dysregulated, as it is driven by the promoter of the 5′ fusion partner. The overall consequence is activation of the downstream mitogen-activated protein kinase (MAPK) pathway.

The Cancer Genome Atlas classifies cutaneous melanoma into four molecular categories [55]. The most prevalent, accounting for approximately 50% of cases, is the BRAF subtype, defined by $BRAF^{V600E}$ mutations [55, 56]. The RAS subtype comprises about 25% of melanomas and includes NRAS mutations (~24%) along with less common HRAS and KRAS hotspot mutations (<1%) [55]. Approximately 10% of melanomas fall under the NF1 subtype, characterized by NF1 mutations, over half of which result in complete loss-of-function through nonsense, frameshift, or splice-site alterations [55]. This subtype often co-occurs with mutations that modestly activate the MAPK/ERK pathway and is more frequently seen in desmoplastic melanoma and in tumors from chronically sun-exposed skin [57, 58]. Melanomas without mutations in BRAF, NRAS/HRAS/KRAS, or NF1 are grouped as triple wild type. This heterogeneous category includes tumors with GNAQ or GNA11 mutations (well-established in uveal melanoma and blue-nevus type melanoma), KIT mutations (common in acral and mucosal melanomas), and genomic rearrangements involving BRAF or RAF1. Because BRAF is constitutively expressed in melanocytic lesions, immunohistochemistry is not specific for detecting BRAF fusions. Instead, genomic techniques such as FISH or NGS are required for accurate identification.

With the increasing routine use of genomic testing, it has become evident that melanocytic neoplasms harboring BRAF or NRAS mutations exist along a spectrum from benign to malignant and can closely resemble Spitz neoplasms in their histomorphology. These lesions have been referred to as BRAF-mutated Spitzoid (BAMS) lesions [59].

Spitz neoplasms with BRAF fusions most commonly present clinically as pink papules on the extremities, particularly in young females. These lesions can be compound or intradermal, with a range of different patterns including plaque-like, wedge-shaped, or nodular forms. They are primarily composed of large epithelioid melanocytes featuring abundant amphophilic cytoplasm, vesicular, pleomorphic nuclei, and prominent nucleoli. Cytologic atypia is often moderate to severe, with common mitotic figures (Fig. 10.7). Among the various fusion subtypes of Spitz tumors, BRAF and MAP 3K8 (as explained above) are associated with the most significant cytologic atypia. BRAF-fused Spitz tumors are characteristically described as having a superficial sheet-like dermal component, which is more cellular, and a less cellular base with a prominent desmoplastic reaction, often lacking melanocytic maturation. Due to these atypical histologic features, these neoplasms are usually classified as atypical Spitz tumor or, sometimes, as Spitz melanoma. Some atypical histological features, such as ulceration or increased mitotic activity, may be acceptable in a true Spitz tumor with a fusion driver. However, the same features in a BRAF-mutated neoplasm would be more concerning [60]. Therefore, immunohistochemistry for $BRAF^{V600E}$ or genomic studies can be crucial in resolving some of these cases [60].

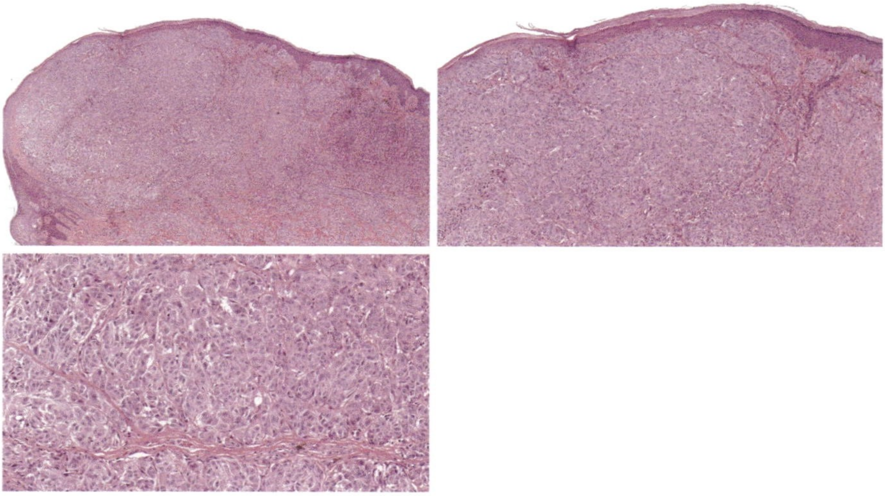

Fig. 10.7 BRAF-mutated Spitz tumor: This is an intradermal tumor with nodular growth. It is composed of large epithelioid melanocytes with abundant amphophilic cytoplasm and vesicular, pleomorphic nuclei. Note the upper portion of the tumor with a superficial sheet-like dermal component, which is more cellular (original magnifications x20, x100, x200)

TERT Promoter Mutation

Telomerase activity plays a critical role in tumor development and cancer progression. This activity, essential for maintaining telomeric DNA during cell replication, is regulated by the telomerase reverse transcriptase (TERT) gene. Mutations in the promoter region of the TERT gene are common in a variety of cancers, including melanoma, where their reported prevalence ranges from 17% to 71%. These alterations represent a key oncogenic mechanism by driving sustained telomerase expression. In normal somatic cells, progressive telomere shortening occurs with each cell division due to the end-replication problem, eventually leading to replicative senescence or apoptosis. TERT counteracts this telomere erosion by adding TTAGGG repeats to the ends of chromosomes, thereby maintaining telomere length and allowing cells to evade senescence.

The challenge of predicting the risk of hematogenous metastasis in patients with AST has led to considerable research. Many studies have proposed a histopathologic grading system to stratify risk in pediatric AST, such as age ≥10 years, presence of ulceration, and mitotic activity greater than 5/mm^2—as being associated with subsequent development of extranodal metastasis [12, 61]. Studies have observed that TERT promoter mutations are associated with adverse histopathologic features, including increased mitotic activity and ulceration. It is well established that Spitzoid tumors arising in prepubertal children (under 10 years of age), even when exhibiting histological features suggestive of malignancy, almost never progress to distant metastasis [62]. This observation has been validated in cases where there is absence of TERT promoter mutations in tumors from younger patients, although the biological basis for this age-related difference remains unclear.

TERT promoter mutational status may also support risk stratification of ASTs and Spitz melanomas, especially given that lymph node metastasis alone is not a reliable predictor of extranodal spread or mortality. Studies have shown that the presence of hotspot TERT promoter mutations is more commonly associated with Spitz melanomas than with AST [63]. In cases of metastatic Spitz melanoma with a fatal outcome, RT-PCR has revealed markedly elevated TERT mRNA expression. In contrast, TERT mRNA was either undetectable or present at low levels in cases of ASTs [63, 64]. In these cases, tumors with wild-type TERT promoter mutation remained free of distant metastasis after a median follow-up of 32.5 months [12]. This observation was supported by other studies in pediatric patients, where wild-type TERT promoter tumors did not progress beyond lymph node involvement [65, 66]. Additionally, in cases of ASTs with TERT promoter hotspot mutations have been linked to patients age ≥10 years, mitotic rate > 5/mm^2, and the presence of ulceration.

References

1. van Dijk MC, Bernsen MR, Ruiter DJ. Analysis of mutations in B-RAF, N-RAS, and H-RAS genes in the differential diagnosis of Spitz nevus and spitzoid melanoma. Am J Surg Pathol. 2005;29(9):1145–51.
2. van Engen-van Grunsven AC, van Dijk MC, Ruiter DJ, Klaasen A, Mooi WJ, Blokx WA. HRAS-mutated Spitz tumors: a subtype of Spitz tumors with distinct features. Am J Surg Pathol. 2010;34(10):1436–41.
3. Bastian BC, LeBoit PE, Hamm H, Brocker EB, Pinkel D. Chromosomal gains and losses in primary cutaneous melanomas detected by comparative genomic hybridization. Cancer Res. 1998;58(10):2170–5.
4. Bastian BC, LeBoit PE, Pinkel D. Mutations and copy number increase of HRAS in Spitz nevi with distinctive histopathological features. Am J Pathol. 2000;157(3):967–72.
5. Lezcano CM, Yeh I, Eslamdoost N, et al. Expanding the spectrum of microscopic and cytogenetic findings associated with Spitz Tumors with 11p gains. Am J Surg Pathol. 2021;45(2):277–85.
6. Wiesner T, He J, Yelensky R, et al. Kinase fusions are frequent in Spitz tumours and spitzoid melanomas. Nat Commun. 2014;5:3116.
7. Busam KJ, Kutzner H, Cerroni L, Wiesner T. Clinical and pathologic findings of Spitz nevi and atypical Spitz tumors with ALK fusions. Am J Surg Pathol. 2014;38(7):925–33.
8. Saraggi D, Salmaso R, Zamuner C, et al. Prevalence of ALK gene alterations among the spectrum of plexiform spitzoid lesions. J Am Acad Dermatol. 2018;79(4):728–35.
9. Newman S, Fan L, Pribnow A, et al. Clinical genome sequencing uncovers potentially targetable truncations and fusions of MAP 3K8 in spitzoid and other melanomas. Nat Med. 2019;25(4):597–602.
10. Chung CT, Marrano P, Swanson D, Dickson BC, Thorner PS. Fusion of ALK to the melanophilin gene MLPH in pediatric spitz nevi. Hum Pathol. 2019;87:57–64.
11. Kastnerova L, Martinek P, Grossmann P, et al. A clinicopathological study of 29 spitzoid melanocytic lesions with ALK fusions, including novel fusion variants, accompanied by

fluorescence in situ hybridization analysis for chromosomal copy number changes, and both TERT promoter and next-generation sequencing mutation analysis. Am J Dermatopathol. 2020;42(8):578–92.
12. Lee S, Barnhill RL, Dummer R, et al. TERT promoter mutations are predictive of aggressive clinical behavior in patients with spitzoid melanocytic neoplasms. Sci Rep. 2015;5:11200.
13. Yeh I, de la Fouchardiere A, Pissaloux D, et al. Clinical, histopathologic, and genomic features of Spitz tumors with ALK fusions. Am J Surg Pathol. 2015;39(5):581–91.
14. Amin SM, Haugh AM, Lee CY, et al. A comparison of morphologic and molecular features of BRAF, ALK, and NTRK1 fusion spitzoid neoplasms. Am J Surg Pathol. 2017;41(4):491–8.
15. Kiuru M, Jungbluth A, Kutzner H, Wiesner T, Busam KJ. Spitz tumors: comparison of histological features in relationship to immunohistochemical staining for ALK and NTRK1. Int J Surg Pathol. 2016;24(3):200–6.
16. Brown RA, Wang JY, Raghavan SS, et al. ALK-positive compound Spitz nevus with extensive perineural and intraneural neurotropism. J Cutan Pathol. 2021;48(1):154–9.
17. Niu X, Chuang JC, Berry GJ, Wakelee HA. Anaplastic lymphoma kinase testing: IHC vs. FISH vs. NGS. Curr Treat Options in Oncol. 2017;18(12):71.
18. Quan VL, Zhang B, Zhang Y, et al. Integrating next-generation sequencing with morphology improves prognostic and biologic classification of spitz neoplasms. J Invest Dermatol. 2020;140(8):1599–608.
19. Gerami P, Kim D, Compres EV, et al. Clinical, morphologic, and genomic findings in ROS1 fusion Spitz neoplasms. Mod Pathol. 2021;34(2):348–57.
20. Donati M, Kastnerova L, Martinek P, et al. Spitz tumors with ROS1 fusions: a clinicopathological study of 6 cases, including FISH for chromosomal copy number alterations and mutation analysis using next-generation sequencing. Am J Dermatopathol. 2020;42(2):92–102.
21. Perron E, Pissaloux D, Neub A, et al. Unclassified sclerosing malignant melanomas with AKAP9-BRAF gene fusion: a report of two cases and review of BRAF fusions in melanocytic tumors. Virchows Arch. 2018;472(3):469–76.
22. Ross JS, Wang K, Chmielecki J, et al. The distribution of BRAF gene fusions in solid tumors and response to targeted therapy. Int J Cancer. 2016;138(4):881–90.
23. Quan VL, Zhang B, Mohan LS, et al. Activating structural alterations in MAPK genes are distinct genetic drivers in a unique subgroup of Spitzoid neoplasms. Am J Surg Pathol. 2019;43(4):538–48.
24. Houlier A, Pissaloux D, Masse I, et al. Melanocytic tumors with MAP 3K8 fusions: report of 33 cases with morphological-genetic correlations. Mod Pathol. 2020;33(5):846–57.
25. Cesinaro AM, Gallo G, Manfredini S, Maiorana A, Bettelli SR. ROS1 pattern of immunostaining in 11 cases of spitzoid tumour: comparison with histopathological, fluorescence in-situ hybridisation and next-generation sequencing analysis. Histopathology. 2021;79(6):966–74.
26. VandenBoom T, Quan VL, Zhang B, et al. Genomic fusions in pigmented spindle cell nevus of reed. Am J Surg Pathol. 2018;42(8):1042–51.
27. Manea CA, Badiu DC, Ploscaru IC, et al. A review of NTRK fusions in cancer. Ann Med Surg (Lond). 2022;79:103893.
28. Creancier L, Vandenberghe I, Gomes B, et al. Chromosomal rearrangements involving the NTRK1 gene in colorectal carcinoma. Cancer Lett. 2015;365(1):107–11.
29. Pekova B, Sykorova V, Mastnikova K, et al. NTRK fusion genes in thyroid carcinomas: clinicopathological characteristics and their impacts on prognosis. Cancers (Basel). 2021;13(8):1932.
30. Yeh I, Busam KJ, McCalmont TH, et al. Filigree-like rete ridges, lobulated nests, rosette-like structures, and exaggerated maturation characterize Spitz tumors with NTRK1 fusion. Am J Surg Pathol. 2019;43(6):737–46.
31. Kervarrec T, Pissaloux D, Tirode F, et al. Morphologic features in a series of 352 spitz melanocytic proliferations help predict their oncogenic drivers. Virchows Arch. 2022;480(2):369–82.
32. Goto K, Pissaloux D, Tirode F, de la Fouchardiere A. Spitz nevus with a novel TFG-NTRK2 fusion: the first case report of NTRK2-rearranged Spitz/Reed nevus. J Cutan Pathol. 2021;48(9):1193–6.

33. Scarfo F, Brunetto E, Magliacane G, Pecciarini L, Ferrara G, Rizzo N. Spitz spindle cell/reed nevus with SQSTM1::NTRK2 fusion and atypical features in an older male patient: a case report and review of literature. J Cutan Pathol. 2025;52(5):367–73.
34. Mansour B, Vanecek T, Kastnerova L, Nosek D, Kazakov DV, Donati M. Spitz tumor with SQSTM1::NTRK2 fusion: a clinicopathological study of 5 cases. Am J Dermatopathol. 2023;45(5):306–10.
35. Phillips GS, Mengden-Koon S, Dhossche J, et al. Atypical Spitz tumor with SQSTM1::NTRK2 fusion: report of a case with unique spindled cell features. J Cutan Pathol. 2024;51(3):198–204.
36. de la Fouchardiere A, Tee MK, Peternel S, et al. Fusion partners of NTRK3 affect subcellular localization of the fusion kinase and cytomorphology of melanocytes. Mod Pathol. 2021;34(4):735–47.
37. Marchio C, Scaltriti M, Ladanyi M, et al. ESMO recommendations on the standard methods to detect NTRK fusions in daily practice and clinical research. Ann Oncol. 2019;30(9):1417–27.
38. Hung YP, Fletcher CDM, Hornick JL. Evaluation of pan-TRK immunohistochemistry in infantile fibrosarcoma, lipofibromatosis-like neural tumour and histological mimics. Histopathology. 2018;73(4):634–44.
39. Lee CY, Sholl LM, Zhang B, et al. Atypical spitzoid neoplasms in childhood: a molecular and outcome study. Am J Dermatopathol. 2017;39(3):181–6.
40. Yeh I, Lang UE, Durieux E, et al. Combined activation of MAP kinase pathway and beta-catenin signaling cause deep penetrating nevi. Nat Commun. 2017;8(1):644.
41. Nikolaev SI, Rimoldi D, Iseli C, et al. Exome sequencing identifies recurrent somatic MAP 2K1 and MAP 2K2 mutations in melanoma. Nat Genet. 2011;44(2):133–9.
42. Hodis E, Watson IR, Kryukov GV, et al. A landscape of driver mutations in melanoma. Cell. 2012;150(2):251–63.
43. Brown NA, Furtado LV, Betz BL, et al. High prevalence of somatic MAP 2K1 mutations in BRAF V600E-negative Langerhans cell histiocytosis. Blood. 2014;124(10):1655–8.
44. Sasaki H, Hikosaka Y, Okuda K, et al. MEK1 gene mutation in Japanese lung adenocarcinoma patients. Mol Med Rep. 2009;2(2):153–5.
45. Marks JL, Gong Y, Chitale D, et al. Novel MEK1 mutation identified by mutational analysis of epidermal growth factor receptor signaling pathway genes in lung adenocarcinoma. Cancer Res. 2008;68(14):5524–8.
46. Shin SY, Lee ST, Kim HJ, et al. BRAF V600E and MAP 2K1 mutations in hairy cell leukemia and splenic marginal zone lymphoma cases. Ann Lab Med. 2015;35(2):257–9.
47. Andritsos LA, Grieselhuber NR, Anghelina M, et al. Trametinib for the treatment of IGHV4-34, MAP 2K1-mutant variant hairy cell leukemia. Leuk Lymphoma. 2018;59(4):1008–11.
48. Gounder MM, Solit DB, Tap WD. Trametinib in histiocytic sarcoma with an activating MAP 2K1 (MEK1) mutation. N Engl J Med. 2018;378(20):1945–7.
49. Donati M, Nosek D, Waldenback P, et al. MAP 2K1-mutated melanocytic neoplasms with a SPARK-like morphology. Am J Dermatopathol. 2021;43(6):412–7.
50. Sunshine JC, Kim D, Zhang B, et al. Melanocytic neoplasms with MAP 2K1 in frame deletions and spitz morphology. Am J Dermatopathol. 2020;42(12):923–31.
51. Donati M, Goutas D, Pissaloux D, et al. Clinical, morphologic, and genomic findings in Spitz Tumors with RET fusion: a series of 31 cases. Mod Pathol. 2025;38(5):100740.
52. Kim D, Compres EV, Zhang B, et al. A series of RET fusion Spitz neoplasms with plaque-like silhouette and dyscohesive nesting of epithelioid melanocytes. Am J Dermatopathol. 2021;43(4):243–51.
53. Newman S, Pappo A, Raimondi S, Zhang J, Barnhill R, Bahrami A. Pathologic characteristics of Spitz melanoma with MAP 3K8 fusion or truncation in a pediatric cohort. Am J Surg Pathol. 2019;43(12):1631–7.
54. Patel P, Hagstrom M, Sharma N, et al. Clinical, morphologic, and molecular features of MAP 3K8 rearranged Spitz neoplasms: a retrospective study documenting that Bonafide Spitz melanomas are rare. Am J Surg Pathol. 2024;48(4):437–46.

55. Cancer Genome Atlas N. Genomic classification of cutaneous melanoma. Cell. 2015;161(7):1681–96.
56. Curtin JA, Fridlyand J, Kageshita T, et al. Distinct sets of genetic alterations in melanoma. N Engl J Med. 2005;353(20):2135–47.
57. Krauthammer M, Kong Y, Bacchiocchi A, et al. Exome sequencing identifies recurrent mutations in NF1 and RASopathy genes in sun-exposed melanomas. Nat Genet. 2015;47(9):996–1002.
58. Wiesner T, Kiuru M, Scott SN, et al. NF1 mutations are common in desmoplastic melanoma. Am J Surg Pathol. 2015;39(10):1357–62.
59. Gerami P, Chen A, Sharma N, et al. BRAF mutated and morphologically spitzoid tumors, a subgroup of melanocytic neoplasms difficult to distinguish from true Spitz neoplasms. Am J Surg Pathol. 2024;48(5):538–45.
60. Long GV, Wilmott JS, Capper D, et al. Immunohistochemistry is highly sensitive and specific for the detection of V600E BRAF mutation in melanoma. Am J Surg Pathol. 2013;37(1):61–5.
61. Spatz A, Calonje E, Handfield-Jones S, Barnhill RL. Spitz tumors in children: a grading system for risk stratification. Arch Dermatol. 1999;135(3):282–5.
62. Paradela S, et al. Prognostic factors for melanoma in children and adolescents: a clinicopathologic, single-center study of 137 patients. Cancer. 2010;116(18):4334–44. https://doi.org/10.1002/cncr.25222.
63. Lee S, Opresko P, Pappo A, Kirkwood JM, Bahrami A. Association of TERT promoter mutations with telomerase expression in melanoma. Pigment Cell Melanoma Res. 2016;29(3):391–3.
64. Motaparthi K, Kim J, Andea AA, et al. TERT and TERT promoter in melanocytic neoplasms: current concepts in pathogenesis, diagnosis, and prognosis. J Cutan Pathol. 2020;47(8):710–9.
65. Lu C, Zhang J, Nagahawatte P, et al. The genomic landscape of childhood and adolescent melanoma. J Invest Dermatol. 2015;135(3):816–23.
66. Wu G, Barnhill RL, Lee S, et al. The landscape of fusion transcripts in spitzoid melanoma and biologically indeterminate spitzoid tumors by RNA sequencing. Mod Pathol. 2016;29(4):359–69.

Chapter 11
Congenital Melanocytic Nevi and Associated Lesions: Proliferative Nodules and Melanoma

Pavandeep Gill

Introduction

Congenital melanocytic nevi (CMN) are rare, benign, neural crest-derived melanocytic proliferations. They can present at birth or within the first year of life (i.e., late or tardive CMN) [1]. These lesions grow in proportion to the child and are categorized based on their maximal projected adult size as small, medium/intermediate, large, or giant (see Table 11.1) [1, 2]. Other classification schemes are based on features such as the ease of surgical removal of the CMN, anatomical distribution, number of satellite nevi, morphological features, and surface area involved [1, 2]. CMN likely result from the unregulated growth of melanoblasts during the migration of these cells from the neural crest to the skin, early on in the embryonic or fetal periods [3]. CMN affect approximately 1%–3% of newborn infants, and giant CMN are even less common, affecting less than 1 in 20,000 neonates [3–7].

Categorization of CMN is necessary to allow for risk stratification, as large and giant CMN have an increased risk of developing melanoma compared to small and medium CMN [8–11]. While overall pediatric melanomas are rare and represent only 1%–3% of pediatric malignancies, a high proportion of these childhood melanomas have been reported to be associated with giant CMN and, in a smaller proportion, with small or medium CMN or with acquired melanocytic nevi [4, 12, 13]. In addition to large or giant size, the location of the CMN on the trunk and its association with multiple satellite nevi have been reported as increased risk factors for the development of melanoma [8, 12–15]. Multiple medium-sized CMN are also

P. Gill (✉)
University of Calgary, Department of Pathology and Laboratory Medicine, Calgary, AB, Canada

Alberta Precision Laboratories, Diagnostic and Scientific Center, Calgary, AB, Canada
e-mail: pavandeep.gill@albertaprecisionlabs.ca

V. G. Prieto, C. A. Torres-Cabala (eds.), *Precision Molecular Pathology of Melanocytic Lesions*, Molecular Pathology Library,
https://doi.org/10.1007/978-3-032-18222-7_11

Table 11.1 Categorization of congenital melanocytic nevi based on their projected diameter in adults

Category	Sub-category	Diameter (mm)
Small	–	Less than 15
Medium/intermediate	M1	15–100
	M2	100–200
Large	L1	200–300
	L2	300–400
Giant	G1	400–600
	G2	Greater than 600

associated with an increased risk of melanoma [13]. Melanomas arising in large or giant CMN typically occur before puberty, whereas those in small CMN occur after puberty [4, 8, 13, 16]. Melanomas arising in CMN can be aggressive and have potential for recurrence and metastases, and are associated with an overall poor survival [3, 4, 10, 12, 17, 18]. Melanomas can arise in patients with large or giant CMN despite prior attempts at surgical removal or dermabrasion of the CMN [8, 12, 15, 19–21].

The probability of developing benign nodular proliferations (i.e., proliferative nodules) in large or giant CMN is actually much higher than the probability of developing melanoma [22]. It has been proposed that the risk of melanoma arising in CMN may actually have been overestimated in the past literature due to the misdiagnosis of proliferative nodules as melanomas [12, 23]. Proliferative nodules, compared to melanomas, have an indolent clinical course with eventual stabilization or regression after a period of time [3, 17, 18, 24, 25]. However, reliable distinction of proliferative nodules from melanomas arising in CMN can be difficult.

CMN can be associated with neurological abnormalities of the central nervous system, termed "CMN syndrome" (OMIM 137550), previously known as neurocutaneous melanosis [11, 15, 26]. Neurological abnormalities include benign and malignant melanocytic and non-melanocytic lesions and symptoms such as hydrocephalus and seizures [13, 26–29]. Symptomatic neurological disease and central nervous system melanomas have been reported to have a high risk of mortality [4, 5, 14, 29, 30]. Early routine magnetic resonance imaging-based central nervous system screening has been reported to be the best predictor of adverse outcomes in children with risk factors for CMN syndrome [26, 30]. Rarely, patients with CMN may have melanomas at sites other than the skin and central nervous system, including lymph nodes and the retroperitoneum [9, 30]. Other non-melanocytic tumors, such as rhabdomyosarcoma, have also been described in CMN [5, 14, 31]. Non-cutaneous melanomas and non-melanocytic tumors arising in CMN are beyond the scope of this chapter and will not be discussed further.

The remainder of this chapter will focus on the clinical, histological, immunohistochemical, and molecular features of conventional CMN, proliferative nodules, and cutaneous melanomas arising in CMN.

Clinical Features

Congenital Melanocytic Nevi

In general, CMN present as well-demarcated, round to oval-shaped, variably pigmented lesions [1]. They are often associated with hypertrichosis [14]. Their clinical appearance may change with age, becoming progressively darker with raised areas and increased hair [1, 11, 14]. Visible pigmentary or nodular change in a CMN usually prompts a biopsy for histologic evaluation [25]. CMN may have smooth, papular, rugose, pebbly, verrucous, or cerebriform surfaces [1]. Small CMN can be clinically indistinguishable from commonly acquired nevi. There is a higher prevalence of CMN in females [10, 14].

CMN have a wide anatomical distribution, with the trunk and extremities being more common than the head and neck [14, 32, 33]. "Kissing nevus" or the divided nevus of the eyelid occurs on adjacent parts of the upper and lower eyelids and appears as a single lesion when the eyelids are closed [34]. It is postulated that these CMN develop between the 9th and 20th weeks of gestation when the eyelids are fused [34]. There are also nevus spilus-type CMN with a large café-au-lait macular background and superimposed multiple clustered small and medium CMN [35]. The café-au-lait background may not be visible at birth [35]. Multiple CMN may be seen in a single patient [14]. Large and giant CMN are usually associated with other smaller CMN, called satellite nevi [1, 5, 10, 14, 32, 33]. For large or giant "garment--type" CMN, terms such as "bathing trunk," "vest," "shoulder-sleeve," "stocking," or "glove" have been used to describe their anatomic distribution. Up to 80% of the skin surface area can be covered in nevi in the most severe cases [5]. Large and multiple CMN can be associated with pruritus, skin fragility, bleeding, and superficial infections [36–39]. Limb atrophy can be seen with giant CMN [40, 41]. High serum S100 protein levels have been found to be associated with larger size, increased number, greater depth, and increased cellularity of CMN [42].

On dermoscopy, CMN may demonstrate reticular networks, globules, dots, focal network thickening, perifollicular hypopigmentation, target networks with globules, dots, or blood vessels, target and haloed globules, milia-like cysts, and hypertrichosis [43].

Proliferative Nodules Arising in Congenital Melanocytic Nevi

Proliferative nodules (Fig. 11.1) can have variable clinical appearances and can occur congenitally or at any time after birth [25]. They demonstrate small size, well-demarcated borders, round or oval shape, a smooth and sometimes shiny surface, and can vary from pale to black in color [5, 24, 25]. They can be soft or somewhat firm, but not hard, and may occasionally be ulcerated [22–25]. Proliferative nodules with neuroid overgrowth may be larger, demonstrate poorly defined edges, round or

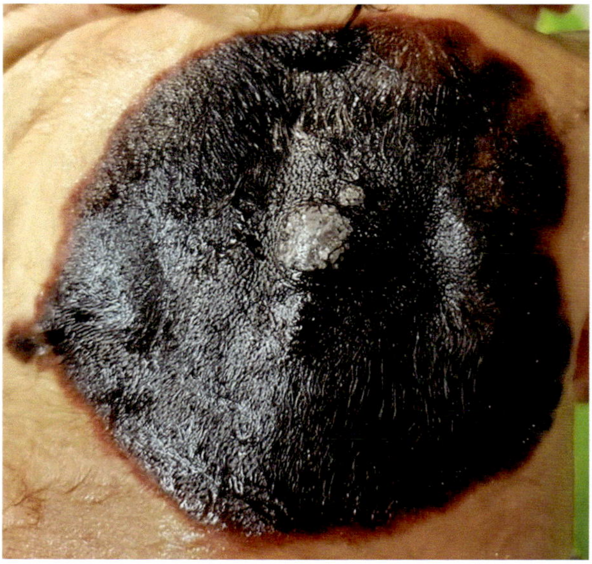

Fig. 11.1 A giant congenital melanocytic nevus with brown to black coloration and hypertrichosis demonstrating a central fibrotic area, consistent with a proliferative nodule. (Reprinted with permission from Gill et al. [44])

ovoid/fusiform shape, less pigment than the surrounding CMN or pink to red color, and are soft or lipoma-like, sometimes becoming pendulous [5]. Proliferative nodules can undergo spontaneous regression and demonstrate softening or a decrease in size and pigmentation, or remain as long-standing, stable lesions [24, 25]. There may be multiple proliferative nodules in a single CMN [22, 25, 45].

Melanomas Arising in Congenital Melanocytic Nevi

Melanomas arising in CMN (Fig. 11.2) can present as new, growing, deeply seated, solitary nodules that may demonstrate color variation, ulceration, bleeding, pruritus, pain, and necrosis [22, 46]. Detection using the ABCDE criteria (asymmetry, irregular borders, multiple colors, diameter greater than 6 mm, and evolution/enlargement) may be challenging given the benign changes that can also occur in CMN in young patients [47]. Dermoscopy can demonstrate features concerning for malignancy, including an atypical network, irregular pigment dots or globules, irregular blotches, and a blue-white veil [46, 47]. Local lymphadenopathy secondary to metastasis has been reported as a presenting feature for melanomas arising in CMN [5]. A rare, fatal, metastatic congenital melanoma in a giant CMN has been described [48]. Noteworthy is that proliferative nodules and melanomas can arise concurrently in a CMN [49].

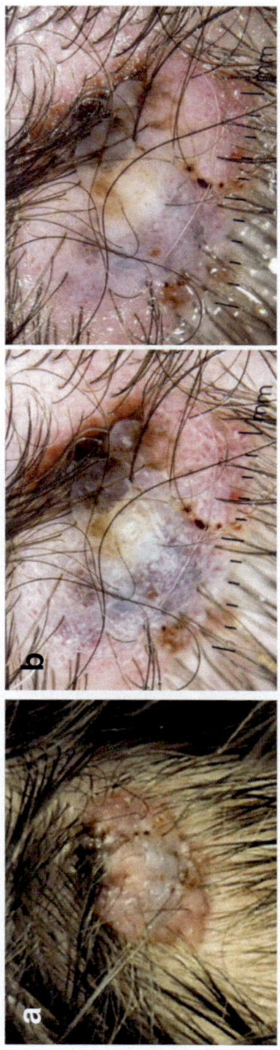

Fig. 11.2 (**a**) Clinical image of a melanoma arising in a congenital melanocytic nevus on the scalp of a young adult. (**b**) Dermatoscopic images: Left, polarized dermatoscopic image (10× magnification) showing multiple shiny white lines, polymorphous vessels, and an atypical pigment network. Right: non-polarized dermatoscopic image (10× magnification) showing polymorphous vessels and an atypical pigment network. (Images and dermoscopy figure legend courtesy of Dr. Justin Chia, Division of Dermatology, University of Calgary, Calgary, Alberta, Canada)

Histological Features

Congenital Melanocytic Nevi

CMN are composed of small, uniform, nevoid melanocytes that extend throughout the lower two-thirds of the dermis and into the subcutis (Fig. 11.3) [1]. The melanocytes percolate singly or as cords of cells through the collagen bundles of the reticular dermis and extend around and within hair follicles, arrector pili muscles, sebaceous glands, eccrine apparatus, nerves, and subcutaneous tissue [1]. Angiotropism can be observed [50, 51]. Maturation with depth is present. Small to giant CMN all share these histologic features, although the findings may be more pronounced in larger CMN. Occasionally, there may be epithelioid or spindled cytology or neurotized and blue nevus-like areas. CMN can demonstrate junctional, dermal, or compound morphology [52]. The junctional component can occasionally demonstrate atypical features similar to a dysplastic nevus [1, 22, 32]. Low central pagetoid scatter is common in CMN excised from newborns in the first year of life [1]. In the nevus spilus-type of CMN, the café-au-lait areas demonstrate mild hyperpigmentation and melanocytic hyperplasia in the epidermis and a few scattered,

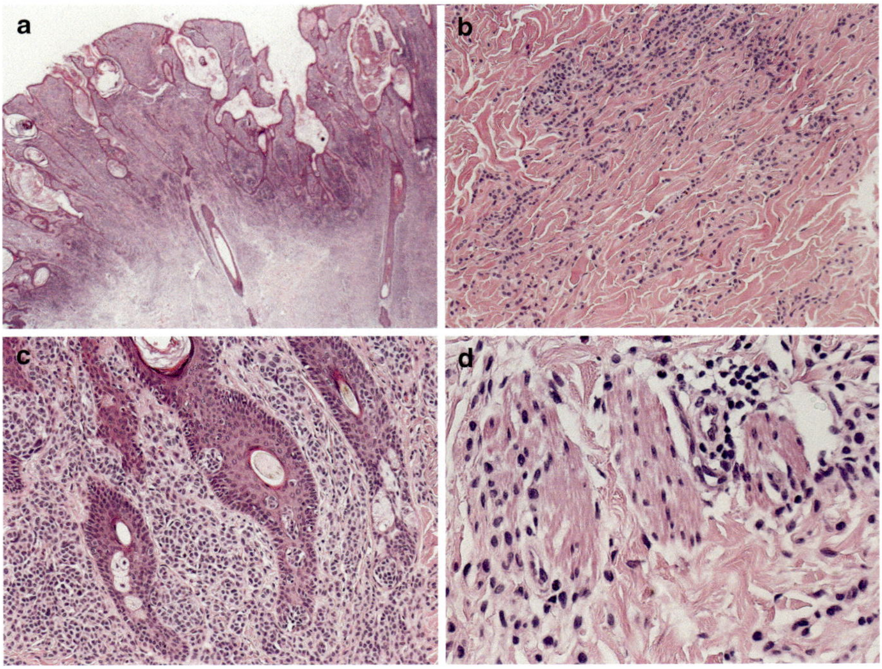

Fig. 11.3 (**a**) A compound congenital melanocytic lesion with hyperkeratosis, acanthosis, and papillomatosis. (**b**) Nevoid melanocytes percolate singly and as cords through collagen bundles into the deep dermis. Appendageal ensheathment and occasional involvement, including (**c**) involvement of hair follicles and (**d**) arrector pili muscles, is seen (H&E)

spindle-shaped cells in the dermis [53]. CMN can demonstrate decreasing cellularity over time [52]. The presence of increased mast cells has been associated with pruritus in large and giant CMN [54].

Proliferative Nodules Arising in Congenital Melanocytic Nevi

On histologic examination (Fig. 11.4), proliferative nodules are ill-defined, nodular, cellular lesions with pushing but nondestructive borders, readily noted at low-power magnification [5, 24, 25]. Melanocytes composing the proliferative nodule may be enlarged, are monomorphic, can demonstrate spindled or epithelioid morphology, and lack prominent cytologic atypia [24, 25]. The melanocytes of the proliferative nodule blend and mix with the adjacent melanocytes of the CMN, imparting a smooth and imperceptible transition between the two components [1, 24, 25]. Mitotic activity is usually low [1, 22, 24, 25]. Necrosis and a significant inflammatory infiltrate are usually absent [1, 24, 25]. Maturation is present. There may be neural or mesenchymal differentiation and cellular blue nevus-like features [5, 22, 24, 55]. Neuroid overgrowth areas are composed of spindle cell aggregates in a myxoid stroma without significant atypia or mitotic activity [5].

Some proliferative nodules may demonstrate atypical features such as sharp demarcation, expansile growth, high cellularity, increased cellular atypia, epidermal effacement, necrosis, hemorrhage, some pagetoid scatter, and ulceration [25, 56,

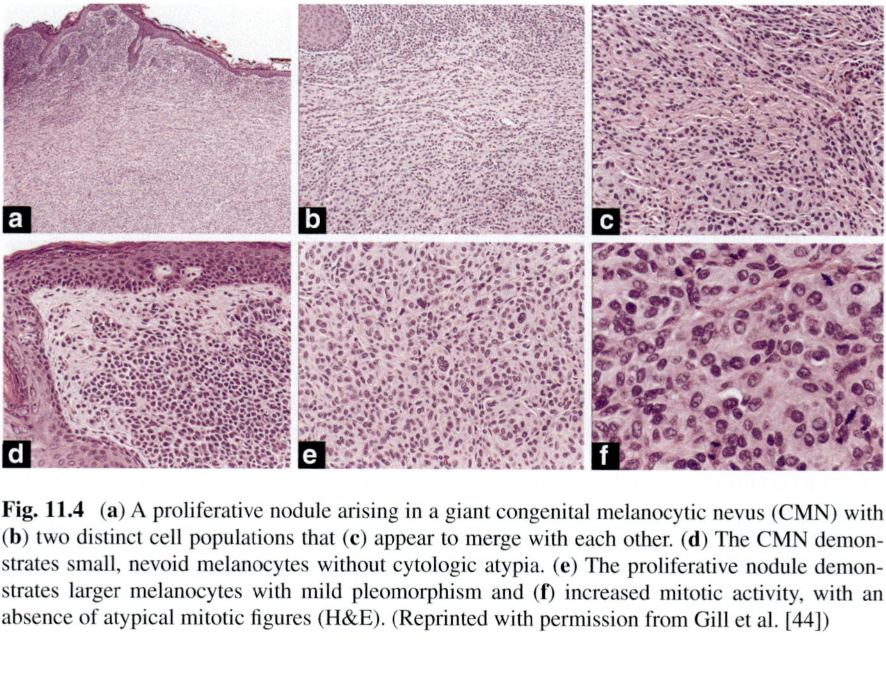

Fig. 11.4 (**a**) A proliferative nodule arising in a giant congenital melanocytic nevus (CMN) with (**b**) two distinct cell populations that (**c**) appear to merge with each other. (**d**) The CMN demonstrates small, nevoid melanocytes without cytologic atypia. (**e**) The proliferative nodule demonstrates larger melanocytes with mild pleomorphism and (**f**) increased mitotic activity, with an absence of atypical mitotic figures (H&E). (Reprinted with permission from Gill et al. [44])

57]. There may be pronounced mitotic activity, but atypical mitotic figures are not identified [56–58].

Melanomas Arising in Congenital Melanocytic Nevi

Histologically, melanomas arising in large or giant CMN (Fig. 11.5) present as sharply demarcated, cellular, expansile, and destructive nodules in the dermis and/or subcutis that may be separated from the epidermis by a grenz zone [1, 12, 16, 22]. These lesions often demonstrate a high Breslow thickness at the time of diagnosis [4]. Cytomorphologically, lesional cells demonstrate cellular and/or nuclear enlargement, marked pleomorphism, prominent nucleoli, and abundant mitotic activity, including the presence of atypical mitotic figures [12, 16, 22]. Maturation is not identified. Large zones of necrosis and ulceration may be present [22]. Lesional cells may demonstrate epithelioid, spindled, or small round blue cell cytology [1, 12, 16]. There may be areas resembling malignant blue nevus, malignant epithelioid schwannoma, and rhabdomyosarcomatous differentiation [1, 59]. Melanomas

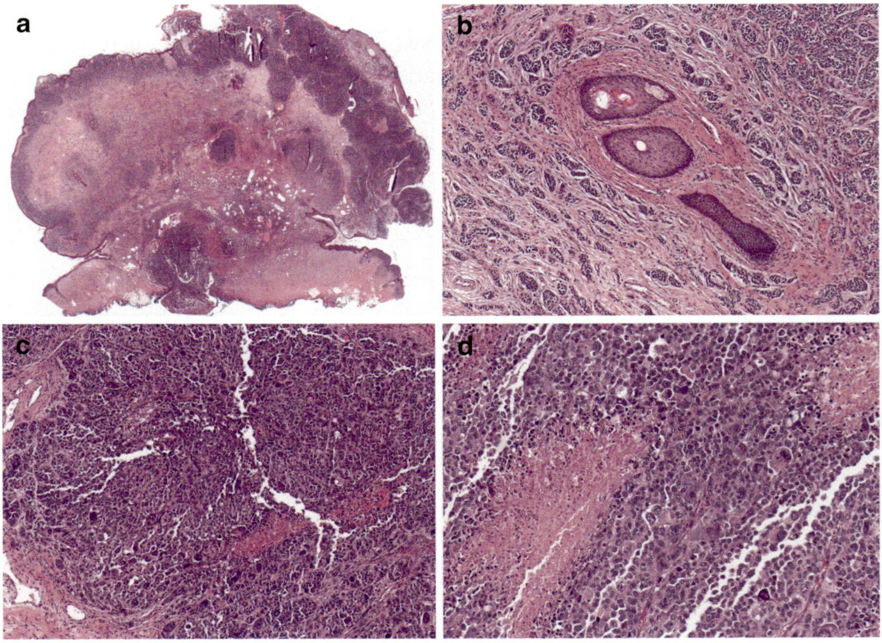

Fig. 11.5 (**a**) Low power examination of a melanoma arising in a congenital melanocytic nevus (CMN). (**b**) The CMN is composed of small, bland nevoid melanocytes extending along adnexal structures. (**c**) The melanoma component demonstrates a destructive expansile nodule with necrosis and (**d**) markedly atypical melanocytes (H&E). (Images courtesy of Dr. Woo Cheal Cho, Department of Anatomical Pathology, University of Texas MD Anderson Cancer Center, Houston, Texas, United States of America)

arising in small CMN usually originate in the epidermis and resemble conventional superficial spreading or nodular melanomas [1, 16, 22].

Immunohistochemical Features

CMN and proliferative nodules express melanocytic markers, such as SOX10, S100, MelanA/Mart1, and tyrosinase [25]. Associated melanomas can lose expression of melanocytic markers. CMN can demonstrate decreasing expression of HMB45 over time [52]. HMB45 may demonstrate diffuse expression or even no expression in melanomas [12]. Varying literature on CD117 expression patterns in CMN and proliferative nodules have been reported with conflicting findings [25, 57]. p16 expression may be retained or absent in CMN and melanomas [12, 17, 25]. Proliferative nodules usually retain p16 expression and typically demonstrate a low Ki67 proliferative index and PHH3 expression [17, 25, 57]. However, atypical proliferative nodules may demonstrate an increased Ki67 proliferative index and PHH3 expression [57, 58]. Melanomas may demonstrate either an increased or a low Ki67 proliferative index [12, 17].

Immunohistochemistry has been traditionally thought to be of limited use in differentiating proliferative nodules from melanomas arising in CMN [12, 17]. However, recently, markers of epigenetic modification have been found to be useful for this purpose. High levels of 5-hydroxymethylcytosine expression have been reported in proliferative nodules and giant CMN compared to an absence of expression in melanoma [60]. Retained normal expression of H3K27me3 has been shown in medium to large CMN and proliferative nodules arising in CMN, while significantly reduced expression of H3K27me3 has been shown in melanomas arising in medium to large CMN in children [61]. PReferentially expressed Antigen in MElanoma (PRAME) may have some utility in distinguishing between proliferative nodules and melanomas in CMN as well, but needs further investigation [44, 62].

Molecular Findings

Congenital Melanocytic Nevi

Large or giant or multiple CMN develop in utero as a result of postzygotic somatic mutations, leading to mosaicism [5]. The mutations can hit multipotent progenitor cells if early enough in development, potentially leading to the development of multiple cutaneous CMN and sometimes to the involvement of other organ systems [5]. The variation in size, number, and distribution of CMN is determined by the cellular lineage commitment at the time of the mutation onset. In patients with multiple CMN, the same mutation has been found in different CMN in the skin and in melanocytic and non-melanocytic lesions of the central nervous system, but not in unaffected tissues [5].

The most common mutations in large or giant CMN are in *NRAS* (80% of cases), with p.Q61K and p.Q61R being the most common [5, 12, 57, 63–67]. A phenotypic difference between these two mutations has not been seen [5]. *NRAS* mutations have been reported to be associated with increased hypertrichosis [66]. *NRAS* p.Q61H, p.G13R, and p.Q61L mutations have usually been associated with CMN with a nevus spilus phenotype [5, 35, 53, 63]. Rare *MAP 2K1* mutation has been detected in a nevus spilus-type CMN without apparent background café-au-lait pigmentation and multiple associated melanomas [68]. *BRAF* mutations have been less commonly demonstrated in large CMN [5, 64, 66, 67]. When present, *BRAF* mutations have been reported to be associated with scattered, extensive, dermal, and subcuticular nodules [66]. Medium CMN can show either *NRAS* or, less commonly, *BRAF* mutations, and multiple medium CMN are typically associated with *NRAS* mutations [5, 66, 67, 69]. Acquired or small CMN typically demonstrate *BRAF* mutations, but may also less commonly demonstrate *NRAS* mutations [12, 64, 69]. Other mutations that have been described in CMN include *KRAS, HRAS, APC, MET, MC1R, TP53, EGFR, PIK3CA,* and *GNAQ* [5, 57, 63]. There may be a role for germline *MC1R* variants in patients with a family history of CMN and a more severe cutaneous phenotype [70].

Fusion transcripts have been identified in CMN without somatic *NRAS* or *BRAF* mutations. Studies have shown some large/giant CMN to harbor *BRAF, ALK, RAF1,* and *RASGRF2* fusions [39, 59, 63, 71–74]. CMN with mosaic *BRAF* fusions have been found to be associated with a more hyperproliferative phenotype, innumerable satellite nevi, intense pruritus, often hairless appearance, and a desmoplastic and fibrotic stroma [75, 76].

Chromosomal aberrations or copy number changes are usually not seen in CMN [18, 67].

Proliferative Nodules and Melanomas Arising in Congenital Melanocytic Nevi

Melanomas and proliferative nodules arising in CMN can demonstrate distinct chromosomal aberrations, and therefore, molecular genetic analysis for DNA copy number changes may be useful in clinically and histologically ambiguous cases [18]. Comparative genomic hybridization (CGH) allows genome-wide detection of DNA copy number changes and demonstrates either no detectable cytogenetic aberrations or whole chromosomal copy number changes (either gains or losses) in proliferative nodules (Fig. 11.6) [18]. In contrast, melanomas arising in CMN may

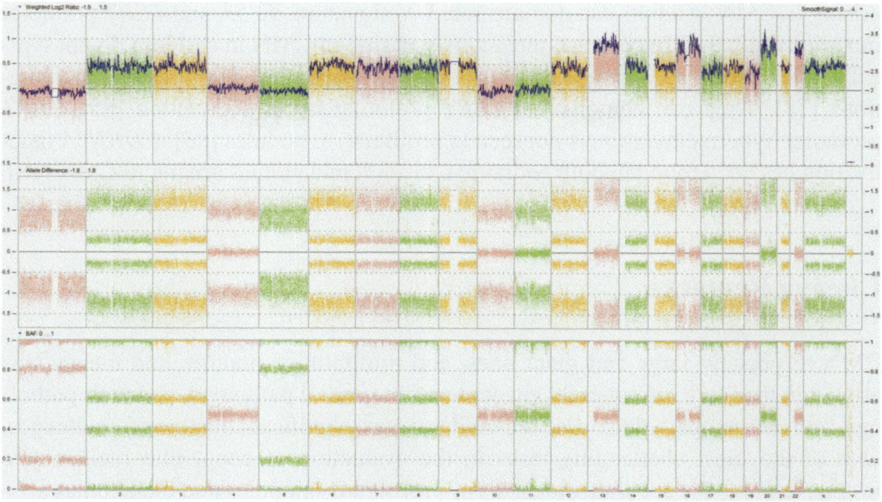

Fig. 11.6 Chromosomal microarray profile (OncoScan CNV Assay, Thermo Fisher Scientific, Waltham, Massachusetts) from a proliferative nodule arising in a congenital nevus. Top panel: Copy number data displayed on the weighted Log_2 ratio plot. Middle panel: Allele data displayed on the allele difference plot. Bottom panel: B allele frequency (BAF) plot for chromosomes 1–22, X, and Y, from left to right. This proliferative nodule demonstrates a near triploid baseline copy number. There is whole chromosomal loss of chromosomes 1 and 5 with corresponding loss of heterozygosity, whole chromosomal loss of chromosomes 4, 10, and 11 with retained heterozygosity, and whole chromosomal gains of chromosomes 13, 16, 20, and 22. (Reprinted with permission from Gill et al. [44])

demonstrate numerous complex, structural chromosomal aberrations, including partial copy number gains or losses [18, 22]. However, there are exceptions to this copy-number pattern in benign and malignant lesions [22, 77]. Fluorescence in situ hybridization (FISH) analysis may demonstrate numerical and/or structural chromosomal abnormalities in melanomas compared to the adjacent CMN, and while a 4-probe FISH analysis may have limited value, a more extensive FISH analysis could be useful for differentiating proliferative nodules from melanoma [12, 17]. In atypical proliferations arising in CMN with controversial CGH findings, the addition of FISH has been shown to demonstrate utility in making a diagnosis [77].

Mutational analyses of proliferative nodules arising in CMN have demonstrated *NRAS*, *BRAF*, *KRAS*, and *GNAQ* mutations [57, 65]. *NRAS* mutations are more common in proliferative nodules arising in giant CMN, and *BRAF* mutations are more common in proliferative nodules arising in small and medium CMN [57].

Mutational analysis of melanomas arising in CMN has also frequently demonstrated *NRAS* mutations [78–82]. *SMARCA2*, *BRAF*^{V600E}, and *PTEN* mutations and *ZEB2:ALK* and *AGK:BRAF* fusions have also been reported [74, 82, 83]. Melanomas arising in CMN in adults can demonstrate UV signature, *TP53,* and *TERT* promoter mutations [82, 84]. In contrast, melanomas arising in CMN in children do not typically demonstrate UV-induced mutations or UV-signature *TERT* promoter mutations [78]. They can demonstrate *TERT* promoter hypermethylation [85]. *TERT* promoter hypermethylation is not seen in proliferative nodules [85]. *CDKN2A* inactivation has been found in both pediatric and adult melanomas arising in CMN [78].

Closing Remarks

CMN, especially large and giant ones, and proliferative nodules and melanomas arising in them are infrequently encountered in general pathology, pediatric pathology, and dermatopathology practices and can pose significant diagnostic challenges. One of the most challenging tasks in the evaluation of congenital melanocytic lesions remains the accurate diagnosis of proliferative nodules and melanomas arising in these lesions, especially in those cases with ambiguous features. For reference, a summary of the key differences discussed in this chapter between proliferative nodules and melanomas arising in CMN is provided in Table 11.2. Congenital nevi and their associated lesions are rare, and our understanding of their clinical, histological, and immunohistochemical features and molecular pathogenesis continues to evolve.

Table 11.2 Summary of the key clinical, histopathological, immunohistochemical, and molecular differences between proliferative nodules and melanomas developing in congenital melanocytic nevi (CMN)

	Clinical features	Histological features	Immunohistochemical findings	Molecular findings
Proliferative nodules	Higher probability of development in CMN compared to melanomas Generally have an indolent clinical course with eventual stabilization or regression Can be multiple May demonstrate some overlapping clinical features with melanomas, including ulceration	Lesional cells blend with adjacent CMN Usually mild cytologic atypia Low mitotic index Absence of atypical mitotic figures Absence of necrosis Lack pagetoid scatter Demonstrate maturation Atypical proliferative nodules may have overlapping histological features with melanomas	Limited value in differentiating from melanomas Usually low Ki67 proliferative index May demonstrate expression of 5-hydroxymethylcytosine and H3K27me3 Utility of PRAME needs further exploration	No detectable cytogenetic aberrations or usually *whole* chromosomal copy number changes (gains or losses) on comparative genomic hybridization, with rare exceptions Lack *TERT* promoter hypermethylation or mutations
Melanomas	Lower probability of development in CMN compared to proliferative nodules Generally aggressive clinical course with potential for recurrence and metastases Usually single, but may present concurrently with proliferative nodules Can be associated with ulceration and necrosis	Typically have more exaggerated histologic features than those seen in atypical proliferative nodules Demonstrate well--circumscribed, expansile nodules with destructive growth Severe cytologic atypia Numerous mitotic figures, including atypical forms Presence of necrosis Presence of pagetoid scatter Lack of maturation	Limited value in differentiating from proliferative nodules Often markedly elevated Ki67 proliferative index May demonstrate reduced expression of 5-hydroxymethylcytosine and H3K27me3 Utility of PRAME needs further exploration	Usually complex, structural chromosomal aberrations, including *partial* copy number gains or losses on comparative genomic hybridization, with rare exceptions Can demonstrate *TERT* promoter hypermethylation or mutations

Acknowledgments The author thanks Dr. Andrea Bakker (Department of Pathology and Laboratory Medicine, University of Calgary, Calgary, Alberta, Canada) for providing the cases of CMN photographed in Fig. 11.3.

Competing Interests The author has no conflicts of interest to declare that are relevant to the content of this chapter.

References

1. Tannous ZS, Mihm MC, Sober AJ, Duncan LM. Congenital melanocytic nevi: clinical and histopathologic features, risk of melanoma, and clinical management. J Am Acad Dermatol. 2005;52(2):197–203. https://doi.org/10.1016/j.jaad.2004.07.020.
2. Krengel S, Scope A, Dusza SW, Vonthein R, Marghoob AA. New recommendations for the categorization of cutaneous features of congenital melanocytic nevi. J Am Acad Dermatol. 2013;68(3):441–51. https://doi.org/10.1016/j.jaad.2012.05.043.
3. Viana ACL, Gontijo B, Vasques BF. Giant congenital melanocytic nevus. An Bras Dermatol. 2013;88(6):863–78. https://doi.org/10.1590/abd1806-4841.20132233.
4. Jen M, Murphy M, Grant-Kels JM. Childhood melanoma. Clin Dermatol. 2009;27(6):529–36. https://doi.org/10.1016/j.clindermatol.2008.09.011.
5. Kinsler VA, O'Hare P, Bulstrode N, et al. Melanoma in congenital melanocytic naevi. Br J Dermatol. 2017;176(5):1131–43. https://doi.org/10.1111/bjd.15301.
6. Alper J, Holmes LB, Mihm MC. Birthmarks with serious medical significance: nevocullular nevi, sebaceous nevi, and multiple café au lait spots. J Pediatr. 1979;95(5 Pt 1):696–700. https://doi.org/10.1016/s0022-3476(79)80713-1.
7. Alper JC, Holmes LB. The incidence and significance of birthmarks in a cohort of 4,641 newborns. Pediatr Dermatol. 1983;1(1):58–68. https://doi.org/10.1111/j.1525-1470.1983.tb01093.x.
8. Vourc'h-Jourdain M, Martin L, Barbarot S. Large congenital melanocytic nevi: therapeutic management and melanoma risk: a systematic review. J Am Acad Dermatol. 2013;68(3):493–8. https://doi.org/10.1016/j.jaad.2012.09.039.
9. Marghoob AA, Schoenbach SP, Kopf AW, Orlow SJ, Nossa R, Bart RS. Large congenital melanocytic nevi and the risk for the development of malignant melanoma. A prospective study. Arch Dermatol. 1996;132(2):170–5. http://www.ncbi.nlm.nih.gov/pubmed/8629825
10. Ruiz-Maldonado R, Tamayo L, Laterza AM, Durán C. Giant pigmented nevi: clinical, histopathologic, and therapeutic considerations. J Pediatr. 1992;120(6):906–11. https://doi.org/10.1016/s0022-3476(05)81958-4.
11. Kinsler VA, Birley J, Atherton DJ. Great Ormond Street Hospital for Children Registry for congenital melanocytic naevi: prospective study 1988-2007. Part 1-epidemiology, phenotype and outcomes. Br J Dermatol. 2009;160(1):143–50. https://doi.org/10.1111/j.1365-2133.2008.08849.x.
12. Lacoste C, Avril M-F, Frassati-Biaggi A, et al. Malignant melanoma arising in patients with a large congenital melanocytic naevus: retrospective study of 10 cases with cytogenetic analysis. Acta Derm Venereol. 2015;95(6):686–90. https://doi.org/10.2340/00015555-2049.
13. Neuhold JC, Friesenhahn J, Gerdes N, Krengel S. Case reports of fatal or metastasizing melanoma in children and adolescents: a systematic analysis of the literature. Pediatr Dermatol. 2015;32(1):13–22. https://doi.org/10.1111/pde.12400.
14. Alikhan A, Ibrahimi OA, Eisen DB. Congenital melanocytic nevi: where are we now? Part I. Clinical presentation, epidemiology, pathogenesis, histology, malignant transformation, and neurocutaneous melanosis. J Am Acad Dermatol. 2012;67(4):495.e1–17. quiz 512–514. https://doi.org/10.1016/j.jaad.2012.06.023.

15. Bett BJ. Large or multiple congenital melanocytic nevi: occurrence of cutaneous melanoma in 1008 persons. J Am Acad Dermatol. 2005;52(5):793–7. https://doi.org/10.1016/j.jaad.2005.02.024.
16. Paradela S, Fonseca E, Prieto VG. Melanoma in children. Arch Pathol Lab Med. 2011;135(3):307–16. https://doi.org/10.5858/2009-0503-RA.1.
17. Vergier B, Laharanne E, Prochazkova-Carlotti M, et al. Proliferative nodules vs melanoma arising in giant congenital melanocytic nevi during childhood. JAMA Dermatol. 2016;152(10):1147–51. https://doi.org/10.1001/jamadermatol.2016.2667.
18. Bastian BC, Xiong J, Frieden IJ, et al. Genetic changes in neoplasms arising in congenital melanocytic nevi: differences between nodular proliferations and melanomas. Am J Pathol. 2002;161(4):1163–9. https://doi.org/10.1016/S0002-9440(10)64393-3.
19. Coughlin CC, Council ML, Gru AA, Fields RC, Bayliss SJ. Malignant melanoma arising at the site of a previously excised giant congenital melanocytic nevus. JAMA Dermatol. 2014;150(1):100–1. https://doi.org/10.1001/jamadermatol.2013.5775.
20. Zutt M, Kretschmer L, Emmert S, Haenssle H, Neumann C, Bertsch HP. Multicentric malignant melanoma in a giant melanocytic congenital nevus 20 years after dermabrasion in adulthood. Dermatologic Surg. 2003;29(1):99–101. discussion 101. https://doi.org/10.1046/j.1524-4725.2003.29007.x.
21. Dragieva G, Hafner J, Künzi W, et al. Malignant melanoma in a large congenital melanocytic nevus 9 years after dermabrasion in childhood. Dermatology. 2006;212(2):208–9. https://doi.org/10.1159/000090666.
22. Yélamos O, Arva NC, Obregon R, et al. A comparative study of proliferative nodules and lethal melanomas in congenital nevi from children. Am J Surg Pathol. 2015;39(3):405–15. https://doi.org/10.1097/PAS.0000000000000351.
23. Leech SN, Bell H, Leonard N, et al. Neonatal giant congenital nevi with proliferative nodules: a clinicopathologic study and literature review of neonatal melanoma. Arch Dermatol. 2004;140(1):83–8. https://doi.org/10.1001/archderm.140.1.83.
24. Xu X, Bellucci KSW, Elenitsas R, Elder DE. Cellular nodules in congenital pattern nevi. J Cutan Pathol. 2004;31(2):153–9. https://doi.org/10.1111/j.0303-6987.2004.00156.x.
25. Herron MD, Vanderhooft SL, Smock K, Zhou H, Leachman SA, Coffin C. Proliferative nodules in congenital melanocytic nevi: a clinicopathologic and immunohistochemical analysis. Am J Surg Pathol. 2004;28(8):1017–25. https://doi.org/10.1097/01.pas.0000126785.61609.6e.
26. Waelchli R, Aylett SE, Atherton D, Thompson DJ, Chong WK, Kinsler VA. Classification of neurological abnormalities in children with congenital melanocytic naevus syndrome identifies magnetic resonance imaging as the best predictor of clinical outcome. Br J Dermatol. 2015;173(3):739–50. https://doi.org/10.1111/bjd.13898.
27. Ramaswamy V, Delaney H, Haque S, Marghoob A, Khakoo Y. Spectrum of central nervous system abnormalities in neurocutaneous melanocytosis. Dev Med Child Neurol. 2012;54(6):563–8. https://doi.org/10.1111/j.1469-8749.2012.04275.x.
28. Kadonaga JN, Frieden IJ. Neurocutaneous melanosis: definition and review of the literature. J Am Acad Dermatol. 1991;24(5 Pt 1):747–55. https://doi.org/10.1016/0190-9622(91)70115-i.
29. Hale EK, Stein J, Ben-Porat L, et al. Association of melanoma and neurocutaneous melanocytosis with large congenital melanocytic naevi—results from the NYU-LCMN registry. Br J Dermatol. 2005;152(3):512–7. https://doi.org/10.1111/j.1365-2133.2005.06316.x.
30. Bittencourt FV, Marghoob AA, Kopf AW, Koenig KL, Bart RS. Large congenital melanocytic nevi and the risk for development of malignant melanoma and neurocutaneous melanocytosis. Pediatrics. 2000;106(4):736–41. https://doi.org/10.1542/peds.106.4.736.
31. Pitjadi TM, Wadee R, Grayson W. Rhabdomyosarcoma arising in a giant congenital melanocytic naevus: case report and literature review. Dermatopathology. 2019;6(2):91–8. https://doi.org/10.1159/000496337.
32. Yun SJ, Kwon OS, Han JH, et al. Clinical characteristics and risk of melanoma development from giant congenital melanocytic naevi in Korea: a nationwide retrospective study. Br J Dermatol. 2012;166(1):115–23. https://doi.org/10.1111/j.1365-2133.2011.10636.x.

33. Chen AC-C, McRae MY, Wargon O. Clinical characteristics and risks of large congenital melanocytic naevi: a review of 31 patients at the Sydney Children's Hospital. Australas J Dermatol. 2012;53(3):219–23. https://doi.org/10.1111/j.1440-0960.2012.00897.x.
34. Hamming N. Anatomy and embryology of the eyelids: a review with special reference to the development of divided nevi. Pediatr Dermatol. 1983;1(1):51–8. https://doi.org/10.1111/j.1525-1470.1983.tb01092.x.
35. Kinsler VA, Krengel S, Riviere J-B, et al. Next-generation sequencing of nevus spilus-type congenital melanocytic nevus: exquisite genotype-phenotype correlation in mosaic RASopathies. J Invest Dermatol. 2014;134(10):2658–60. https://doi.org/10.1038/jid.2014.195.
36. Feng J, Sethi A, Reyes-Múgica M, Antaya R. Life-threatening blood loss from scratching provoked by pruritus in the bulky perineal nevocytoma variant of giant congenital melanocytic nevus in a child. J Am Acad Dermatol. 2005;53(2 Suppl 1):S139–42. https://doi.org/10.1016/j.jaad.2004.12.040.
37. Price HN, Schaffer JV. Congenital melanocytic nevi-when to worry and how to treat: facts and controversies. Clin Dermatol. 2010;28(3):293–302. https://doi.org/10.1016/j.clindermatol.2010.04.004.
38. Neuhaus K, Landolt M, Vojvodic M, et al. Surgical treatment of children and youth with congenital melanocytic nevi: self- and proxy-reported opinions. Pediatr Surg Int. 2020;36(4):501–12. https://doi.org/10.1007/s00383-020-04633-z.
39. Mir A, Agim NG, Kane AA, Josephs SC, Park JY, Ludwig K. Giant congenital melanocytic nevus treated with trametinib. Pediatrics. 2019;143(3):e20182469. https://doi.org/10.1542/peds.2018-2469.
40. Itin PH, Lautenschlager S. Lower and upper extremity atrophy associated with a giant congenital melanocytic nevus. Pediatr Dermatol. 1998;15(4):287–9. https://doi.org/10.1046/j.1525-1470.1998.1998015287.x.
41. Skidmore RA, Ivker RA, Resnick SD. Upper extremity atrophy associated with a giant congenital melanocytic nevus. Pediatr Dermatol. 1995;12(3):272–4. https://doi.org/10.1111/j.1525-1470.1995.tb00176.x.
42. Tomás-Velázquez A, López-Gutiérrez JC, Reyes-Múgica M, et al. Serum levels of S-100 protein are directly proportional to the size, number, thickness and degree of cellularity of congenital melanocytic nevi. J Am Acad Dermatol. 2023;89(5):1074–7. https://doi.org/10.1016/j.jaad.2023.06.059.
43. Changchien L, Dusza SW, Agero ALC, et al. Age- and site-specific variation in the dermoscopic patterns of congenital melanocytic nevi: an aid to accurate classification and assessment of melanocytic nevi. Arch Dermatol. 2007;143(8):1007–14. https://doi.org/10.1001/archderm.143.8.1007.
44. Gill P, Prieto VG, Austin MT, Giubellino A, Torres-Cabala CA. Diagnostic utility of PRAME in distinguishing proliferative nodules from melanoma in giant congenital melanocytic nevi. J Cutan Pathol. 2021;48(11):1410–5. https://doi.org/10.1111/cup.14091.
45. Aoyagi S, Akiyama M, Mashiko M, Shibaki A, Shimizu H. Extensive proliferative nodules in a case of giant congenital naevus. Clin Exp Dermatol. 2008;33(2):125–7. https://doi.org/10.1111/j.1365-2230.2007.02542.x.
46. Zeglinski-Spinney A, Kirchhof MG. Melanoma in a congenital melanocytic nevus. CMAJ. 2024;196(18):E625. https://doi.org/10.1503/cmaj.240037.
47. Alos L, Carrasco A, Teixidó C, et al. Melanoma on congenital melanocytic nevi. Pathol Res Pract. 2024;256:155262. https://doi.org/10.1016/j.prp.2024.155262.
48. Schneiderman H, Wu AY, Campbell WA, et al. Congenital melanoma with multiple prenatal metastases. Cancer. 1987;60(6):1371–7. https://doi.org/10.1002/1097-0142(19870915)60:6<1371::aid-cncr2820600635>3.0.co;2-0.
49. Feito-Rodríguez M, de Lucas-Laguna R, Bastian BC, et al. Nodular lesions arising in a large congenital melanocytic naevus in a newborn with eruptive disseminated Spitz naevi. Br J Dermatol. 2011;165(5):1138–42. https://doi.org/10.1111/j.1365-2133.2011.10502.x.

50. Barnhill RL, Chastain MA, Jerdan MS, Lebbé C, Janin A, Lugassy C. Angiotropic neonatal congenital melanocytic nevus: how extravascular migration of melanocytes may explain the development of congenital nevi. Am J Dermatopathol. 2010;32(5):495–9. https://doi.org/10.1097/DAD.0b013e3181c6afce.
51. Kokta V, Hung T, Al Dhaybi R, Lugassy C, Barnhill RL. High prevalence of angiotropism in congenital melanocytic nevi: an analysis of 53 cases. Am J Dermatopathol. 2013;35(2):180–3. https://doi.org/10.1097/DAD.0b013e318260908c.
52. Gassenmaier M, Häfner H-M, Hahn M, Kofler L, Wagner NB, Forchhammer S. Histological and immunohistochemical changes of congenital melanocytic nevi with age. Am J Dermatopathol. 2021;43(10):707–13. https://doi.org/10.1097/DAD.0000000000001894.
53. Krengel S, Widmer DS, Kerl K, Levesque MP, Schiestl C, Weibel L. Naevus spilus-type congenital melanocytic naevus associated with a novel NRAS codon 61 mutation. Br J Dermatol. 2016;174(3):642–4. https://doi.org/10.1111/bjd.14105.
54. Salgado CM, Silver RB, Bauer BS, et al. Skin of patients with large/giant congenital melanocytic nevi shows increased mast cells. Pediatr Dev Pathol. 2014;17(3):198–203. https://doi.org/10.2350/14-02-1444-OA.1.
55. Mancianti ML, Clark WH, Hayes FA, Herlyn M. Malignant melanoma simulants arising in congenital melanocytic nevi do not show experimental evidence for a malignant phenotype. Am J Pathol. 1990;136(4):817–29. http://www.ncbi.nlm.nih.gov/pubmed/2327470
56. de Vooght A, Vanwijck R, Gosseye S, Bayet B. Pseudo-tumoral proliferative nodule in a giant congenital naevus. Br J Plast Surg. 2003;56(2):164–7. https://doi.org/10.1016/s0007-1226(03)00090-0.
57. Phadke PA, Rakheja D, Le LP, et al. Proliferative nodules arising within congenital melanocytic nevi: a histologic, immunohistochemical, and molecular analyses of 43 cases. Am J Surg Pathol. 2011;35(5):656–69. https://doi.org/10.1097/PAS.0b013e31821375ea.
58. Nguyen TLT, Theos A, Kelly DR, Busam K, Andea AA. Mitotically active proliferative nodule arising in a giant congenital melanocytic nevus: a diagnostic pitfall. Am J Dermatopathol. 2013;35(1):16–21. https://doi.org/10.1097/DAD.0b013e318265fe12.
59. Baltres A, Salhi A, Houlier A, et al. Malignant melanoma with areas of rhabdomyosarcomatous differentiation arising in a giant congenital nevus with RAF1 gene fusion. Pigment Cell Melanoma Res. 2019;32(5):708–13. https://doi.org/10.1111/pcmr.12785.
60. Pavlova O, Fraitag S, Hohl D. 5-Hydroxymethylcytosine expression in proliferative nodules arising within congenital nevi allows differentiation from malignant melanoma. J Invest Dermatol. 2016;136(12):2453–61. https://doi.org/10.1016/j.jid.2016.07.015.
61. Busam KJ, Shah KN, Gerami P, Sitzman T, Jungbluth AA, Kinsler V. Reduced H3K27me3 expression is common in nodular melanomas of childhood associated with congenital melanocytic nevi but not in proliferative nodules. Am J Surg Pathol. 2017;41(3):396–404. https://doi.org/10.1097/PAS.0000000000000769.
62. Boutko A, Hagstrom M, Lampley N, et al. PRAME immunohistochemical expression and TERT promoter mutational analysis as ancillary diagnostic tools for differentiating proliferative nodules from melanoma arising in congenital nevi. Am J Dermatopathol. 2023;45(7):437–47. https://doi.org/10.1097/DAD.0000000000002357.
63. Martins da Silva V, Martinez-Barrios E, Tell-Martí G, et al. Genetic abnormalities in large to giant congenital nevi: beyond NRAS mutations. J Invest Dermatol. 2019;139(4):900–8. https://doi.org/10.1016/j.jid.2018.07.045.
64. Charbel C, Fontaine RH, Malouf GG, et al. NRAS mutation is the sole recurrent somatic mutation in large congenital melanocytic nevi. J Invest Dermatol. 2014;134(4):1067–74. https://doi.org/10.1038/jid.2013.429.
65. Bauer J, Curtin JA, Pinkel D, Bastian BC. Congenital melanocytic nevi frequently harbor NRAS mutations but no BRAF mutations. J Invest Dermatol. 2007;127(1):179–82. https://doi.org/10.1038/sj.jid.5700490.

66. Salgado CM, Basu D, Nikiforova M, et al. BRAF mutations are also associated with neurocutaneous melanocytosis and large/giant congenital melanocytic nevi. Pediatr Dev Pathol. 2015;18(1):1–9. https://doi.org/10.2350/14-10-1566-OA.1.
67. Dessars B, De Raeve LE, Morandini R, et al. Genotypic and gene expression studies in congenital melanocytic nevi: insight into initial steps of melanotumorigenesis. J Invest Dermatol. 2009;129(1):139–47. https://doi.org/10.1038/jid.2008.203.
68. Muthiah S, Polubothu S, Husain A, Oliphant T, Kinsler VA, Rajan N. A mosaic variant in MAP 2K1 is associated with giant naevus spilus-type congenital melanocytic naevus and melanoma development. Br J Dermatol. 2020;183(4):760–1. https://doi.org/10.1111/bjd.19118.
69. Ichii-Nakato N, Takata M, Takayanagi S, et al. High frequency of BRAFV600E mutation in acquired nevi and small congenital nevi, but low frequency of mutation in medium-sized congenital nevi. J Invest Dermatol. 2006;126(9):2111–8. https://doi.org/10.1038/sj.jid.5700366.
70. Kinsler VA, Abu-Amero S, Budd P, et al. Germline melanocortin-1-receptor genotype is associated with severity of cutaneous phenotype in congenital melanocytic nevi: a role for MC1R in human fetal development. J Invest Dermatol. 2012;132(8):2026–32. https://doi.org/10.1038/jid.2012.95.
71. Dessars B, De Raeve LE, El Housni H, et al. Chromosomal translocations as a mechanism of BRAF activation in two cases of large congenital melanocytic nevi. J Invest Dermatol. 2007;127(6):1468–70. https://doi.org/10.1038/sj.jid.5700725.
72. Molho-Pessach V, Hartshtark S, Merims S, et al. Giant congenital melanocytic naevus with a novel CUX1-BRAF fusion mutation treated with trametinib. Br J Dermatol. 2022;187(6):1052–4. https://doi.org/10.1111/bjd.21851.
73. Houlier A, Pissaloux D, Tirode F, et al. RASGRF2 gene fusions identified in a variety of melanocytic lesions with distinct morphological features. Pigment Cell Melanoma Res. 2021;34(6):1074–83. https://doi.org/10.1111/pcmr.13004.
74. Perkins IU, Tan SY, McCalmont TH, et al. Melanoma in infants, caused by a gene fusion involving the anaplastic lymphoma kinase (ALK). Pigment Cell Melanoma Res. 2024;37(1):6–14. https://doi.org/10.1111/pcmr.13115.
75. Roy SF, Agim NG, Mir A, et al. Congenital melanocytic nevi initiated by BRAF fusion oncogene with firmness, pruritus, and desmoplastic stroma. Br J Dermatol. 2025;193:232–9. https://doi.org/10.1093/bjd/ljaf061.
76. Martin SB, Polubothu S, Bruzos AL, et al. Mosaic BRAF fusions are a recurrent cause of congenital melanocytic nevi targetable by MAPK pathway inhibition. J Invest Dermatol. 2024;144(3):593–600.e7. https://doi.org/10.1016/j.jid.2023.06.213.
77. Machan S, Molina-Ruiz AM, Fernández-Aceñero MJ, et al. Metastatic melanoma in association with a giant congenital melanocytic nevus in an adult: controversial CGH findings. Am J Dermatopathol. 2015;37(6):487–94. https://doi.org/10.1097/DAD.0000000000000152.
78. Lu C, Zhang J, Nagahawatte P, et al. The genomic landscape of childhood and adolescent melanoma. J Invest Dermatol. 2015;135(3):816–23. https://doi.org/10.1038/jid.2014.425.
79. Bansal N, Das M, Chatterjee U, Mallick MG, Arora N, Mishra DK. NRAS mutant melanoma arising in a giant congenital melanocytic nevus in an infant. Indian J Pathol Microbiol. 2021;64(2):402–5. https://doi.org/10.4103/IJPM.IJPM_38_20.
80. Lalor L, Busam K, Shah K. Prepubertal melanoma arising within a medium-sized congenital melanocytic nevus. Pediatr Dermatol. 2016;33(6):e372–4. https://doi.org/10.1111/pde.12961.
81. Kiyohara T, Takata M, Itoh H, et al. Malignant melanoma arising from an NRAS-mutated medium-sized congenital melanocytic nevus. J Dermatol. 2012;39(12):1034–5. https://doi.org/10.1111/j.1346-8138.2012.01542.x.
82. Hanrahan GB, Tsibris HC. Mutational landscape and tumour mutational burden in adults with malignant melanoma arising from congenital naevi. Br J Dermatol. 2024;191(4):627–30. https://doi.org/10.1093/bjd/ljae214.

83. Xie Y, Zhou Z, Deng D, Liu Y. Malignant melanoma arising from giant congenital melanocytic nevus with SMARCA2 gene mutation. Asian J Surg. 2024;47(7):3320–1. https://doi.org/10.1016/j.asjsur.2024.03.171.
84. Ricci C, Ambrosi F, Grillini M, et al. Next-generation sequencing revealing TP53 mutation as potential genetic driver in dermal deep-seated melanoma arising in giant congenital nevus in adult patients: a unique case report and review of the literature. J Cutan Pathol. 2020;47(12):1164–9. https://doi.org/10.1111/cup.13802.
85. Fan Y, Lee S, Wu G, et al. Telomerase expression by aberrant methylation of the TERT promoter in melanoma arising in giant congenital nevi. J Invest Dermatol. 2016;136(1):339–42. https://doi.org/10.1038/JID.2015.374.

Chapter 12
Molecular Biomarkers Applied to Treatment of Melanoma Patients

Riyad N. H. Seervai, Woo Cheal Cho, and Jonathan L. Curry

BRAF

BRAF is a cytoplasmic serine/threonine protein kinase encoded by the *BRAF* oncogene located on chromosome 7q34. Activation of BRAF (or the other RAF isoforms ARAF and CRAF) activates the mitogen-associated protein kinase (MAPK) signaling pathway via phosphorylation of the downstream targets MEK (MAPK/ERK Kinase) and ERK (extracellular signal-regulated kinase) [1]. *BRAF* mutations leading to constitutive MAPK activation and uncontrolled cell growth and proliferation are the most common genetic alterations in cutaneous melanomas, seen in 40–60% of cases [2–4]. The most common mutation involving *BRAF* is substitution of glutamic acid for valine at amino acid 600 (V600E), which represents 70–80% of gene alterations [2] and mimics phosphorylation of neighboring T599 threonine and S602 serine residues in the activation segment of the wild-type BRAF protein [5]. *BRAF* V600E is associated with superficial spreading (low-cumulative sun damage [CSD]) melanoma, younger age of onset, and sites lacking chronic sun damage (e.g., extremities) [6, 7]. Melanomas harboring this constitutively active mutant

R. N. H. Seervai
Department of Dermatology, Oregon Health & Science University, Portland, OR, USA
e-mail: seervai@ohsu.edu

W. C. Cho
Department of Anatomical Pathology, The University of Texas MD Anderson Cancer Center, Houston, TX, USA
e-mail: wcho@mdanderson.org

J. L. Curry (✉)
Department of Anatomical Pathology and Translational Molecular Pathology, Section of Dermatopathology, The University of Texas MD Anderson Medical Center, Houston, TX, USA
e-mail: jlcurry@mdanderson.org

V. G. Prieto, C. A. Torres-Cabala (eds.), *Precision Molecular Pathology of Melanocytic Lesions*, Molecular Pathology Library,
https://doi.org/10.1007/978-3-032-18222-7_12

protein have a >400-fold increase in kinase activity compared with those with wild-type *BRAF* [2, 5]. Other known *BRAF* mutations are V600K (10–30%) associated with older age and sites associated with chronic sun damage (e.g., head and neck) [6, 8], V600R (3–7%) associated with older age, male predominance, and ulceration, and V600M [9, 10]. *BRAF* mutations are also found in >80% of benign acquired melanocytic nevi [11, 12]. They were previously thought to be absent in congenital melanocytic nevi [13], although studies have identified rare *BRAF* mutations and gene fusions [14–16]. Sequencing studies have shown alterations in *BRAF* are oncogenic driver mutations in both acquired nevi and melanomas [17, 18] with additional genetic alterations, such as *CDKN2A* inactivation and *TERT* promoter mutation, contributing to evolution and progression of the latter [17, 19, 20]. The genetic evolution of acral melanomas shows an "inverted order" in which *BRAF* mutations are a later event, perhaps explaining why treatments of this subtype are met with limited success [21]. *BRAF* V600E and other MAP kinase mutations are rarely seen in clear cell sarcomas [22], and lack of diffuse PRAME (PReferentially expressed Antigen in Melanoma) expression is a useful immunophenotypic feature distinguishing these lesions from melanomas [23].

Immunohistochemistry (IHC) testing for BRAF V600E has become a standard procedure for predicting *BRAF* mutation status in melanoma. The anti–BRAF V600E monoclonal antibody (clone VE1) exhibits a high sensitivity and specificity of 92–100% when compared with detection of the same mutation by gene sequencing in primary and metastatic melanoma samples [24–30]. Our group has shown that increased labeling intensity is significantly associated with *BRAF* V600E mutation, and that homogeneous IHC staining in melanomas with epithelioid morphology (Fig. 12.1a, b) has a 99% specificity and 98% positive predictive value but 85% sensitivity [31]. Inclusion of a heterogeneous staining pattern improves the sensitivity (96%) with a slight decrease in specificity (96%). BRAF V600E IHC can aid in diagnosing undifferentiated or dedifferentiated melanomas with ambiguous morphology and loss of other melanoma markers (Fig. 12.2a, b) [32–34], particularly in cases in which the original melanoma already had that mutation. The cellular localization of BRAF V600E staining can have prognostic implications. Predominantly

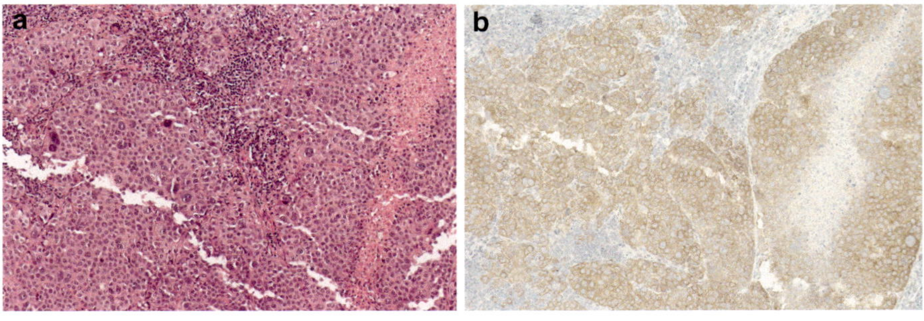

Fig. 12.1 Metastatic melanoma exhibiting epithelioid morphology (**a**, hematoxylin and eosin, original magnification ×200). There is diffuse and homogeneous expression of BRAF V600E (clone VE1) (**b**, immunohistochemistry, original magnification ×200) in the tumor cells

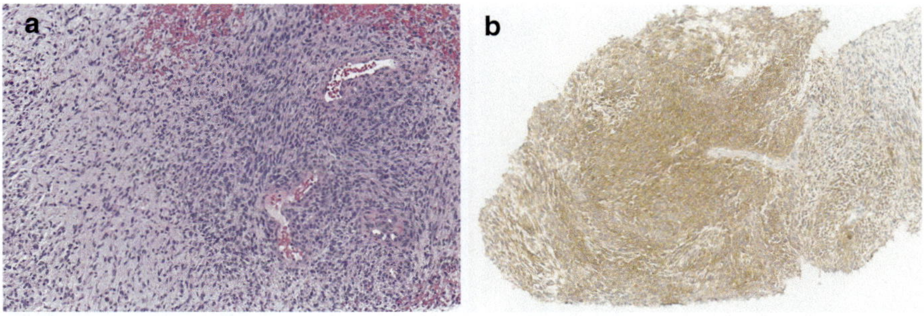

Fig. 12.2 Dedifferentiated melanoma (**a**, hematoxylin and eosin, original magnification ×200). Dedifferentiated melanomas often completely lack immunoreactivity for melanocytic cocktail (HMB45, MART1, tyrosinase). Note the diffuse expression of BRAF V600E (clone VE1) (**b**, immunohistochemistry, original magnification ×200) in this tumor, supporting the diagnosis of melanoma. The tumor cells in this case were additionally positive for MiTF (rare, scattered cells)

nuclear expression of BRAF V600E is associated with aggressive features, including lymphovascular and perineural invasion, advanced tumor stage, depth of invasion, lymph node metastasis, and is possibly even associated with resistance to targeted therapy [35, 36].

Challenges with interpretation of BRAF V600E IHC expression can arise in the setting of heavily pigmented lesions. In such cases, use of Giemsa as a counterstain creates contrast between melanin pigment (that turns dark green with Giemsa) and diaminobenzidine used in IHC (brown) (Fig. 12.3a–c) [37]. Use of a red chromogen detection agent and melanin depigmentation [38] are other alternatives to improve the accuracy of IHC interpretation. However, bleaching techniques may alter tissue antigenicity, and laboratories utilizing this technique will need to have processes validated and standardized to minimize aberrant tissue labeling [39]. The peptide sequence used to generate VE1 anti–BRAF V600E antibody shares homology with axonemal dynein heavy chains DNAH2, DNAH7, and DNAH12 [40], which might result in labeling of ciliated structures. This likely explains why BRAF V600E IHC is a reliable test in melanoma and papillary thyroid carcinoma, but not in colorectal carcinoma [41]. Furthermore, cross-reactivity of BRAF IHC with arrector pili muscle and vascular walls (Fig. 12.4) may be observed in the skin. When present, BRAF V600E expression in these structures tends to be weaker in intensity than in BRAF-mutated melanoma cells. Decalcification of tumor samples (especially in the context of bone metastasis) can lead to failure of BRAF V600E IHC and false negative results [42]. Finally, there are rare cases in which BRAF V600E expression is positive by IHC but molecular analysis fails to show the corresponding gene mutation [43, 44]. This scenario is most likely due to inadequate tissue sampling, tissue necrosis, or decalcification of tissue samples. In one case, a patient with metastatic melanoma of unknown primary with wild-type *BRAF* on genetic analysis of a bone marrow biopsy (the sample was decalcified), who progressed on immunotherapy, was found to have IHC immunoreactivity using the VE1 antibody. The patient had significant improvement after switching to BRAF inhibitor therapy, thus supporting

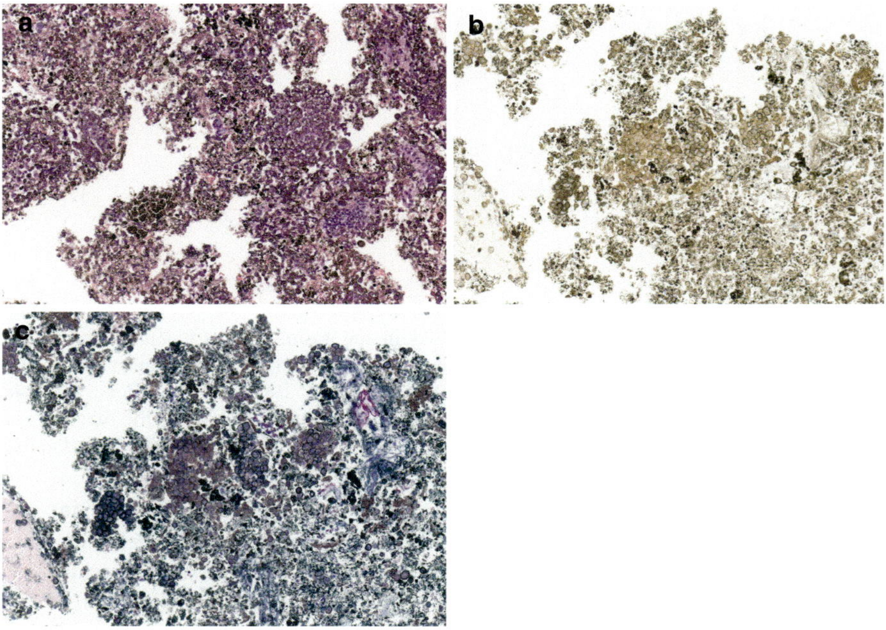

Fig. 12.3 Metastatic melanoma with heavy pigmentation (**a**, hematoxylin and eosin). In cases where melanoma cells are densely pigmented, both peritumoral melanophages and intracytoplasmic melanin pigment within tumor cells can make interpretation of BRAF V600E IHC (**b**, clone VE1, immunohistochemistry, original magnification ×200) challenging. Giemsa counterstaining of BRAF V600E IHC (**c**, histochemical, original magnification ×200) provides a clear contrast between true BRAF V600E expression (brown) in tumor cells and background melanin pigment (dark green)

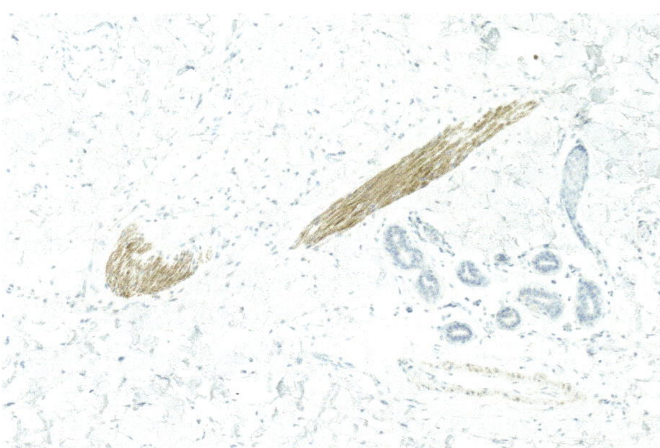

Fig. 12.4 BRAF V600E cross-reactivity in non-tumor cells within the skin. BRAF V600E (clone VE1) immunoreactivity (original magnification ×200) is observed in both the arrector pili muscles (center) and the vascular walls (bottom right, below the eccrine glands)

the interpretation of a positive *BRAF* V600E mutation [45]. Additionally, heterogeneous and weak immunoreactivity for BRAF V600E (clone VE1) can be seen in rare cases of melanomas with other *BRAF* mutations, especially V600K (Fig. 12.5)

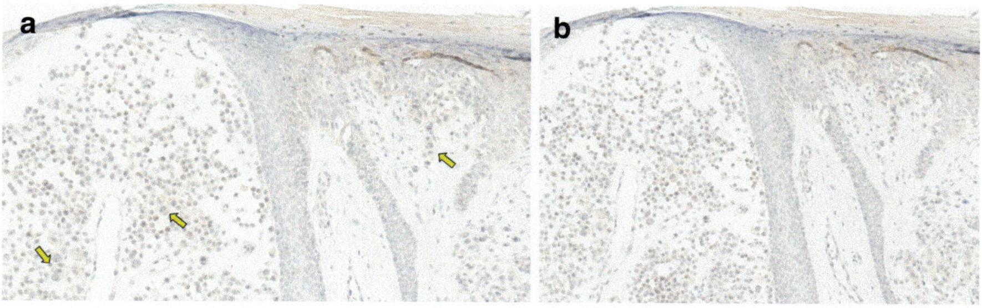

Fig. 12.5 Non-*BRAF* V600E-mutated melanoma weakly expressing BRAF V600E (clone VE1) (**a**) arrows, (**b**) original magnification ×200. This pattern of immunoreactivity is often observed in melanomas harboring a *BRAF V600K* mutation, which in this case was subsequently confirmed by molecular studies

[31]. As such, further workup or testing of additional/alternative samples is recommended in the setting of clinically, histologically, or genetically ambiguous or discordant cases.

NRAS

NRAS is a small GTP-binding protein encoded by the *NRAS* oncogene on chromosome 1p13.2. Together with other members of the RAS family (HRAS and KRAS), it mediates growth and survival via transduction of the MAPK and phosphatidyl inositol 3 kinase (PI3K) pathways [1, 46]. Mutations in the oncogene decrease RAS GTPase activity and result in a constitutively active GTP-bound signaling protein [18, 46, 47]. *NRAS* Q61K and Q61R mutations occur in up to 20% of melanoma cases and are associated with chronic sun damage and a nodular subtype [7, 48–50]. These mutations are also seen in congenital melanocytic nevi, suggesting a role for additional mutagenesis independent of UV radiation in *NRAS*-mutant melanomas [13, 51]. Studies have shown melanomas harboring mutated *NRAS* have a poor prognosis, including central nervous system involvement of metastases and worse overall survival [52–55].

Detection of NRAS Q61R biomarker expression with IHC using an anti–NRAS Q61R monoclonal antibody (clone SP174) has 92–100% sensitivity and 99–100% specificity in primary and metastatic melanomas with *NRAS* Q61R mutation [28, 30, 56–58]. An anti–NRAS Q61L monoclonal antibody (clone 26193) is less accurate in detecting the corresponding *NRAS* Q61L mutation, with sensitivity of 82.6% and specificity of 96.2% [28]. Cross-reactivity of the SP174 antibody with HRAS and KRAS Q61R mutant proteins [59], most likely due to high sequence homology of the N-terminal catalytic domain of the RAS family [60], is a potential pitfall in its use for biomarker identification in *RAS*-mutated melanomas. Similar cross-reactivity has been noted in colorectal and medullary thyroid carcinomas [61, 62]. Additionally, the SP174 antibody shows immunoreactivity in PRAME-negative,

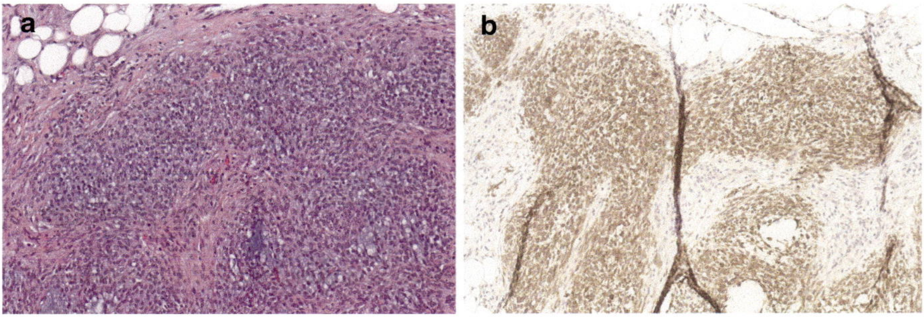

Fig. 12.6 Metastatic dedifferentiated melanoma (**a**, hematoxylin and eosin, original magnification ×200) showing strong and diffuse expression of RAS Q61R (**b**, immunohistochemistry, original magnification ×200). In this case, the tumor cells were focally positive for MiTF, while largely lacking immunoreactivity for other melanocytic markers such as HMB45, MART1, and tyrosinase. Subsequent molecular analysis confirmed the presence of an *NRAS* Q61R mutation, with a variant allele frequency of 88%

11p-amplified, *NRAS* Q61R-negative Spitz nevi in which *HRAS* Q61R mutation was confirmed by sequencing [63]. Lastly, similar to BRAF V600E IHC, RAS Q61R IHC is also useful in confirming the diagnosis of dedifferentiated or undifferentiated melanoma (Fig. 12.6a, b), particularly when expression of other melanocytic markers—such as HMB45, MART1, tyrosinase, and MiTF—is absent or minimal.

C-KIT

c-KIT (also known as mast cell growth factor, CD117) is a membrane-associated receptor tyrosine kinase encoded by the *KIT* proto-oncogene on chromosome 4q12. It is a primary effector of growth factor signaling via the MAPK and PI3K pathways [64, 65]. The role of c-KIT as a mediator of melanocyte migration is underscored by loss-of-function mutations in the KIT pathway leading to piebaldism [66, 67]. Studies showing c-KIT signaling antagonizes melanocyte proliferation [68, 69] and its expression is lost in the setting of tumor progression and metastasis [70–73] suggested it might function as a tumor suppressor in melanoma. Since then, oncogenic *KIT* mutations and copy number variations have been identified in melanomas of acral (9–59%), mucosal (15–22%), and chronic sun-damaged (2–31%) sites [74–78]. Mutations involving *KIT* are a later event, arising after tumorigenesis in acral melanomas [21], and appear to be mutually exclusive from alterations in *BRAF* or *NRAS* [18]. c-KIT L576P substitution (exon 11) affecting the juxtamembrane domain is the most common alteration in melanoma and promotes dimerization and constitutive activation [74, 77, 79]. Substitution at K642E (exon 13) affecting the first kinase domain is weakly activating and has oncogenic potential in the context of additional *KIT* mutations [74]. Collectively, *KIT* exon 11 and 13 alterations are likely susceptible to imatinib and other tyrosine kinase inhibitors [74, 77, 79, 80]. Mutations in exon 17 affecting the second c-KIT kinase domain (D816V/Y and D820Y) are resistant to treatment with imatinib in melanoma [79] and other cancer types [81, 82]. Alterations in *KIT* are associated with improved progression-free survival in vulvovaginal melanoma but have no impact on overall survival [53, 83, 84]. In Asian populations, presence of *KIT* alterations is associated with worse survival compared with wild-type melanomas [85–87]. It is likely these differences reflect the prognostic implications of different *KIT* mutations [79].

c-KIT biomarker expression with IHC using a polyclonal rabbit anti–CD117 antibody has a low specificity, owing largely to the fact that the in situ and junctional component of primary melanomas are almost always positive regardless of *KIT* mutation status [88, 89]. Analysis of canine oral melanoma has also shown IHC positivity in 86% of samples with no evidence of *KIT* mutation [90]. c-KIT IHC expression in the invasive component has a 100% and 96.6% negative predictive value for *KIT* mutation in acral and mucosal melanomas with <5% and <50% positive tumor cells, respectively (Fig. 12.7a, b) [88]. The intensity of IHC expression in the invasive component of melanoma has a correspondingly high negative predictive value. In this study, KIT IHC expression was retained in metastases compared with primary tumors in the four matched samples. Other studies have shown decreased KIT biomarker expression in melanoma metastases [73, 91]. KIT IHC expression is seen with frequency in melanomas and nevi (including Spitz and atypical acral nevi) [73, 92–94]; however, dermal IHC positivity might help distinguish melanomas from compound or intradermal nevi [95]. Overall, unlike with BRAF V600E and RAS Q61R IHCs, IHC for KIT expression has utility in excluding *KIT* mutations in melanomas rather than acting as an indicator of tyrosine kinase inhibitor response in these tumors.

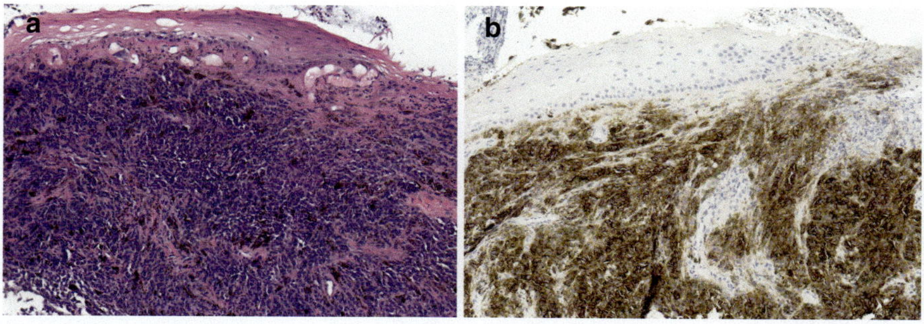

Fig. 12.7 Anorectal mucosal melanoma (**a**, hematoxylin and eosin, original magnification ×200) demonstrating strong and diffuse expression of c-KIT (**b**, immunohistochemistry, original magnification ×200). Although c-KIT protein expression is typically not specific for underlying molecular alterations, subsequent molecular analysis in this case confirmed the presence of *KIT* N822Y and *KIT* M618L mutations, with variant allele frequencies of 29% and 30%, respectively, along with a copy number gain of 4q12 involving the *KIT* gene

PTEN

Phosphatase and tensin homologue (PTEN) is a lipid phosphatase encoded by the *PTEN* tumor suppressor gene on chromosome 10q23. PTEN function and activity varies based on its intracellular localization [96, 97]. In the cytoplasm, PTEN antagonizes the PI3K signaling pathway by dephosphorylating phosphatidylinositol 3,4,5-triphosphate (PIP3) and AKT [98, 99] and acts as a scaffolding protein to promote calcium-mediated apoptosis [100]. Nuclear PTEN controls genomic stability in a phosphatase-independent manner through interaction with centromere proteins, DNA repair proteins, and histone modifiers [101–104]. PTEN activity is lost in melanomas through mutation and deletion of the *PTEN* gene [105] or via epigenetic/posttranslational regulation [106–108]. *PTEN* mutations or deletions are a later event associated with advanced primary or metastatic melanomas [20, 109]. These alterations are also associated with poor prognosis, with decreased overall survival [110] and resistance to BRAF inhibitors [111, 112] and immunotherapy [113–115].

Loss of PTEN biomarker expression by IHC has been defined as less than 10% tumor cell immunoreactivity compared with an internal endothelial cell positive control (Fig. 12.8a, b) [110]. A heterogeneous "clonal-like" pattern with distinct negative foci has been described in 6–10% of cases (Fig. 12.9a, b) [115, 116]. These tumors are associated with an immunosuppressive phenotype, with decreased CD8+ T-cell infiltration into the PTEN-negative tumor regions [115, 117]. Loss of PTEN IHC expression has not been shown to correlate strongly with *PTEN* genetic alterations, although 7/8 (87.5%) of cases with confirmed alterations by sequencing or FISH showed aberrant (negative or clonal-like) PTEN expression [116]. Quantitative analysis has shown decreased PTEN IHC expression in tumors with Breslow depth >2 cm, suggesting it may serve as a surrogate for tumor invasion [118] (although this observation would be apparent on examination of routine H&E-stained slides). Additionally, subcellular localization of PTEN by IHC might have clinical implications, with uniformly strong cytoplasmic expression noted in benign melanocytic

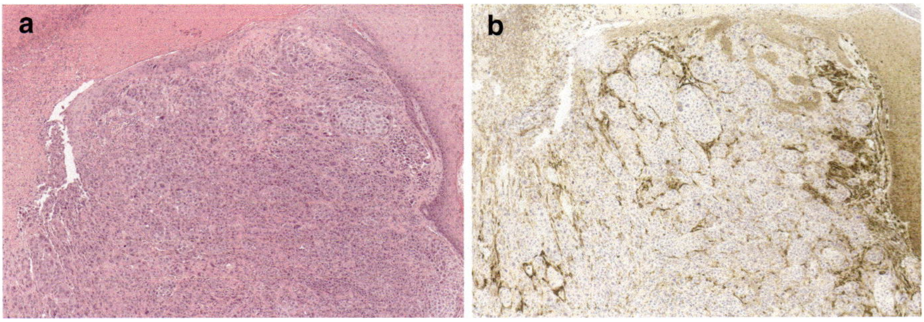

Fig. 12.8 Metastatic melanoma (**a**, hematoxylin and eosin, original magnification ×100) with absence of PTEN expression (**b**, immunohistochemistry, original magnification ×100). Molecular analysis revealed *PTEN* C304* mutation along with other somatic mutations, including *BRAF* V600E, *BTK*, *CDKN2A*, *PIK3CB*, and *TERT* promoter mutations

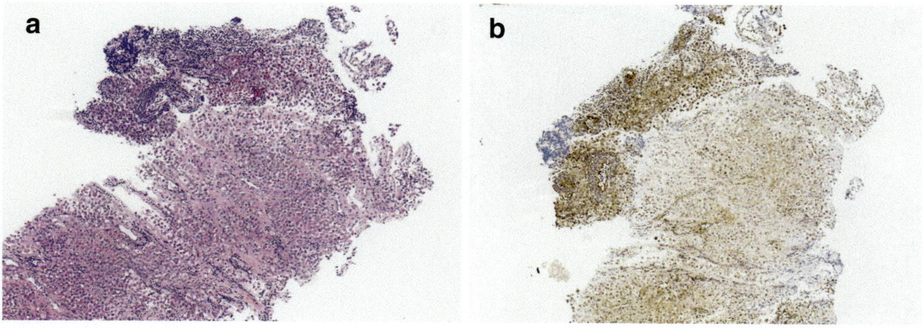

Fig. 12.9 Metastatic melanoma (**a**, hematoxylin and eosin, original magnification ×100) exhibiting a heterogeneous pattern of PTEN expression (**b**, immunohistochemistry, original magnification ×100). In this case, subsequent molecular analysis did not reveal any alterations involving *PTEN*. Instead, the melanoma harbored other somatic mutations, including *ARID2*, *AXL*, *HDAC9*, and *IL7R* mutations

nevi [119] and positive cytoplasmic PTEN expression associated with better disease-free survival [116].

PD-L1

Programmed cell death ligand-1 (PD-L1, also known as B7-H1 and CD274) is a part of the B7 family of T-cell co-inhibitory transmembrane glycoproteins. PD-L1 interaction with the programmed cell death receptor-1 (PD-1) has an immunosuppressive effect by inhibiting T-cell proliferation and survival, promoting their differentiation to regulatory T-cells, and inducing apoptosis [120, 121]. PD-L1 expression has been reported in primary, satellite, in-transit, and metastatic melanomas of all subtypes, including cutaneous (both with high and low cumulative damage (35–62%), acral (31%), mucosal (44%), and uveal (10%) melanomas, and is associated with presence of tumor-infiltrating lymphocytes [122, 123]. Targeting the PD-1/PD-L1 axis with immune checkpoint inhibitor (ICI) immunotherapy has revolutionized the treatment of melanoma, and positive PD-L1 expression is associated with improved response to ICIs [124–126].

PD-L1 biomarker IHC expression can be detected with multiple different antibodies. Although some of these antibodies reportedly had different quantitative results, a study using standardized methodology reported similar results for the most commonly used antibodies [127]. IHC detection of PD-L1 with a rabbit monoclonal anti-PD-L1 antibody (clone 28-8) [128–130] is FDA-approved as a complementary diagnostic test to assess candidacy for ICI therapy. Macrophages may also exhibit membranous labeling with PD-L1 IHC, and distinction from PD-L1-positive melanoma cells may be challenging. Multiplex IHC staining with PD-L1 and SOX10 may be deployed to mitigate the interpretation of inflammatory cells as positive tumor cells [131]. There are several different scoring systems for

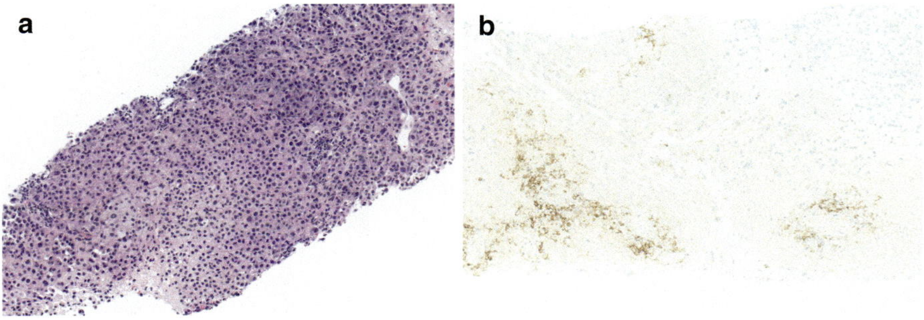

Fig. 12.10 Metastatic melanoma (**a**, hematoxylin and eosin, original magnification ×200) demonstrating approximately 1–2% membranous expression of PD-L1 (**b**, clone 28-8, immunohistochemistry, original magnification ×200), based on the tumor proportion score

determining PD-L1 IHC positivity: the tumor proportion score measures tumor cell expression only (Fig. 12.10a, b), the combined proportion score measures tumor and immune cell expression, and the melanoma score measures the proportion of all positive cells in relation to the tumor but excluding the surrounding stroma [132–134]. Most studies have used a 1% cut-off to determine PD-L1 IHC positivity [125, 135], largely due to the suggestion that patients with <1% expression may benefit from combination ICI therapy versus monotherapy for those with >1% expression [136]. Other studies have proposed a 5% cutoff to define positivity [137, 138]. As such, the clinical utility of PD-L1 IHC assessment and interpretation of PD-L1 scoring in melanoma is still a matter of debate [139].

BAP1

BRCA1-associated protein 1 (BAP1) is a ubiquitin C-terminal hydroxylase (deubiquitinase) enzyme encoded by the *BAP1* tumor suppressor gene on chromosome 3p21.1. It maintains genome stability through regulation of chromatin architecture, gene transcription, and DNA repair, and is also involved in metabolic processes (e.g., apoptosis and ferroptosis), cell differentiation, and development [140, 141]. Germline *BAP1* mutations lead to a BAP1-tumor predisposition syndrome (BAP1-TPS) with increased susceptibility to cutaneous and uveal melanoma, mesothelioma, and renal cell carcinoma [142–146]. These patients sporadically develop benign BRAF V600E-positive melanocytic neoplasms called BAP1-inactivated melanocytic tumors (BIMTs) or "BAPomas" in the setting of biallelic *BAP1* loss [147–149]. Details regarding BAP-1 inactivated melanocytoma are discussed elsewhere in this book. There are rare cases of melanomas arising from BIMTs [150]. Somatic *BAP1* mutations have also been identified in cutaneous and metastasizing uveal melanomas in the absence of BAP1-TPS, and these mutations are associated with a higher risk of metastasis [151–153]. Sequencing studies have shown *BAP1* mutations are secondary drivers of uveal melanoma, associated with monosomy 3, and are early events typically preceding metastatic dissemination [154]. They generally occur exclusive from *SF3B1* and *EIF1AX* mutations, which are seen in uveal melanomas with disomy 3 [155]. Histone deacetylase (HDAC) inhibitors have been shown to reverse the effect of BAP1 depletion in uveal melanoma cells [156], and HDAC4 has emerged as a promising candidate for targeted therapy in *BAP1*-mutant uveal melanoma [157].

BAP1 IHC expression can be detected with a mouse monoclonal anti-BAP1 antibody (sc-28383, clone C-4) and is lost in 43–51% primary and 77% metastatic uveal melanoma samples [158–162]. Low *BAP1 gene* expression and loss of disomy 3 correlate with decreased/absent IHC expression [161, 163, 164], and loss of BAP1 immunoreactivity has 88% sensitivity and 97% specificity compared with *BAP1* mutation analysis [160]. All these studies have shown that loss of nuclear BAP1 IHC expression is associated with aggressive uveal melanomas, higher risk of metastasis, and worse survival [158–163]. Low nuclear BAP1 IHC also correlates with gene expression profiling (GEP) class 2 and is equally accurate in predicting metastasis [164, 165]. A cutoff of ≥25% loss of BAP1 immunoreactivity has been determined to be a reliable predictor of poor prognosis, similar to predominant (≥50%) loss of BAP1 IHC expression and more reliable than chromosome 3 loss of heterozygosity [166]. HDAC inhibitor therapy might thus be suitable for patients with ≥25% loss of BAP1 biomarker expression by IHC. There are a few cases with loss of nuclear BAP1 expression in which cytoplasmic expression is retained in a diffuse or "focal perinuclear" pattern, most likely sequestered within the Golgi apparatus [159, 167].

Overall, loss of BAP1 biomarker IHC expression is a reliable predictor of *BAP1* mutation status, monosomy 3, and metastasis in uveal melanoma. The association between BAP1 IHC and these outcomes is negatively impacted by brachytherapy, most likely due to changes in tissue antigenicity and radiation-induced epigenetic changes [168], which is a potential pitfall of this analysis in previously irradiated uveal melanoma samples.

GNAQ/GNA11

The *GNAQ* gene on chromosome 9q21.2 and its paralogue *GNA11* on chromosome 19p13.3 encode the GNAQ (alpha-q) and GNA11 (alpha-11) subunits of heterotrimeric G-proteins. Somatic mutations in *GNAQ/GNA11* exon 5 (Q209L/P) and less commonly exon 4 (R183C/H) alter the GNAQ/GNA11 RAS-like switch I and II domains, leading to decreased GTPase activity and a constitutively active state [169]. These and other mutations are the most common alterations in uveal melanoma (80–90%), melanocytic proliferations of the central nervous system (37–42%), blue nevi and melanoma blue nevus type (50–83%), and nevi of Ota (15%) [170–175]. A subset of *GNAQ/GNA11*-mutated nonuveal melanomas has also been identified and thought to represent a subset of melanomas clinically and genetically distinct from cutaneous and uveal melanoma [176]. Details regarding *GNAQ* and

GNA11 mutations in blue nevi and melanomas arising in blue nevi are discussed elsewhere in this book.

GNAQ and *GNA11* mutations are mutually exclusive driver mutations in uveal melanoma [154, 173] and contribute to melanomagenesis via activation of the MAP kinase and Hippo signaling pathways [177–179]. *GNAQ* mutations are one of the earliest events in uveal melanomas, and loss of heterozygosity has been observed with progression, while *GNA11* mutations are more frequent in metastatic uveal melanoma samples and loss of heterozygosity is not seen [154, 173]. The prognostic implications of these mutations have been a matter of debate: some studies have shown *GNA11* mutation is associated with metastasis and worse disease-specific survival [180–182], while others have shown no impact of *GNAQ* or *GNA11* mutations on metastasis or survival [171, 183–187].

Detection of GNA11 expression by IHC with a rabbit polyclonal anti-GNA11 antibody (sc-394, clone D-17) has been studied in the context of DNA methylation and *GNA11* gene silencing in breast cancer [188]. Similarly, decreased GNAQ IHC expression with a rabbit polyclonal anti-GNAQ antibody (ab75825) is associated with poor survival in pancreatic tumors [189]. Studies in feline iris melanoma have shown higher GNAQ/GNA11 labeling intensity compared with control eyes [190], although mutation analysis has not identified *GNAQ/GNA11* mutations in feline ocular melanomas [191]. There are no studies investigating the utility of GNAQ/GNA11 IHC expression as a surrogate for *GNAQ/GNA11* mutation in human uveal melanoma samples.

ALK

Anaplastic lymphoma kinase (ALK, also known as CD246) is a receptor tyrosine kinase belonging to the insulin receptor superfamily, encoded by the *ALK* gene on chromosome 2p23. *ALK* gene rearrangements resulting in fusion with *tropomyosin-3* (*TPM3::ALK*) and *dynactin-1* (*DCTN1::ALK*) are seen in 10% of Spitz melanocytic neoplasms, including Spitz nevi, atypical Spitz tumors (most commonly), and Spitz melanomas [192]. ALK fusions are associated with a plexiform/fascicular growth pattern of fusiform dermal melanocytes and generally lack epithelioid morphology, although some tumors with *TMP3::ALK* fusions can have a higher proportion of large, pleomorphic epithelioid melanocytes. [193–196]. A novel *SLC20A1::ALK* fusion has been reported in a Spitz melanoma lacking a plexiform morphology [197]. Increased *ALK* copy number has also been reported in a Spitzoid melanoma with a similar plexiform growth pattern [198]. Finally, a subset of primary and metastatic cutaneous melanomas expresses a novel ALK isoform from a de novo alternative transcription initiation (ATI) site in intron 19 (ALK^{ATI}), with increased ALK expression independent of *ALK* gene rearrangements [199, 200]. ALK translocations and ALK^{ATI} are associated with increased kinase activity and activation of the MAPK and PI3K pathways, and this signaling is suppressed by the ALK inhibitors crizotinib and ceritinib [192, 199, 200].

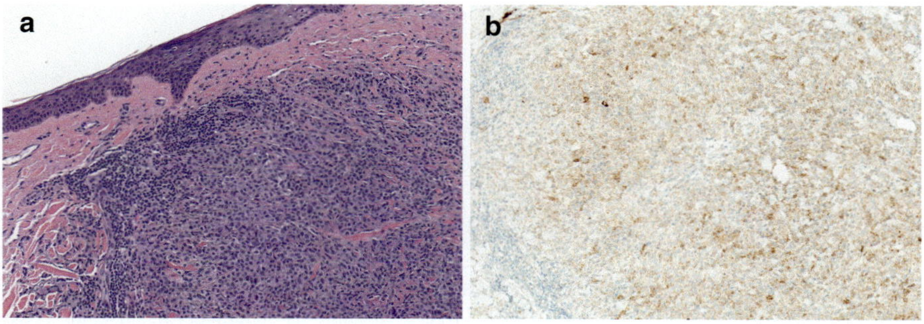

Fig. 12.11 Nodular melanoma (**a**, hematoxylin and eosin, original magnification ×100) showing patchy ALK expression (**b**, immunohistochemistry, original magnification ×200). Molecular analysis revealed a tumor mutational burden of 53 mut/Mb and *ALK G893R* and *ALK R557C* somatic mutations. There were also *BRAF D594N, PTCH1, ROS1,* and other somatic mutations in addition to *TERT* promoter mutation

Detection of ALK biomarker expression by IHC with a rabbit monoclonal anti–ALK antibody (clone D5F3) has high specificity and sensitivity for *ALK* alterations in melanocytic neoplasms (Fig. 12.11a, b), including melanomas. Tumor cells from samples with *ALK* rearrangements show ALK immunoreactivity on IHC, and conversely, cases without *ALK* rearrangements do not show expression on IHC [192–194]. Staining can be helpful in appreciating the infiltrative growth pattern at the peripheral and deep margins of the tumor. Membranous immunoreactivity has been seen in a Spitz nevus with *EHBP1::ALK* fusion, suggesting the fusion partner might determine localization of the chimeric protein [201]. ALK^{ATI}-positive tumors show nuclear and cytoplasmic IHC expression [199], and strong diffuse cytoplasmic IHC positivity has ~100% specificity and 52% sensitivity in detecting ALK^{ATI} [202]. Similarly, primary and metastatic melanoma samples with IHC positivity but no *ALK* rearrangements on molecular analysis all harbor the ALK^{ATI} variant [200]. A study assessing ALK IHC in metastatic melanomas showed ALK expression is enriched in *NRAS* Q61K/R-mutated samples and is associated with better disease-specific survival in patients with *NRAS* mutations [203]. Use of a commercially available Ventana ALK (D5F3) CDx assay is FDA-approved as a standalone test for *ALK* rearrangements in lung cancer, with lower cost and superior accuracy compared with FISH in predicting response and survival to crizotinib in patients with advanced tumors [204]. Similar studies are needed to determine the comparative cost-effectiveness and accuracy of ALK IHC in melanocytic lesions.

NTRK

Neutrotropic tropomyosin receptor kinase-1 (NTRK1) and NTRK3 are receptor tyrosine kinases encoded by the *NTRK1* and *NTRK3* genes on chromosomes 1q23.1 and 15q25.3, respectively. *NTRK1/3* fusions are seen in up to 16% of Spitz

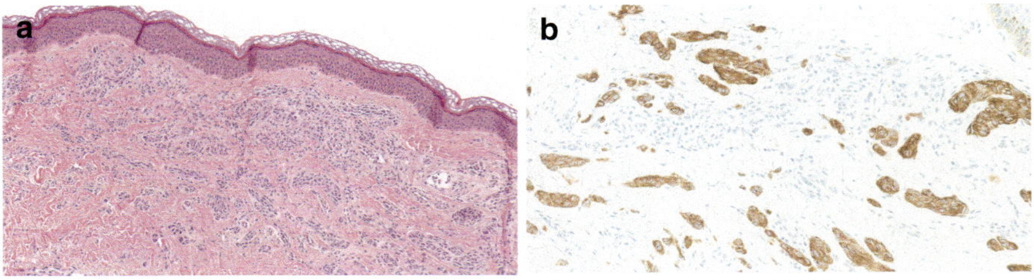

Fig. 12.12 *NTRK1*-rearranged Spitz melanoma (**a**, hematoxylin and eosin, original magnification ×100) showing diffuse and strong expression of TRK (**b**, immunohistochemistry against pan-TRK, original magnification ×200). In addition to the *NTRK1* gene rearrangement, this melanoma also exhibited multiple copy number aberrations, including gains of 1q, 7, 11p, and 22q, as well as loss of 1q

melanocytic neoplasms, including Spitz and Reed nevi, atypical spitzoid neoplasms, and Spitz melanomas, and show a predominantly epithelioid morphology [192, 205–207]. The gene fusions are also seen in 2.5% of acral melanomas and <1% of non-acral cutaneous and mucosal melanomas of non-Spitz lineage [208, 209]. Targeted therapy with the pan-TRK inhibitors larotrectinib and entrectinib (which also inhibit ROS1 and ALK) has shown efficacy in these tumors [210, 211].

Detection of NTRK biomarker expression by IHC with a rabbit monoclonal anti–NTRK antibody (clone EPR17341) has a 79–100% sensitivity for detecting *NTRK1-3* translocations across multiple tumor types, and ~100% sensitivity and specificity in melanoma samples tested (Fig. 12.12a, b) [212]. A different antibody (clone A7H6R) is less specific as IHC-positive samples did not show *NTRK* rearrangements on FISH analysis [213]. Studies in other tumor types have also shown different staining patterns between these antibodies, with some concluding FISH is the preferred modality over IHC for detecting *NTRK* fusions [214–217]. IHC expression in *NTRK*-rearranged lesions is predominantly cytoplasmic with or without nuclear staining, and there are no cases of membrane-localized immunoreactivity [205, 218, 219].

TERT

Telomerase reverse transcriptase (TERT), encoded by the *TERT* gene on chromosome 5p15, is the catalytic subunit of the telomerase enzyme that maintains telomere length during replication. *TERT* amplifications are the most frequent genetic alterations in acral melanoma, seen in 70% of tumors and occurring at the earliest stages in progression [21] and associated with poor prognosis and progression to metastasis [220, 221]. *TERT* promoter (*TERT*-p) mutations are rare in acral melanomas [21, 222] but are commonly seen in primary and metastatic cutaneous melanomas and may co-occur with *BRAF* and *CDKN2A* mutations [223–225]. The heterogeneity of *TERT*-p contributes to differences in histology, clinical presentation, and prognosis in melanoma patients [226, 227]. Studies have shown *TERT*-p mutations are associated with better survival in patients receiving BRAF and MEK inhibitor therapy [228], while other *TERT*-p mutations and TERT expression are indicators of poor prognosis and resistance to MAPK inhibitory therapy [229–231]. Given *TERT* promoter activation is a key step in the progression of MAPK-mutated melanomas [232], targeting TERT expression is a potential therapeutic strategy in these patients [233].

Detection of TERT biomarker expression by IHC with a rabbit monoclonal anti-TERT antibody (clone Y182) shows a positive correlation between immunoreactivity and copy number amplification [234]. Positive staining has ~100% sensitivity and negative predictive value for detecting these alterations; however, its utility is limited by a low specificity (57%) and positive predictive value (38%) [234]. Our group has also shown that TERT immunoreactivity in acral melanomas is cytoplasmic (Fig. 12.13) and has higher intensity than other acral nevi, but it does not correlate with survival [235]. TERT IHC expression in cutaneous melanoma with a rabbit polyclonal antibody (600-401-252) has a 70% sensitivity and 35% specificity, with no correlation between immunoreactivity and mutation status, but a significant association between positive expression and worse survival [236]. Another study identified higher levels of nucleolar TERT expression in benign nevi and an increase in "melanoma-like" non-nucleolar expression in dysplastic nevi, primary melanomas, and metastases [237]. Here too, expression did not correlate with *TERT* promoter mutation status.

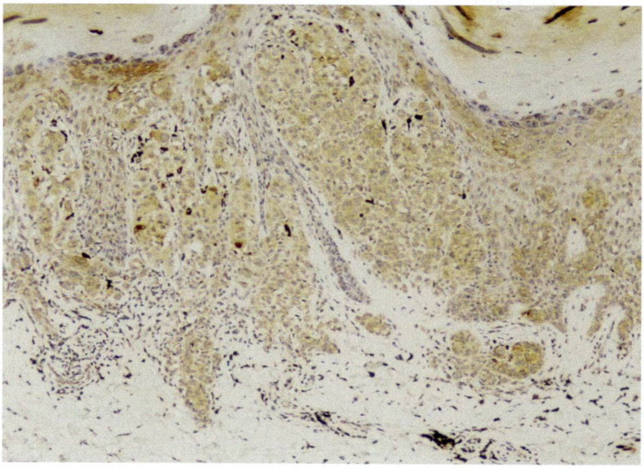

Fig. 12.13 Acral melanoma showing diffuse TERT expression by immunohistochemistry (original magnification ×100)

Summary

As this chapter demonstrates, immunohistochemistry for biomarker expression has implications for prognosis and selection of targeted therapy in mutation-specific melanoma patients. A summary of the genes discussed is below.

1. *BRAF*: IHC has high sensitivity and specificity for detecting *BRAF* V600 mutations and can be a useful tool both in selecting targeted anti-BRAF therapies and in identifying undifferentiated melanomas with desmoplastic morphology and loss of other tumor markers.
2. *NRAS*: IHC has high sensitivity and specificity for detecting Q61R mutations, less so for Q61L mutations due to cross-reactivity.
3. *C-KIT*: IHC is less accurate in predicting the presence of *KIT* mutations, but loss of immunoreactivity has a high negative predictive value in excluding mutations in acral and mucosal melanomas.
4. *PTEN*: Negative or "clonal-like" IHC expression may be associated with *PTEN* alterations, and decreased expression may be associated with increased depth of invasion. Strong cytoplasmic IHC expression may be associated with better disease-free survival.
5. PD-L1: IHC expression has been FDA-approved as an independent test for predicting response to immune checkpoint inhibitor therapy. The cutoff for PD-L1 positivity (1% or 5%) is debated.
6. *BAP1*: Loss of IHC expression is a reliable predictor of *BAP1* mutation, monosomy of chromosome 3, and in metastasis of uveal melanoma.
7. *GNAQ/GNA11*: IHC expression is associated with poor survival in pancreatic tumors, but there are no studies assessing the utility of this test as a surrogate for *GNAQ* or *GNA11* mutations in uveal melanoma.
8. *ALK*: IHC expression has high sensitivity and specificity for *ALK* alterations, including gene fusions, copy number increase, or $\mathit{ALK}^{\mathrm{ATI}}$.
9. *NTRK*: IHC expression has high sensitivity and specificity for detecting fusions; however, this may be clone-dependent.
10. *TERT*: IHC expression has high sensitivity but low specificity for detecting gene amplifications or promoter mutations. Additionally, IHC is unlikely to capture the genetic heterogeneity associated with *TERT*-p mutations.

As discussed in this chapter, the accuracy of assessing biomarker expression by IHC is impacted by a variety of factors, such as sample preparation (e.g., decalcification of *BRAF*-positive tumors), pigmentation, or previous therapy (e.g., brachytherapy for *BAP1*-negative uveal melanomas). It is important for pathologists and clinicians to be aware of these potential pitfalls when utilizing these tests that have significant clinical implications in melanoma patients.

References

1. Buscà R, et al. Ras mediates the cAMP-dependent activation of extracellular signal-regulated kinases (ERKs) in melanocytes. EMBO J. 2000;19(12):2900–10.
2. Davies H, et al. Mutations of the BRAF gene in human cancer. Nature. 2002;417(6892):949–54.
3. Hayward NK, et al. Whole-genome landscapes of major melanoma subtypes. Nature. 2017;545(7653):175–80.
4. Brose MS, et al. BRAF and RAS mutations in human lung cancer and melanoma. Cancer Res. 2002;62(23):6997–7000.
5. Wan PT, et al. Mechanism of activation of the RAF-ERK signaling pathway by oncogenic mutations of B-RAF. Cell. 2004;116(6):855–67.
6. Kim SY, et al. Metaanalysis of BRAF mutations and clinicopathologic characteristics in primary melanoma. J Am Acad Dermatol. 2015;72(6):1036–46.e2.
7. Pracht M, et al. Prognostic and predictive values of oncogenic BRAF, NRAS, c-KIT and MITF in cutaneous and mucous melanoma. J Eur Acad Dermatol Venereol. 2015;29(8):1530–8.
8. Bucheit AD, et al. Clinical characteristics and outcomes with specific BRAF and NRAS mutations in patients with metastatic melanoma. Cancer. 2013;119(21):3821–9.
9. Comito F, et al. Clinical characteristics and treatment outcomes of non-V600 E/K BRAF mutant melanoma patients: a single-institution experience. Melanoma Res. 2022;32(6):477–84.
10. Malkhasyan KA, et al. The clinical characteristics of melanoma with BRAF V600R mutation: a case series study. Melanoma Res. 2020;30(1):107–12.
11. Colebatch AJ, et al. Molecular genomic profiling of melanocytic nevi. J Invest Dermatol. 2019;139(8):1762–8.
12. Pollock PM, et al. High frequency of BRAF mutations in nevi. Nat Genet. 2003;33(1):19–20.
13. Bauer J, et al. Congenital melanocytic nevi frequently harbor NRAS mutations but no BRAF mutations. J Invest Dermatol. 2007;127(1):179–82.
14. Martin SB, et al. Mosaic BRAF fusions are a recurrent cause of congenital melanocytic nevi targetable by MAPK pathway inhibition. J Invest Dermatol. 2024;144(3):593–600.e7.
15. Martins da Silva V, et al. Genetic abnormalities in large to giant congenital Nevi: beyond NRAS mutations. J Invest Dermatol. 2019;139(4):900–8.
16. Roy SF, et al. Congenital melanocytic nevi initiated by BRAF fusion oncogene with firmness, pruritus, and desmoplastic stroma. Br J Dermatol. 2025;193(2):232–9.
17. Erdmann-Pham DD, et al. Tracing cancer evolution and heterogeneity using Hi-C. Nat Commun. 2023;14(1):7111.
18. Hodis E, et al. A landscape of driver mutations in melanoma. Cell. 2012;150(2):251–63.
19. Gadal S, et al. Tumorigenesis driven by BRAFV600E requires secondary mutations that overcome it's feedback Inhibition of RAC1 and migration. Cancer Res. 2025;85(9):1611–27.
20. Shain AH, et al. The genetic evolution of melanoma from precursor lesions. N Engl J Med. 2015;373(20):1926–36.
21. Wang M, et al. The genetic evolution of acral melanoma. Nat Commun. 2024;15(1):6146.
22. Negri T, et al. Receptor tyrosine kinase pathway analysis sheds light on similarities between clear-cell sarcoma and metastatic melanoma. Genes Chromosom Cancer. 2012;51(2):111–26.
23. Raghavan SS, et al. Diffuse PRAME expression is highly specific for malignant melanoma in the distinction from clear cell sarcoma. J Cutan Pathol. 2020;47(12):1226–8.
24. Busam KJ, et al. Immunohistochemical analysis of BRAF(V600E) expression of primary and metastatic melanoma and comparison with mutation status and melanocyte differentiation antigens of metastatic lesions. Am J Surg Pathol. 2013;37(3):413–20.
25. Feller JK, Yang S, Mahalingam M. Immunohistochemistry with a mutation-specific monoclonal antibody as a screening tool for the BRAFV600E mutational status in primary cutaneous malignant melanoma. Mod Pathol. 2013;26(3):414–20.
26. Lo MC, et al. A UK feasibility and validation study of the VE1 monoclonal antibody immunohistochemistry stain for BRAF-V600E mutations in metastatic melanoma. Br J Cancer. 2016;115(2):223–7.

27. Long GV, et al. Immunohistochemistry is highly sensitive and specific for the detection of V600E BRAF mutation in melanoma. Am J Surg Pathol. 2013;37(1):61–5.
28. Kakavand H, et al. BRAF(V600E) and NRAS(Q61L/Q61R) mutation analysis in metastatic melanoma using immunohistochemistry: a study of 754 cases highlighting potential pitfalls and guidelines for interpretation and reporting. Histopathology. 2016;69(4):680–6.
29. Corean JLE, et al. Bone marrow findings in metastatic melanoma, including role of BRAF immunohistochemistry. Int J Lab Hematol. 2019;41(4):550–60.
30. Uguen A, et al. Dual NRASQ61R and BRAFV600E mutation-specific immunohistochemistry completes molecular screening in melanoma samples in a routine practice. Hum Pathol. 2015;46(11):1582–91.
31. Tetzlaff MT, et al. Utility of BRAF V600E immunohistochemistry expression pattern as a surrogate of BRAF mutation status in 154 patients with advanced melanoma. Hum Pathol. 2015;46(8):1101–10.
32. Kamata M, et al. A case of dedifferentiated melanoma with lymph node metastasis where molecular biological tests were useful for diagnosis. Cureus. 2022;14(1):e21644.
33. Rothrock AT, et al. BRAF V600E immunohistochemistry as a useful tool in the diagnosis of melanomas with ambiguous morphologies and immunophenotypes. J Cutan Pathol. 2023;50(3):223–9.
34. Uguen A, et al. NRASQ61R and BRAFV600E mutation-specific immunohistochemistry is a helpful tool to diagnose metastatic undifferentiated/dedifferentiated melanomas. Am J Surg Pathol. 2016;40(7):1004–5.
35. Abd Elmageed ZY, et al. Prognostic role of BRAF(V600E) cellular localization in melanoma. J Am Coll Surg. 2018;226(4):526–37.
36. Beleaua MA, et al. Relevance of BRAF subcellular localization and its interaction with KRAS and KIT mutations in skin melanoma. Int J Mol Sci. 2021;22(21)
37. Ravishankar S, et al. Giemsa is the optimal counterstain for immunohistochemical detection of BRAF V600E mutation status in pigmented melanomas. J Cutan Pathol. 2016;43(8):722–4.
38. Liu CH, et al. An optimized melanin depigmentation method for histopathological and immunohistochemical staining of formalin-fixed paraffin-embedded tissues. Int J Surg Pathol. 2024;32(4):679–83.
39. Prieto VG, Shea CR. Use of immunohistochemistry in melanocytic lesions. J Cutan Pathol. 2008;35(Suppl 2):1–10.
40. Jones RT, et al. Cross-reactivity of the BRAF VE1 antibody with epitopes in axonemal dyneins leads to staining of cilia. Mod Pathol. 2015;28(4):596–606.
41. Estrella JS, et al. Assessment of BRAF V600E status in colorectal carcinoma: tissue-specific discordances between immunohistochemistry and sequencing. Mol Cancer Ther. 2015;14(12):2887–95.
42. Bourhis A, Le Flahec G, Uguen A. Decalcification can cause the failure of BRAF molecular analyses and anti-BRAFV600E VE1 immunohistochemistry. Pathol Int. 2019;69(4):219–23.
43. Jabbar KJ, et al. Comparison of next-generation sequencing mutation profiling with BRAF and IDH1 mutation-specific immunohistochemistry. Am J Surg Pathol. 2015;39(4):454–61.
44. Capper D, et al. Immunohistochemical testing of BRAF V600E status in 1,120 tumor tissue samples of patients with brain metastases. Acta Neuropathol. 2012;123(2):223–33.
45. Rapisuwon S, et al. Discordance between cobas BRAF V600 testing and VE1 immunohistochemistry in a melanoma patient with bone marrow metastases. Am J Dermatopathol. 2016;38(9):687–9.
46. Rodriguez-Viciana P, et al. Phosphatidylinositol-3-OH kinase as a direct target of Ras. Nature. 1994;370(6490):527–32.
47. Hall A, et al. Identification of transforming gene in two human sarcoma cell lines as a new member of the ras gene family located on chromosome 1. Nature. 1983;303(5916):396–400.
48. Curtin JA, et al. Distinct sets of genetic alterations in melanoma. N Engl J Med. 2005;353(20):2135–47.

49. Jiveskog S, et al. N-ras mutations are common in melanomas from sun-exposed skin of humans but rare in mucosal membranes or unexposed skin. J Invest Dermatol. 1998;111(5):757–61.
50. Chiappetta C, et al. BRAF and NRAS mutations are heterogeneous and not mutually exclusive in nodular melanoma. Appl Immunohistochem Mol Morphol. 2015;23(3):172–7.
51. Charbel C, et al. NRAS mutation is the sole recurrent somatic mutation in large congenital melanocytic nevi. J Invest Dermatol. 2014;134(4):1067–74.
52. Jakob JA, et al. NRAS mutation status is an independent prognostic factor in metastatic melanoma. Cancer. 2012;118(16):4014–23.
53. Wróblewska JP, et al. Prognostic roles of BRAF, KIT, NRAS, IGF2R and SF3B1 mutations in mucosal melanomas. Cells. 2021;10(9)
54. Heppt MV, et al. Prognostic significance of BRAF and NRAS mutations in melanoma: a German study from routine care. BMC Cancer. 2017;17(1):536.
55. Yan J, et al. Prognostic role of NRAS isoforms in Chinese melanoma patients. Melanoma Res. 2019;29(3):263–9.
56. Ilie M, et al. Immunohistochemistry as a potential tool for routine detection of the NRAS Q61R mutation in patients with metastatic melanoma. J Am Acad Dermatol. 2015;72(5):786–93.
57. Massi D, et al. Immunohistochemistry is highly sensitive and specific for the detection of NRASQ61R mutation in melanoma. Mod Pathol. 2015;28(4):487–97.
58. Dias-Santagata D, Su Y, Hoang MP. Immunohistochemical detection of NRASQ61R mutation in diverse tumor types. Am J Clin Pathol. 2016;145(1):29–34.
59. Felisiak-Gołąbek A, et al. SP174 antibody lacks specificity for NRAS Q61R and cross-reacts with HRAS and KRAS Q61R mutant proteins in malignant melanoma. Appl Immunohistochem Mol Morphol. 2018;26(1):40–5.
60. Hancock JF. Ras proteins: different signals from different locations. Nat Rev Mol Cell Biol. 2003;4(5):373–84.
61. Jhuang JY, et al. NRASQ61R immunohistochemistry detects both NRASQ61R and KRASQ61R mutations in colorectal cancer. Pathology. 2017;49(4):387–90.
62. Reagh J, et al. NRASQ61R mutation-specific immunohistochemistry also identifies the HRASQ61R mutation in medullary thyroid cancer and may have a role in triaging genetic testing for MEN2. Am J Surg Pathol. 2017;41(1):75–81.
63. Parra O, et al. Cross-reactivity of NRASQ61R antibody in a subset of Spitz nevi with 11p gain: a potential confounding factor in the era of pathway-based diagnostic approach. Hum Pathol. 2021;112:35–47.
64. Duensing A, et al. Mechanisms of oncogenic KIT signal transduction in primary gastrointestinal stromal tumors (GISTs). Oncogene. 2004;23(22):3999–4006.
65. Bosbach B, et al. Direct engagement of the PI3K pathway by mutant KIT dominates oncogenic signaling in gastrointestinal stromal tumor. Proc Natl Acad Sci USA. 2017;114(40):E8448–e8457.
66. Giebel LB, Spritz RA. Mutation of the KIT (mast/stem cell growth factor receptor) protooncogene in human piebaldism. Proc Natl Acad Sci USA. 1991;88(19):8696–9.
67. Spritz RA, et al. Novel mutations of the KIT (mast/stem cell growth factor receptor) proto-oncogene in human piebaldism. J Invest Dermatol. 1993;101(1):22–5.
68. Alexeev V, Yoon K. Distinctive role of the cKit receptor tyrosine kinase signaling in mammalian melanocytes. J Invest Dermatol. 2006;126(5):1102–10.
69. Zakut R, et al. KIT ligand (mast cell growth factor) inhibits the growth of KIT-expressing melanoma cells. Oncogene. 1993;8(8):2221–9.
70. Huang S, et al. Enforced c-KIT expression renders highly metastatic human melanoma cells susceptible to stem cell factor-induced apoptosis and inhibits their tumorigenic and metastatic potential. Oncogene. 1996;13(11):2339–47.
71. Montone KT, et al. Proto-oncogene c-kit expression in malignant melanoma: protein loss with tumor progression. Mod Pathol. 1997;10(9):939–44.
72. Natali PG, et al. Progression of human cutaneous melanoma is associated with loss of expression of c-kit proto-oncogene receptor. Int J Cancer. 1992;52(2):197–201.

73. Shen SS, et al. Analysis of protein tyrosine kinase expression in melanocytic lesions by tissue array. J Cutan Pathol. 2003;30(9):539–47.
74. Curtin JA, et al. Somatic activation of KIT in distinct subtypes of melanoma. J Clin Oncol. 2006;24(26):4340–6.
75. Went PT, et al. Prevalence of KIT expression in human tumors. J Clin Oncol. 2004;22(22):4514–22.
76. Ashida A, et al. Pathological activation of KIT in metastatic tumors of acral and mucosal melanomas. Int J Cancer. 2009;124(4):862–8.
77. Beadling C, et al. KIT gene mutations and copy number in melanoma subtypes. Clin Cancer Res. 2008;14(21):6821–8.
78. Doma V, et al. KIT mutation incidence and pattern of melanoma in central Europe. Pathol Oncol Res. 2020;26(1):17–22.
79. Jung S, et al. Clinical and genomic correlates of imatinib response in melanomas with KIT alterations. Br J Cancer. 2022;127(9):1726–32.
80. Antonescu CR, et al. L576P KIT mutation in anal melanomas correlates with KIT protein expression and is sensitive to specific kinase inhibition. Int J Cancer. 2007;121(2):257–64.
81. Frost MJ, et al. Juxtamembrane mutant V560GKit is more sensitive to Imatinib (STI571) compared with wild-type c-kit whereas the kinase domain mutant D816VKit is resistant. Mol Cancer Ther. 2002;1(12):1115–24.
82. Beghini A, et al. In vivo differentiation of mast cells from acute myeloid leukemia blasts carrying a novel activating ligand-independent C-kit mutation. Blood Cells Mol Dis. 1998;24(2):262–70.
83. Cui C, et al. Multifactorial analysis of prognostic factors and survival rates among 706 mucosal melanoma patients. Ann Surg Oncol. 2018;25(8):2184–92.
84. Dias-Santagata D, et al. KIT mutations and CD117 overexpression are markers of better progression-free survival in vulvar melanomas. Br J Dermatol. 2017;177(5):1376–84.
85. Jin SA, et al. BRAF mutations and KIT aberrations and their clinicopathological correlation in 202 Korean melanomas. J Invest Dermatol. 2013;133(2):579–82.
86. Kong Y, et al. Large-scale analysis of KIT aberrations in Chinese patients with melanoma. Clin Cancer Res. 2011;17(7):1684–91.
87. Ma X, et al. The clinical significance of c-Kit mutations in metastatic oral mucosal melanoma in China. Oncotarget. 2017;8(47):82661–73.
88. Torres-Cabala CA, et al. Correlation between KIT expression and KIT mutation in melanoma: a study of 173 cases with emphasis on the acral-lentiginous/mucosal type. Mod Pathol. 2009;22(11):1446–56.
89. Willmore-Payne C, et al. Human malignant melanoma: detection of BRAF- and c-kit-activating mutations by high-resolution amplicon melting analysis. Hum Pathol. 2005;36(5):486–93.
90. Brocca G, et al. KIT somatic mutations and immunohistochemical expression in canine oral melanoma. Animals (Basel). 2020;10(12)
91. Sari Aslani F, Geramizadeh B, Dehghanian AR. Comparison of c-Kit expression between primary and metastatic melanoma of skin and mucosa. Med J Islam Repub Iran. 2015;29:203.
92. Giehl KA, et al. Protein expression of melanocyte growth factors (bFGF, SCF) and their receptors (FGFR-1, c-kit) in nevi and melanoma. J Cutan Pathol. 2007;34(1):7–14.
93. Isabel Zhu Y, Fitzpatrick JE. Expression of c-kit (CD117) in Spitz nevus and malignant melanoma. J Cutan Pathol. 2006;33(1):33–7.
94. Park E, et al. Lack of correlation between immunohistochemical expression of CKIT and KIT mutations in atypical acral nevi. Am J Dermatopathol. 2012;34(1):41–6.
95. Pilloni L, et al. The usefulness of c-Kit in the immunohistochemical assessment of melanocytic lesions. Eur J Histochem. 2011;55(2):e20.
96. Song MS, Salmena L, Pandolfi PP. The functions and regulation of the PTEN tumour suppressor. Nat Rev Mol Cell Biol. 2012;13(5):283–96.
97. Lee YR, Chen M, Pandolfi PP. The functions and regulation of the PTEN tumour suppressor: new modes and prospects. Nat Rev Mol Cell Biol. 2018;19(9):547–62.

98. Bu L, et al. PTEN suppresses tumorigenesis by directly dephosphorylating Akt. Signal Transduct Target Ther. 2021;6(1):262.
99. Maehama T, Dixon JE. The tumor suppressor, PTEN/MMAC1, dephosphorylates the lipid second messenger, phosphatidylinositol 3,4,5-trisphosphate. J Biol Chem. 1998;273(22):13375–8.
100. Kuchay S, et al. PTEN counteracts FBXL2 to promote IP3R3- and Ca(2+)-mediated apoptosis limiting tumour growth. Nature. 2017;546(7659):554–8.
101. Bassi C, et al. Nuclear PTEN controls DNA repair and sensitivity to genotoxic stress. Science. 2013;341(6144):395–9.
102. Li AG, et al. Mechanistic insights into maintenance of high p53 acetylation by PTEN. Mol Cell. 2006;23(4):575–87.
103. Shen WH, et al. Essential role for nuclear PTEN in maintaining chromosomal integrity. Cell. 2007;128(1):157–70.
104. Song MS, et al. Nuclear PTEN regulates the APC-CDH1 tumor-suppressive complex in a phosphatase-independent manner. Cell. 2011;144(2):187–99.
105. Aguissa-Touré AH, Li G. Genetic alterations of PTEN in human melanoma. Cell Mol Life Sci. 2012;69(9):1475–91.
106. Ciuffreda L, et al. The mitogen-activated protein kinase (MAPK) cascade controls phosphatase and tensin homolog (PTEN) expression through multiple mechanisms. J Mol Med (Berl). 2012;90(6):667–79.
107. Karreth FA, et al. In vivo identification of tumor- suppressive PTEN ceRNAs in an oncogenic BRAF-induced mouse model of melanoma. Cell. 2011;147(2):382–95.
108. Zhou XP, et al. Epigenetic PTEN silencing in malignant melanomas without PTEN mutation. Am J Pathol. 2000;157(4):1123–8.
109. Shain AH, et al. Genomic and transcriptomic analysis reveals incremental disruption of key signaling pathways during melanoma evolution. Cancer Cell. 2018;34(1):45–55.e4.
110. Bucheit AD, et al. Complete loss of PTEN protein expression correlates with shorter time to brain metastasis and survival in stage IIIB/C melanoma patients with BRAFV600 mutations. Clin Cancer Res. 2014;20(21):5527–36.
111. Catalanotti F, et al. PTEN loss-of-function alterations are associated with intrinsic resistance to BRAF inhibitors in metastatic melanoma. JCO Precis Oncologia. 2017:1.
112. Zuo Q, et al. AXL/AKT axis mediated-resistance to BRAF inhibitor depends on PTEN status in melanoma. Oncogene. 2018;37(24):3275–89.
113. Trujillo JA, et al. Secondary resistance to immunotherapy associated with β-catenin pathway activation or PTEN loss in metastatic melanoma. J Immunother Cancer. 2019;7(1):295.
114. Cabrita R, et al. The role of PTEN loss in immune escape, melanoma prognosis and therapy response. Cancers (Basel). 2020;12(3)
115. Peng W, et al. Loss of PTEN promotes resistance to T cell-mediated immunotherapy. Cancer Discov. 2016;6(2):202–16.
116. Němejcová K, et al. Comprehensive analysis of PTEN in primary cutaneous melanoma. Folia Biol (Praha). 2020;66(1):7–16.
117. Chagani S, et al. Multiplatform analysis of intratumoral PTEN heterogeneity in melanoma. J Invest Dermatol. 2023;143(9):1779–1787.e1.
118. Sun Z, Arnouk H. Phosphatase and Tensin Homolog (PTEN) expression as a surrogate biomarker correlated with the depth of invasion in cutaneous malignant melanoma. Cureus. 2023;15(9):e45295.
119. Tsao H, Mihm MC Jr, Sheehan C. PTEN expression in normal skin, acquired melanocytic nevi, and cutaneous melanoma. J Am Acad Dermatol. 2003;49(5):865–72.
120. Iwai Y, et al. Involvement of PD-L1 on tumor cells in the escape from host immune system and tumor immunotherapy by PD-L1 blockade. Proc Natl Acad Sci USA. 2002;99(19):12293–7.
121. Merelli B, et al. Targeting the PD1/PD-L1 axis in melanoma: biological rationale, clinical challenges and opportunities. Crit Rev Oncol Hematol. 2014;89(1):140–65.

122. Kaunitz GJ, et al. Melanoma subtypes demonstrate distinct PD-L1 expression profiles. Lab Investig. 2017;97(9):1063–71.
123. Taube JM, et al. Colocalization of inflammatory response with B7-h1 expression in human melanocytic lesions supports an adaptive resistance mechanism of immune escape. Sci Transl Med. 2012;4(127):127ra37.
124. Ellebaek E, et al. PD-L1 is a biomarker of real-world clinical outcomes for anti-CTLA-4 plus anti-PD-1 or anti-PD-1 monotherapy in metastatic melanoma. Eur J Cancer. 2024;198
125. Larkin J, et al. Five-year survival with combined nivolumab and ipilimumab in advanced melanoma. N Engl J Med. 2019;381(16):1535–46.
126. Wolchok JD, et al. Final, 10-year outcomes with nivolumab plus ipilimumab in advanced melanoma. N Engl J Med. 2025;392(1):11–22.
127. Sunshine JC, et al. PD-L1 expression in melanoma: a quantitative immunohistochemical antibody comparison. Clin Cancer Res. 2017;23(16):4938–44.
128. Koppel C, et al. Optimization and validation of PD-L1 immunohistochemistry staining protocols using the antibody clone 28-8 on different staining platforms. Mod Pathol. 2018;31(11):1630–44.
129. Krigsfeld GS, et al. Analysis of real-world PD-L1 IHC 28-8 and 22C3 pharmDx assay utilisation, turnaround times and analytical concordance across multiple tumour types. J Clin Pathol. 2020;73(10):656–64.
130. Phillips T, et al. Development of a diagnostic programmed cell death 1-ligand 1 immunohistochemistry assay for nivolumab therapy in melanoma. Appl Immunohistochem Mol Morphol. 2018;26(1):6–12.
131. Pineda-Reyes J, et al. Dual PD-L1/SOX10 immunohistochemistry combined with digital imaging enhances stratification accuracy of patients with metastatic melanoma. Am J Surg Pathol. 2024;48(12):1551–6.
132. Darmon-Novello M, et al. Harmonization of programmed death-ligand 1 immunohistochemistry and mRNA expression scoring in metastatic melanoma: a multicentre analysis. Histopathology. 2022;80(7):1091–101.
133. Daud AI, et al. Programmed death-ligand 1 expression and response to the anti-programmed death 1 antibody pembrolizumab in melanoma. J Clin Oncol. 2016;34(34):4102–9.
134. Marletta S, et al. Atlas of PD-L1 for pathologists: indications, scores, diagnostic platforms and reporting systems. J Pers Med. 2022;12(7)
135. Yoneta D, et al. Difference in immunohistochemical findings among anti-PD-L1 antibodies and their relationships with CD4+ and CD8+ T cells in Japanese melanoma patients. Int J Clin Oncol. 2022;27(8):1364–71.
136. Wolchok JD, et al. Overall survival with combined nivolumab and ipilimumab in advanced melanoma. N Engl J Med. 2017;377(14):1345–56.
137. Carbognin L, et al. Differential activity of nivolumab, pembrolizumab and MPDL3280A according to the tumor expression of Programmed Death-Ligand-1 (PD-L1): sensitivity analysis of trials in melanoma, lung and genitourinary cancers. PLoS One. 2015;10(6):e0130142.
138. Formica V, et al. PD-L1 thresholds predict efficacy of immune checkpoint inhibition in first-line treatment of advanced gastroesophageal adenocarcinoma. A systematic review and meta-analysis of seven phase III randomized trials. ESMO Open. 2024;9(11)
139. Fiorentino V, et al. Programmed cell death ligand 1 immunohistochemical expression and cutaneous melanoma: a controversial relationship. Int J Mol Sci. 2024;25(1)
140. Elsayed AM, et al. An overview of BAP1 biological functions and current therapeutics. Biochim Biophys Acta Rev Cancer. 2025;1880(2):189267.
141. Kwon J, Lee D, Lee SA. BAP1 as a guardian of genome stability: implications in human cancer. Exp Mol Med. 2023;55(4):745–54.
142. Farley MN, et al. A novel germline mutation in BAP1 predisposes to familial clear-cell renal cell carcinoma. Mol Cancer Res. 2013;11(9):1061–71.
143. Masoomian B, Shields JA, Shields CL. Overview of BAP1 cancer predisposition syndrome and the relationship to uveal melanoma. J Curr Ophthalmol. 2018;30(2):102–9.

144. Njauw CN, et al. Germline BAP1 inactivation is preferentially associated with metastatic ocular melanoma and cutaneous-ocular melanoma families. PLoS One. 2012;7(4):e35295.
145. Popova T, et al. Germline BAP1 mutations predispose to renal cell carcinomas. Am J Hum Genet. 2013;92(6):974–80.
146. Rai K, et al. Comprehensive review of BAP1 tumor predisposition syndrome with report of two new cases. Clin Genet. 2016;89(3):285–94.
147. Busam KJ, et al. Combined BRAF(V600E)-positive melanocytic lesions with large epithelioid cells lacking BAP1 expression and conventional nevomelanocytes. Am J Surg Pathol. 2013;37(2):193–9.
148. Wiesner T, et al. A distinct subset of atypical Spitz tumors is characterized by BRAF mutation and loss of BAP1 expression. Am J Surg Pathol. 2012;36(6):818–30.
149. Wiesner T, et al. Germline mutations in BAP1 predispose to melanocytic tumors. Nat Genet. 2011;43(10):1018–21.
150. Donati M, Šteiner P, Kazakov DV. BAP1-inactivated melanoma arising from BAP1-inactivated melanocytic tumor in a patient with BAP1 germline mutation: a case report and review of the literature. Am J Dermatopathol. 2023;45(2):117–22.
151. Aung PP, et al. Melanoma with Loss of BAP1 expression in patients with no family history of BAP1-associated cancer susceptibility syndrome: a case series. Am J Dermatopathol. 2019;41(3):167–79.
152. Krauthammer M, et al. Exome sequencing identifies recurrent somatic RAC1 mutations in melanoma. Nat Genet. 2012;44(9):1006–14.
153. Harbour JW, et al. Frequent mutation of BAP1 in metastasizing uveal melanomas. Science. 2010;330(6009):1410–3.
154. Shain AH, et al. The genetic evolution of metastatic uveal melanoma. Nat Genet. 2019;51(7):1123–30.
155. Martin M, et al. Exome sequencing identifies recurrent somatic mutations in EIF1AX and SF3B1 in uveal melanoma with disomy 3. Nat Genet. 2013;45(8):933–6.
156. Landreville S, et al. Histone deacetylase inhibitors induce growth arrest and differentiation in uveal melanoma. Clin Cancer Res. 2012;18(2):408–16.
157. Kuznetsoff JN, et al. Dual screen for efficacy and toxicity identifies HDAC inhibitor with distinctive activity spectrum for BAP1-mutant uveal melanoma. Mol Cancer Res. 2021;19(2):215–22.
158. Kalirai H, et al. Lack of BAP1 protein expression in uveal melanoma is associated with increased metastatic risk and has utility in routine prognostic testing. Br J Cancer. 2014;111(7):1373–80.
159. Kennedy S, et al. Prognostic value of BAP1 protein expression in uveal melanoma. Am J Surg Pathol. 2024;48(3):329–36.
160. Koopmans AE, et al. Clinical significance of immunohistochemistry for detection of BAP1 mutations in uveal melanoma. Mod Pathol. 2014;27(10):1321–30.
161. van Essen TH, et al. Prognostic parameters in uveal melanoma and their association with BAP1 expression. Br J Ophthalmol. 2014;98(12):1738–43.
162. Shah AA, Bourne TD, Murali R. BAP1 protein loss by immunohistochemistry: a potentially useful tool for prognostic prediction in patients with uveal melanoma. Pathology. 2013;45(7):651–6.
163. van de Nes JA, et al. Comparing the prognostic value of BAP1 mutation pattern, chromosome 3 status, and BAP1 immunohistochemistry in uveal melanoma. Am J Surg Pathol. 2016;40(6):796–805.
164. Glasgow BJ, McCannel TA. Correlation of immunocytochemistry of BRCA1-associated protein-1 (BAP1) with other prognostic markers in uveal melanoma. Am J Ophthalmol. 2018;189:122–6.
165. See TR, et al. BAP1 immunoreactivity correlates with gene expression class in uveal melanoma. Ocul Oncol Pathol. 2020;6(2):129–37.

166. Cole YC, et al. Correlation between BAP1 localization, driver mutations, and patient survival in uveal melanoma. Cancers (Basel). 2022;14(17)
167. Farquhar N, et al. Patterns of BAP1 protein expression provide insights into prognostic significance and the biology of uveal melanoma. J Pathol Clin Res. 2018;4(1):26–38.
168. Eiger-Moscovich M, et al. BRCA-associated protein1 (BAP1) immunohistochemical stain reliability in postbrachytherapy uveal melanoma enucleation specimens. Indian J Ophthalmol. 2024;72(Suppl 3):S459–s467.
169. Kalinec G, et al. Mutated alpha subunit of the Gq protein induces malignant transformation in NIH 3T3 cells. Mol Cell Biol. 1992;12(10):4687–93.
170. Bauer J, et al. Oncogenic GNAQ mutations are not correlated with disease-free survival in uveal melanoma. Br J Cancer. 2009;101(5):813–5.
171. Koopmans AE, et al. Patient survival in uveal melanoma is not affected by oncogenic mutations in GNAQ and GNA11. Br J Cancer. 2013;109(2):493–6.
172. Van Raamsdonk CD, et al. Frequent somatic mutations of GNAQ in uveal melanoma and blue naevi. Nature. 2009;457(7229):599–602.
173. Van Raamsdonk CD, et al. Mutations in GNA11 in uveal melanoma. N Engl J Med. 2010;363(23):2191–9.
174. Gessi M, et al. GNA11 and N-RAS mutations: alternatives for MAPK pathway activating GNAQ mutations in primary melanocytic tumours of the central nervous system. Neuropathol Appl Neurobiol. 2013;39(4):417–25.
175. Küsters-Vandevelde HV, et al. Activating mutations of the GNAQ gene: a frequent event in primary melanocytic neoplasms of the central nervous system. Acta Neuropathol. 2010;119(3):317–23.
176. Livingstone E, et al. GNAQ and GNA11 mutant nonuveal melanoma: a subtype distinct from both cutaneous and uveal melanoma. Br J Dermatol. 2020;183(5):928–39.
177. Chen X, et al. RasGRP3 mediates MAPK pathway activation in GNAQ mutant uveal melanoma. Cancer Cell. 2017;31(5):685–696.e6.
178. Zuidervaart W, et al. Activation of the MAPK pathway is a common event in uveal melanomas although it rarely occurs through mutation of BRAF or RAS. Br J Cancer. 2005;92(11):2032–8.
179. Feng X, et al. A platform of synthetic lethal gene interaction networks reveals that the GNAQ uveal melanoma oncogene controls the hippo pathway through FAK. Cancer Cell. 2019;35(3):457–472.e5.
180. Griewank KG, et al. Genetic and clinico-pathologic analysis of metastatic uveal melanoma. Mod Pathol. 2014;27(2):175–83.
181. Piaggio F, et al. In uveal melanoma Gα-protein GNA11 mutations convey a shorter disease-specific survival and are more strongly associated with loss of BAP1 and chromosomal alterations than Gα-protein GNAQ mutations. Eur J Cancer. 2022;170:27–41.
182. Staby KM, et al. Prognostic impact of chromosomal aberrations and GNAQ, GNA11 and BAP1 mutations in uveal melanoma. Acta Ophthalmol. 2018;96(1):31–8.
183. Afshar AR, et al. Next-generation sequencing of uveal melanoma for detection of genetic alterations predicting metastasis. Transl Vis Sci Technol. 2019;8(2):18.
184. Decatur CL, et al. Driver mutations in uveal melanoma: associations with gene expression profile and patient outcomes. JAMA Ophthalmol. 2016;134(7):728–33.
185. Psinakis F, et al. Uveal melanoma: GNAQ and GNA11 mutations in a Greek population. Anticancer Res. 2017;37(10):5719–26.
186. Silva-Rodríguez P, et al. Role of somatic mutations and chromosomal aberrations in the prognosis of uveal melanoma in a Spanish Patient Cohort. Acta Ophthalmol. 2021;99(7):e1077–89.
187. Xu X, et al. Oncogenic GNAQ and GNA11 mutations in uveal melanoma in Chinese. PLoS One. 2014;9(10):e109699.
188. Asada K, et al. Reduced expression of GNA11 and silencing of MCT1 in human breast cancers. Oncology. 2003;64(4):380–8.

189. Mann KM, et al. Sleeping Beauty mutagenesis reveals cooperating mutations and pathways in pancreatic adenocarcinoma. Proc Natl Acad Sci USA. 2012;109(16):5934–41.
190. Rushton JG, et al. Protein expression of KIT, BRAF, GNA11, GNAQ and RASSF1 in feline diffuse iris melanomas. Vet J. 2019;249:33–40.
191. Rushton JG, et al. Mutation analysis and gene expression profiling of ocular melanomas in cats. Vet Comp Oncol. 2017;15(4):1403–16.
192. Wiesner T, et al. Kinase fusions are frequent in Spitz tumours and spitzoid melanomas. Nat Commun. 2014;5:3116.
193. Busam KJ, et al. Clinical and pathologic findings of Spitz nevi and atypical Spitz tumors with ALK fusions. Am J Surg Pathol. 2014;38(7):925–33.
194. Yeh I, et al. Clinical, histopathologic, and genomic features of Spitz tumors with ALK fusions. Am J Surg Pathol. 2015;39(5):581–91.
195. Amin SM, et al. A comparison of morphologic and molecular features of BRAF, ALK, and NTRK1 fusion spitzoid neoplasms. Am J Surg Pathol. 2017;41(4):491–8.
196. Kiuru M, et al. Spitz tumors: comparison of histological features in relationship to immunohistochemical staining for ALK and NTRK1. Int J Surg Pathol. 2016;24(3):200–6.
197. Cho WC, Prieto VG, Yang RK. Spitz melanoma with SLC20A1::ALK Fusion: a novel fusion previously undescribed in spitz melanocytic neoplasm. Am J Dermatopathol. 2024;46(10):700–3.
198. Farah M, et al. Spitzoid melanoma with histopathological features of ALK gene rearrangement exhibiting ALK copy number gain: a novel mechanism of ALK activation in spitzoid neoplasia. Br J Dermatol. 2019;180(2):404–8.
199. Wiesner T, et al. Alternative transcription initiation leads to expression of a novel ALK isoform in cancer. Nature. 2015;526(7573):453–7.
200. Busam KJ, et al. Primary and metastatic cutaneous melanomas express ALK through alternative transcriptional initiation. Am J Surg Pathol. 2016;40(6):786–95.
201. Bahrani E, et al. Spitz nevus with EHBP1-ALK fusion and distinctive membranous localization of ALK. J Cutan Pathol. 2022;49(6):584–8.
202. Shah KK, et al. Correlation of novel ALK(ATI) with ALK immunohistochemistry and clinical outcomes in metastatic melanoma. Histopathology. 2020;77(4):601–10.
203. Osella-Abate S, et al. ALK expression favorably impacts the prognosis of NRAS-mutated metastatic melanomas. Oncol Lett. 2018;16(6):7091–6.
204. Uruga H, Mino-Kenudson M. ALK (D5F3) CDx: an immunohistochemistry assay to identify ALK-positive NSCLC patients. Pharmgenomics Pers Med. 2018;11:147–55.
205. Cappellesso R, et al. NTRK gene fusion detection in atypical spitz tumors. Int J Mol Sci. 2021;22(22)
206. Giubellino A, et al. Gene expression profile of benign, intermediate, and malignant spitz and spitzoid melanocytic lesions. Cancers (Basel). 2024;16(10)
207. Wu G, et al. The landscape of fusion transcripts in spitzoid melanoma and biologically indeterminate spitzoid tumors by RNA sequencing. Mod Pathol. 2016;29(4):359–69.
208. Lezcano C, et al. Primary and metastatic melanoma with NTRK fusions. Am J Surg Pathol. 2018;42(8):1052–8.
209. Yeh I, et al. Targeted genomic profiling of acral melanoma. J Natl Cancer Inst. 2019;111(10):1068–77.
210. Drilon A, et al. Efficacy of larotrectinib in TRK fusion-positive cancers in adults and children. N Engl J Med. 2018;378(8):731–9.
211. Drilon A, et al. Safety and antitumor activity of the multitargeted Pan-TRK, ROS1, and ALK inhibitor entrectinib: combined results from two phase I trials (ALKA-372-001 and STARTRK-1). Cancer Discov. 2017;7(4):400–9.
212. Solomon JP, et al. NTRK fusion detection across multiple assays and 33,997 cases: diagnostic implications and pitfalls. Mod Pathol. 2020;33(1):38–46.

213. Bourhis A, et al. Screening for NTRK-rearranged tumors using immunohistochemistry: comparison of 2 different pan-TRK clones in melanoma samples. Appl Immunohistochem Mol Morphol. 2020;28(3):194–6.
214. Bourhis A, et al. Detection of NTRK fusions in glioblastoma: fluorescent in situ hybridisation is more useful than pan-TRK immunohistochemistry as a screening tool prior to RNA sequencing. Pathology. 2022;54(1):55–62.
215. Castillon M, et al. Fluorescent in situ hybridization must be preferred to pan-TRK immunohistochemistry to diagnose NTRK3-rearranged gastrointestinal stromal tumors (GIST). Appl Immunohistochem Mol Morphol. 2021;29(8):626–34.
216. Guibourg B, et al. EPR17341 and A7H6R pan-TRK immunohistochemistry result in highly different staining patterns in a series of salivary gland tumors. Appl Immunohistochem Mol Morphol. 2020;28(9):719–24.
217. Adam J, et al. Multicenter harmonization study of Pan-Trk immunohistochemistry for the detection of NTRK3 fusions. Mod Pathol. 2023;36(8):100192.
218. Cazzato G, et al. LMNA::NTRK1 and PRDX1::NTRK1 atypical spitz tumor: a report of two additional cases with histological, immunohistochemical, and molecular insights. Am J Dermatopathol. 2025;47(1):22–4.
219. Goto K, et al. Spitz nevus with a novel TFG-NTRK2 fusion: the first case report of NTRK2-rearranged Spitz/Reed nevus. J Cutan Pathol. 2021;48(9):1193–6.
220. Diaz A, et al. TERT gene amplification is associated with poor outcome in acral lentiginous melanoma. J Am Acad Dermatol. 2014;71(4):839–41.
221. Ramani NS, et al. TERT amplification but not activation of canonical Wnt/β-catenin pathway is involved in acral lentiginous melanoma progression to metastasis. Mod Pathol. 2020;33(10):2067–74.
222. Liau JY, et al. TERT promoter mutation is uncommon in acral lentiginous melanoma. J Cutan Pathol. 2014;41(6):504–8.
223. Heidenreich B, et al. Telomerase reverse transcriptase promoter mutations in primary cutaneous melanoma. Nat Commun. 2014;5:3401.
224. Horn S, et al. TERT promoter mutations in familial and sporadic melanoma. Science. 2013;339(6122):959–61.
225. Huang FW, et al. Highly recurrent TERT promoter mutations in human melanoma. Science. 2013;339(6122):957–9.
226. Manrique-Silva E, et al. Clinical, histological, and molecular differences in melanoma due to different TERT promoter mutations subtypes. A retrospective cross-sectional study in 684 melanoma patients. Pigm Cell Melanoma Res. 2024;37(3):343–51.
227. Shaughnessy M, et al. Classifying melanoma by TERT promoter mutational status. J Invest Dermatol. 2020;140(2):390–394.e1.
228. Thielmann CM, et al. TERT promoter mutations are associated with longer progression-free and overall survival in patients with BRAF-mutant melanoma receiving BRAF and MEK inhibitor therapy. Eur J Cancer. 2022;161:99–107.
229. Blateau P, et al. TERT promoter mutation as an independent prognostic marker for poor prognosis MAPK inhibitors-treated melanoma. Cancers (Basel). 2020;12(8)
230. Delyon J, et al. TERT expression induces resistance to BRAF and MEK inhibitors in BRAF-mutated melanoma in vitro. Cancers (Basel). 2023;15(11)
231. Sheen YS, Chu CY. Co-occurrence of TERT promotor mutations with BRAF or NRAS alterations correlates with worse prognosis in melanoma. Br J Dermatol. 2021;184(3):390–1.
232. Li Y, et al. Activation of mutant TERT promoter by RAS-ERK signaling is a key step in malignant progression of BRAF-mutant human melanomas. Proc Natl Acad Sci USA. 2016;113(50):14402–7.
233. Reyes-Uribe P, et al. Exploiting TERT dependency as a therapeutic strategy for NRAS-mutant melanoma. Oncogene. 2018;37(30):4058–72.

234. Cho WC, et al. Telomerase reverse transcriptase immunohistochemical expression is sensitive but not specific for TERT gene amplification in acral melanoma. J Cutan Pathol. 2023;50(9):845–51.
235. Cho WC, et al. Telomerase reverse transcriptase protein expression is more frequent in acral lentiginous melanoma than in other types of cutaneous melanoma. Arch Pathol Lab Med. 2021;145(7):842–50.
236. Hugdahl E, et al. Prognostic impact and concordance of TERT promoter mutation and protein expression in matched primary and metastatic cutaneous melanoma. Br J Cancer. 2018;118(1):98–105.
237. Kohli JS, et al. ETS1, nucleolar and non-nucleolar TERT expression in nevus to melanoma progression. Oncotarget. 2017;8(61):104408–17.

Index

V. G. Prieto, C. A. Torres-Cabala (eds.), *Precision Molecular Pathology of Melanocytic Lesions*, Molecular Pathology Library,
https://doi.org/10.1007/978-3-032-18222-7